A Concise Textbook of Psychiatric Mental Health Nursing

(*As per INC Syllabus*)

Visanth VS
MSc (N) RN RM
Assistant Professor
Department of Mental Health Nursing
Hind College of Nursing
Hind Institute of Medical Sciences
Safedabad, Lucknow, Uttar Pradesh

Mallesha S
MSc (N) RN RM
Lecturer
Department of Mental Health Nursing
Hind College of Nursing
Hind Institute of Medical Sciences
Safedabad, Lucknow, Uttar Pradesh

Foreword

Richa Mishra

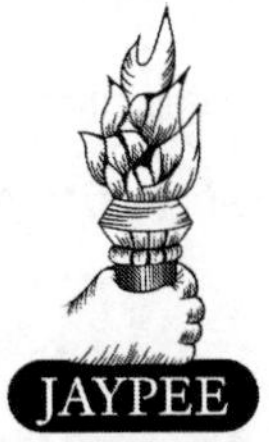

JAYPEE BROTHERS MEDICAL PUBLISHERS
The Health Sciences Publisher
New Delhi | London

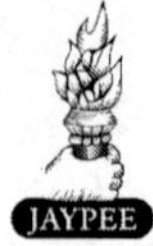

Jaypee Brothers Medical Publishers (P) Ltd

Headquarters
EMCA House
23/23-B, Ansari Road, Daryaganj
New Delhi 110 002, India
Landline: +91-11-23272143, +91-11-23272703
+91-11-23282021, +91-11-23245672
E-mail: jaypee@jaypeebrothers.com

Corporate Office
4838/24, Ansari Road, Daryaganj
New Delhi 110 002, India
Phone: +91-11-43574357
Fax: +91-11-43574314
E-mail: jaypee@jaypeebrothers.com

Overseas Office
J.P. Medical Ltd
83 Victoria Street, London
SW1H 0HW (UK)
Phone: +44 20 3170 8910
E-mail: info@jpmedpub.com

EU GPSR Authorised Representative
Logos Europe, 9 rue Nicolas Poussin
17000, La Rochelle, France
Phone: +33 (0) 6 67 93 73 78
E-mail: contact@logoseurope.eu

Website: www.jaypeebrothers.com
Website: www.jaypeedigital.com

Website: www.jaypeebrothers.com
Website: www.jaypeedigital.com

A Concise Textbook of Psychiatric Mental Health Nursing

First Edition: **2017**

Reprint: **2026**

ISBN: 978-93-86107-01-5

Printed at: Samrat Offset Pvt. Ltd.

Dedicated to

Our Parents, Family
The Nursing Profession
and
Sufferers of Mental Illness

Foreword

It is my privilege to foreword the title *A Concise Textbook of Psychiatric Mental Health Nursing*. The stigma towards mental disorders and mentally ill persons are still in ground. The psychiatric nursing professional can do many things in removing these issues. This title provides comprehensive information regarding various aspects of psychiatric nursing.

The authors designed this book based on Indian Nursing Council (INC) Curriculum and can be used for both undergraduate and postgraduate students. The topics covered in this book helps to provide knowledge for the students and can be effectively apply in their professional practice to provide a standard nursing care.

I congratulate the authors for their effort to publish this book.

Richa Mishra
Chairperson
Hind College of Nursing
Hind Institute of Medical Sciences
Safedabad, Lucknow
Uttar Pradesh

Preface

A Concise Textbook of Psychiatric Mental Health Nursing is a sincere effort made by us and is designed for the undergraduate and postgraduate nursing students. This book is designed exclusively based on Indian Nursing Council (INC) syllabus and is meant for BSc Program even though the other nursing program can be used as a reference guide.

In this book, we have tried to give a comprehensive knowledge regarding various aspects of psychiatric nursing. It attempts to present the essential information on concepts and principles, assessment of mental status, therapeutic communication, various therapies, and mental illnesses with nursing care, legal issues and community mental health nursing.

It is hoped that nursing students, teachers and professional nurses will find this book useful. Their comments and suggestions for the development of this book will be appreciated.

Visanth VS
Mallesha S

Acknowledgments

We thank Almighty, the path of light and the ray of hope, for His grace and endless blessings throughout the preparation of this title.

We are grateful to express the deepest sense of gratitude to Dr Richa Mishra, Chairperson, Hind College of Nursing, Hind Institute of Medical Sciences, Lucknow for her support.

We express our sincere gratitude to Prof (Mrs) Senbagam P, Principal, and Hind College of Nursing for her encouragement.

We also thank Mr Shimil Varghese for contributing *Chapter 1: Introduction* and *Chapter 9: Nursing Management of Patient with Substance use Disorder.*

We take this opportunity to thank Mr Aswini Saini, Assistant Area Manager, Mr Akash Saini, representative of Jaypee Brothers, Lucknow Branch for their encouragement in preparing this book.

We convey our sincere thanks to Jaypee Brothers Medical Publishers (P) Ltd, New Delhi, India for their efforts and suggestions, especially Shri Jitendar P Vij (Group Chairman), Mr Ankit Vij (Group President), Ms Chetna Malhotra Vohra (Associate Director), and Ms Ruby Sharma (Project Manager) for helping us through our idea.

We extend our sincere thanks and gratitude to all who were directly and indirectly helped in successful completion of this book.

Visanth VS
Mallesha S

INC Syllabus

Placement: Third Year

Time: Theory – 90 hours
Practical – 270 hours
Internship – 95 hours (2 weeks)

Course Description: This course is designed for developing an understanding of the modern approach to mental health, identification, prevention and nursing management of common mental health problem with special emphasis on therapeutic interventions for individuals, family and community.

Unit	Time (Hrs)	Learning Objective	Content	Teaching Learning Activity	Assessment Method	Chapter
I	5	• Describe the historical development and current trends in mental health nursing • Describe the epidemiology of mental health problems • Describe the National Mental Health Act, programmes and mental health policy • Discusses the scope of mental health nursing • Describe the concept of normal and abnormal behaviour	**Introduction** • Perspectives of Mental Health and Mental Health Nursing: Evolution of mental health services, treatment and nursing practices • Prevalence and incidence of mental health problems and disorders • Mental Health Act • National Mental Health Policy vis a vis National Health Policy • National Mental Health Programme • Mental health team • Nature and scope of mental health nursing • Role and functions of mental health nurse in various settings and factors affecting the level of nursing practice • Concepts of normal and abnormal behaviour	• Lecture Discussion	• Objective type • Short answer • Assessment of the field visit reports	1
II	5	• Defines the various terms used in Mental Health Nursing	**Principles and Concepts of Mental Health Nursing** • Definition: Mental Health Nursing and terminology used • Classification of mental disorder: ICD	• Lecture discussion • Explain using charts • Review of personality development	• Essay type • Short answer • Objective type	2

Unit	Time (Hrs)	Learning Objective	Content	Teaching Learning Activity	Assessment Method	Chapter
		• Explain the classification of mental disorders • Explain psycho-dynamics of maladaptive behaviour • Discuss the etiological factors, psychopa-thology of mental disorders • Explain the principles and standards of mental health nursing • Describe the conceptual models of mental health nursing	• Review of personality development, defense mechanisms • Maladaptive behaviour of individuals and groups: Stress, crisis and disaster (s) • Etiology: Biopsycho-social factors • Psychopathology of mental disorder: Review of structure and function of brain, limbic system and abnormal neuro-transmission • Principles of mental health nursing • Standards of mental health nursing practice • Conceptual models and the role of nurse: – Existential model – Psychoanalytical models – Behavioural model – Interpersonal model			
III	8	• Describe nature, purpose and process of assessment of mental health status	**Assessment of mental health status** • History taking • Mental status examination • Mini mental status examination • Neurological examination: Review • Investigations: Related bloodchemistry, EEG, CT and MRI • Psychological tests role and responsibilities of nurse	• Lecture discussion • Demonstration • Practice session • Clinical practice	• Short answer • Objective type • Assessment of skills with check list	3
IV	6	• Identify therapeutic communication techniques • Describe therapeutic relationship	**Therapeutic communication and nurse-patient relationship** • Therapeutic communication: Types, techniques, characteristics • Types of relationship • Ethics and responsibilities	• Lecture discussion • Demonstration • Role play • Process recording	• Short answer • Objective type	4

Unit	Time (Hrs)	Learning Objective	Content	Teaching Learning Activity	Assessment Method	Chapter
		• Describe therapeutic impasse and its intervention	• Elements of nurse-patient contract • Review of technique of IPR-Johari window • Goals, phases, tasks, therapeutic techniques • Therapeutic impasse and its intervention			
V	14	• Explain treatment modalities and therapies used in mental disorders and role of the nurse	**Treatment modalities and therapies used in mental disorders** • Psychopharmacology • Psychological therapies: Therapeutic community, psychotherapy-Individual: Psycho-analytical, cognitive and supportive, family, group, behavioural, play, psychodrama, music, dance, recreational and light therapy, relaxation therapies: Yoga, meditation, bio feedback • Alternative system of medicine • Occupational therapy • Physical therapy: Electroconvulsive therapy • Geriatric considerations • Role of nurse in above therapies	• Lecture discussion • Demonstration • Group work • Practice session • Clinical practice	• Essay type • Short answer • Objective type	5
VI	5	• Describe the etiology, psycho-pathology, clinical manifestations, diagnostic criteria and management of patients with Schizophrenia, and other psychotic disorders	**Nursing management of patient with Schizophrenia and psychotic disorders** • Classification: ICD • Etiology, psycho-pathology, types, clinical manifestations, diagnosis • Nursing Assessement-History, physical and mental assessment • Treatment modalities and nursing management of patients with Schizophrenia and other psychotic disorders • Geriatric considerations • Follow-up and home care and rehabilitation	• Lecture discussion • Case discussion • Case presentation • Clinical practice	• Essay type • Short answers • Assessment of patient management problems	6

Unit	Time (Hrs)	Learning Objective	Content	Teaching Learning Activity	Assessment Method	Chapter
VII	5	• Describe the etiology psychopathology, clinical manifestations, diagnostic criteria and management of patients with mood disorders	**Nursing management of patient with mood disorders** • Mood disorders: Bipolar affective disorder, mania depression and dysthamia, etc. • Etiology, psycho-pathology, clinical manifestations, diagnosis • Nursing assessment-History, physical and mental assessment • Treatment modalities and nursing management of patients with mood disorders • Geriatric considerations • Follow-up and home care and rehabilitation	• Lecture discussion • Case discussion • Case presentation • Clinical practice	• Essay type • Short answers • Assessment of patient management problems	7
VIII	8	• Describe the etiology psycho-pathology, clinical manifestations, diagnostic criteria and mangement of patients with neurotic, stress related and somatization disorders	**Nursing management of patient with neurotic, stress related and somatization disorders** • Anxiety disorder, phobias, dissociation and conversion disorder, obsessive compulsive disorder, somatoform disorders, post-traumatic stress disorder • Etiology, psycho-pathology, clinical manifestations, diagnosis • Nursing assessment-History, physcial and mental assessment • Treatment modalities and nursing management of patients with neurotic, stress related and somatization disorders • Geriatric considertions • Follow-up and home care and rehabilitation	• Lecture discussion • Case discussion • Case presentation • Clinical practice	• Essay type • Short answers • Assessment of patient management problems	8
IX	5	• Describe the etiology, psycho-pathology, clinical manifestations,	**Nursing management of patient with substance use disorders** • Commonly used psychotropic substance: Classification	• Lecture discussion • Case discussion • Case presentation	• Essay type • Short answers • Assessment of patient management problems	9

Unit	Time (Hrs)	Learning Objective	Content	Teaching Learning Activity	Assessment Method	Chapter
		diagnostic criteria and management of patients with substance use disorders	forms, routes, action, intoxication and withdrawal • Etiology of dependence: Tolerance, psychological and physical dependence, withdrawal syndrome, diagnosis • Nursing assessment-History, physical, mental assessment and drug assay • Treatment (detoxification antabuse and narcotic antagonist therapy and harm reduction) and nursing management of patients with substance use disorders • Geriaitc considerations • Follow-up and home care and rehabilitation			
X	4	• Describe the etiology, psycho-pathology, clinical manifestations, diagnostic criteria and mangement of patients with personality, sexual and eating disorders	**Nursing management of patient with personality, sexual and eating disorders** • Classification of disorders • Etiology, psycho-pathology, characteristics, diagnosis • Nursing assessment-History, physical and mental assessment • Treatment modalities and nursing management of patients with personality, sexual and eating disorders • Geriatric considerations • Follow-up and home care and rehabilitation	• Lecture discussion • Case discussion • Case presentation • Clinical practice	• Essay type • Short answers • Assessment of patient management problems	10
XI	6	• Describe the etiology, psycho-pathology, clinical	**Nursing management of childhood and adolescent disorders including mental deficiency** • Classification	• Lecture discussion • Case discussion • Case presentation	• Essay type • Short answers • Assessment of patient	11

Unit	Time (Hrs)	Learning Objective	Content	Teaching Learning Activity	Assessment Method	Chapter
		manifestations, diagnostic criteria and management of childhood and adolescent disorders including mental deficiency	• Etiology, psycho-pathology characteristics, diagnosis, Nursing assessmet-History, physical, mental and IQ assessment • Treatment modalities and nursing management of childhood disorders including mental deficiency • Follow-up and home care and rehabilitation	• Clinical practice	management problems	
XII	5	• Describe the etiology psycho-pathology, clinical manifestations, diagnostic criteria and management of organic brain disorders	**Nursing management of organic brain disorders** • Classification: ICD • Etiology, psycho-pathology, clinical features, diagnosis (Parkinson and alzheimers) • Nursing assessment-History, physical, mental and neurological assessment • Treatment modalities and nursing management of organic brain disorders • Geriaitc considerations • Follow-up and home care and rehabilitation	• Lecture discussion • Case discussion • Case presentation • Clinical practice	• Essay type • Short answers • Assessment of patient management problems	12
XIII	6	• Identify psychiatric emergencies and carry out crisis intervention	**Psychiatric emergencies and crisis intervention** • Types of psychiatric emergencies and their management • Stress adaptation model: Stress and stressor, coping, resources and mechanism • Grief: Theories of grieving process, principles, techniques of counselling • Types of crisis • Crisis intervention: Principles, techniques and process • Geriatric consideration • Role and responsibilities of nurse	• Lecture discussion • Demonstration • Practice session • Clinical practice	• Short answers • Objective type	13

Unit	Time (Hrs)	Learning Objective	Content	Teaching Learning Activity	Assessment Method	Chapter
XIV	4	• Explain legal aspects applied in mental health settings and role of the nurse	**Legal issues in Mental Health Nursing** • The Mental Health Act 1987: Act, Sections, Articles and their implication, etc. • Indian Lunacy Act, 1912 • Right of mentally ill clients • Forensic psychiatry • Acts related to narcotic and psychotropic substance and illegal drug trafficking • Admission and discharge procedures • Role and responsibilities of nurse	• Lecture discussion • Case discussion	• Short answers • Objective type	14
XV	4	• Describe the model of preventive psychiatry • Describe community mental health services and role of the nurse	**Community mental health nursing** • Development of community mental health services: • National Mental Health Programme • Institutionalization versus Deinstitutionalization • Model of preventive psychiatry: Levels of prevention • Mental Health services available at the primary, secondary, tertiary levels including rehabilitation and role of nurse • Mental health Agencies: Government and voluntary, National and International • Mental Health nursing issues for special populations: Children, Adolescence, Women, Elderly, Victims of violence and abuse, Handicapped, HIV/AIDS, etc.	• Lecture discussion • Clinical/field practice • Field visits to mental health service agencies	• Short answers • Objective type • Assessment of the field visit reports	15

Contents

1 Introduction

MENTAL HEALTH AND MENTAL ILLNESS

Mental Health

According to WHO, Health is a complete state of physical, mental and social well-being, not merely an absence of disease or infirmity.

Mental health is a state of emotional, psychological and social well-being which is expressed in terms of self-esteem and confidence. It affects the way we think, experience and express and it is essential for making choices, maintaining social relationships and handling stressors.

Box 1.1: Mental health defined

'An adjustment of human beings to the world and to each other with a maximum of effectiveness and happiness'

—*Karl Menninger (1947)*

Mental health is influenced by individual factors, including biologic makeup, autonomy, and independence, self-esteem, capacity for growth and ability to find meaning in life, sense of belonging, reality orientation, and coping or stress management abilities.

The interpersonal factors, such as effective communication, helping others, intimacy, and maintaining a balance of separateness and connectedness and the social/cultural factors are including sense of community, access to resources, intolerance of violence, and support of diversity among people also affect mental health.

Criteria for Good Mental Health

- Adequate contact with reality
- Efficiency in work and play
- Positive self-concept
- Control of thoughts and imagination
- Social acceptance
- A healthy emotional life.

Box 1.2: Indicators of mental health

- Positive attitude towards self.
- Growth, development and the ability for self-actualization.
- Integration.
- Autonomy.
- Adequate control with reality.
- Environmental mastery.

Mental Illness

Mental illness is a condition of behavioral or thinking pattern that results either suffering or an impaired ability to function in normal life. This may be persistent, relapsing and remitting, or occur as a single episode.

Box 1.3: Definition of mental illness

The APA (2000) defines mental disorder as 'a clinically significant behavioral or psychological syndrome or pattern that occurs in an individual and that is associated with present distress or disability or with a significantly increased risk of suffering death, pain, disability or an important loss of freedom'.

Deviant behavior does not necessarily indicate a mental disorder.

Mental Health and Mental Illness Continuum

A primary difference between mental health and mental illness is that everybody has some quantity of mental health all of the time, as in case of physical health, while it is possible that a person can be without a mental illness.

It is possible for a person to have a poor mental health with no mental illness. Despite poor mental health not defined as a disease or an illness, a person with poor mental health often suffer with emotional distress and psychosocial impairment associated with it.

Box 1.4: Mental health and illness continuum

Healthy Normal functioning	**Reacting** Common and reversible problems	**Injured** Significant functional impairment	**Ill** Clinical disorder. Severe and persistent functional Impairment.
Normal mood fluctuations. Takes things in stride. Consistent performance. Normal sleep patterns. Physically and socially active. Usual self-confidence. Comfortable with others.	Irritable/Impatient. Nervousness, sadness, increased worrying. Procrastination, forgetfulness. Trouble sleeping (more often in falling asleep). Lowered energy. Difficulty in relaxing. Intrusive thoughts. Decreased social activity.	Anger, anxiety. Lingering sadness, tearfulness, hopelessness, worthlessness. Preoccupation. Decreased performance in academics or at work. Significantly disturbed sleep (falling asleep and staying asleep). Avoidance of social situations, withdrawal.	Significant difficulty with emotions, thinking high level of anxiety, panic attacks. Depressed mood, feeling overwhelmed. Constant fatigue. Disturbed contact with reality. Significant disturbances in thinking. Suicidal thoughts/ intent/behavior.

Diagram 1.1: Mental health—mental illness continuum

PERSPECTIVES OF MENTAL HEALTH AND MENTAL HEALTH NURSING

Evolution of Mental Health Services, Treatments and Nursing Practices

History of Development of Mental Health Care: Worldwide

It was William Sweetser who referred the term 'mental hygiene' in the mid-19th century, which can be seen as the precursor to modern approaches to focus on promoting positive mental health. Isaac Ray, one of the founders of the American Psychiatric Association (APA), described mental hygiene as an art to preserve the mind against incidents and influences which would inhibit or destroy its energy, quality or development.

Views of madness in the middle ages in Europe used to be a combination of the divine, demoniac and transcendental. Theories of the four humors ***(black bile, yellow bile, phlegm, and blood)*** were used, sometimes separately and sometimes together with theories of evil spirits to describe mental illness.

Arnaldus de Villa Nova (1235–1313) connected 'evil spirit' and Galen-adapted 'four humours' theories and put forward ***trephining*** as a solution to let demons and excess humors escape. Other physical treatment modalities in common use included purges, bloodletting and whipping. Mental illness was often seen as a moral issue, either as a punishment for offense or an assessment of faith and character.

Christian theology recommended various therapies, including fasting and prayer for people disunited from God and exorcism of people possessed by the devil. In this way, although mental disorder was commonly believed to be due to sin, other more prosaic causes were also searched, including diet and alcohol, overwork, and grief.

16th to 18th Centuries

Some psychologically disturbed people may have been sufferer of the occultist-hunts that spread in tides in early modern era. However, those pronounced lunatics were progressively admitted to local correction houses and jails or sometimes to the private madhouses.

Restraints and forceful confinement were used for those people who were judged to be dangerously ill or potentially hostile to themselves, others or equity. The evolution of this group of madhouses has been linked to new plutocrat social relations, which resulted in families no longer being able to or ready to take care of disturbed relatives.

Madness was frequently portrayed in literary works, like the plays of Shakespeare.

By the end of the 17th century, mental illness was progressively viewed as an organic or physical anomaly, no longer involving the spirit or moral responsibility. The insane were typically viewed as aloof wild animals. Harsh treatment methods and restraining in chains was seen as curative, meant to suppress the animal instincts.

There was occasionally a focus on the environment of asylums, from diet to exercise patterns to number of visitors. Owners of the asylums sometimes advertised of their facilities. Treatment modalities used in few public mad houses was also cruel, often secondary to jails. The most vicious and notorious was ***Bedlam*** where at a time people could pay to watch the inmates as a form of entertainment.

Treatments focused on humoral theory then gradually gave away to analogy and phrasings from mechanics and other evolving physical sciences. Multiple new schemes were introduced for the classification of mental illnesses, motivated by evolving systems for the biological classification of organisms and medical classification of diseases.

The term *'crazy'* and insane came to mean mental disorder in this period. The term *'lunacy'*, long used to denote to periodic disturbance, came to be used for insanity. 'Madness', the term previously used to denote crippled or foolish, evolved to mean loss of reasoning or self-control.

The term *'Psychosis'* had varied usage denoting to a condition of the mind or soul. 'Nervous', meaning to wind or twist, meant muscle or vigorous, was used by physiologists to denote to the body's electrochemical signaling process which resulted in coining the term 'nervous system'.

'Obsession', from a Latin word meaning to sit against, previously meant to beset or be owned by an evil spirit, evolved to mean a fixed unchangeable idea that could destroy the mind.

By the end of the 18th century, a moral movement started, that emphasized more humane, social and personalized approaches. Major figures included the Physician *Vincenzo Chiarugi* in Italy, the ex-patient superintendent *Pussin* and the psychologically inclined medic *Philippe Pinel* in revolutionary France; the Quakers in England, led by businessman *William Tuke*; and later, in the United States, campaigner *Dorothea Dix*.

19th Century

The 19th century, in the background of industrialization and population explosion, witnessed a huge expansion of the number and size of asylums in each Western country, a movement known as 'the great confinement' or the 'era of asylum '.

The term 'psychiatry' was formulated as the medical specialization and became more academically entrenched.

20th Century

The 20th century exhibited the evolution of psychoanalysis, which came to the power later. *Kraepelin's* classification attained popularity, including the classification of mood disorders from what would later be termed schizophrenia.

Asylum administrators tried to improve the picture and medical status of their profession. The institutionalized were increasingly referred to as *'patients'* and the asylums were renamed as hospitals. People started referring people as having a *'mental illness'* started from this period in the early 20th century.

Lobotomies, Insulin shock therapy, Electroconvulsive therapy, and the *'neuroleptic'* chlorpromazine came into use mid-century.

A movement against psychiatry came to the existence in the 1960s. Deinstitutionalization progressively occurred in the West, with many psychiatric hospitals being closed down in response to community mental health services.

Various types of psychiatric treatments and medications gradually came into use, like *'psychic energizers'* and *lithium* salts. *Benzodiazepines* obtained widespread popularity in the 1970s for anxiety and depression.

Cognitive behavioral therapy was formulated. During the 1990s, novel *SSRI* antidepressants were some of the most commonly prescribed drugs in the world.

The Diagnostic and Statistical Manual of Mental Disorder (DSM) and then International Statistical Classification of Diseases and Related Health Problems (ICD) accepted new classification, representing a return to a Kraepelin-like descriptive system. The official diagnoses exhibited a large expansion, even though homosexuality was then downgraded and left out in the face of human rights protests.

21st Century

From the year 2002, DSM-5 Research Agenda scientists were called up to contribute with their publication to the theoretical basis for the DSM-5, of which draft criteria are now accessible to the scientific community.

History of Development of Mental Health Care: India

Ancient Hindu and Punjabi manuscripts known as Ramayana and Mahabharata includes fictional characterizations of depression and anxiety states. Mental illnesses were commonly thought to reflect hypothetical metaphysical entities, celestial agents, black magic or witchcraft.

An ancient work known as the *Charaka Samhita,* part of the Hindu medicinal book *'The Ayurveda',* considered ill health as resulting from an inequality among three types of bodily forces called Dosha.

Psychiatry in Precolonial India

During the domination of King Ashoka, many health care facilities were established for people with mental problems. According to Ashoka Samhita, these facilities or hospitals were built with independent enclosures for various curative practices including keeping the inmates and providing treatments available during those times.

A temple at Chengalpattu, Tamil Nadu, contains engravings on the walls belonging to the period of Chola. There are various ancient data regarding propagation of alienation of insane people in Shahdaula's Chauhas in Gujarat and Punjab. Even though there is no much evidence supporting the development of mental health care in the Moghul period, there are some references to some mental health institutions in the period of Mohammad Khilji (1436–1469). There are also some clues of the presence of a mental hospital at Dhar near Mandu, Madhya Pradesh, where Maulana Fazulur Hakim was the physician.

Psychiatry in Colonial India

Mental asylums existed in the British India was a very less obvious form of social control and were greatly influenced by British psychiatry. They were mainly for the British soldiers who were posted in India during that time. The function of such institutions was mainly custodial rather than curative.

Development of mental asylums started during the early colonial period and was more apparent till the first Indian independence revolution was started. The first mental hospital in India was at Bombay which was established in the year of 1745 and was able to accommodate around 30 inmates. In 1795, the first mental hospital which was run by the government was established in Bihar and was aimed at providing custodial services to mentally ill soldiers.

During this period, patients with mania were treated with opium and leeches were used on the mentally ill patients to suck their blood out. Hot baths were also given as a way of treatment. Music was used as a method to calm down the patients. In the community settings, mentally ill patients were taken care by the local communities and the treatment were given by the traditional doctors of Ayurveda and Unani.

After 1914, a new trend of gradual expansion of mental asylums where observed rather than building new projects. One of the important developments in this period is the establishment of India's first psychiatric rehabilitation projects by the Central Institute of Psychiatry. They initiated an occupational therapy for the mentally ill in the year 1922.

Another important change occurred during this period is the increasing awareness about the mental hygiene which paved its way to preventive psychiatry in India. Electroconvulsive Therapy (ECT) in 1943 and Psychosurgery (1947) treatment were started in India.

It was in the year 1946, when the Bhore Committee (Health survey and planning committee) was appointed and surveyed the mental hospitals. They reported many medical and professional inadequacies that were prevalent in the mental health institutions. It also suggested more intensive training for professionals of psychiatry and a separate child psychiatry units in hospitals.

Psychiatry in Independent India

A new era of betterment of mental hospitals started after the independence of India in 1947. The government of India focused primarily upon the formation of ***General hospital psychiatric units*** (GHPUs) rather than building more psychiatric hospitals.

Some new mental institutions, mainly at Delhi, Jaipur, Kottayam and Bengal were added. During Mid-1950s a rapid development in the spread to GHPUs in India was witnessed. In 1957, Dutta Ray started a mental health out-patient service at Irwin Hospital in New Delhi.

By the 1960s, traditional institutions like ***Central institutions of psychiatry (CIP)*** offered a variety of specialized services, like child and adult clinics. Old age, epileptic and neuro psychiatric services were started to fulfill the range of all-inclusive Out-patient Department (OPDs).

Another main innovation in the 1960s was the idea of a day-time hospital. Gradually, alternative accommodations were searched for patients who had recovered from the mental illness, yet could not return to their own families.

With respect to the recommendation of the Bhore committee, AIIMH (All India Institute of Mental Health) was started in 1954, which formed the National Institute of Mental Health and Neurosciences (NIMHANS) in 1974 at Bangalore.

A training program for Primary Health Care was started in 1978–79. In 1978–1984 Indian Council of Medical Research financed and administered a multicenter collective project on 'severe mental morbidity' in Bangalore and Patiala.

Many training programs for psychiatrists, psychologists, social workers, nurses and primary vare doctors were carried out at *Sakalwara,* Karnataka unit during 1981–82. Fighting social stigma and improving the social network of patients were considered as main elements of a useful rehabilitation program.

Box 1.5: Important history glimpses on evolution of mental health care and services

1.	**Sigmund Freud (1856–1939)**	• Father of Psychoanalysis • Structural theory of mind • Topographic theory of mind • '*Interpretation of Dreams*'
2.	**Alfred Adler**	• Importance of feelings of inferiority–the *inferiority complex* • Individual psychology
3.	**Anna Freud (1895–1982)**	• Psychoanalysis • Object Relational Theory • Child Psychiatry
4.	**Erik Erikson (1902–1994)**	• He coined the phrase *identity crisis.* • Erikson's theory of personality -*Theory of psychosocial development*
5.	**Jean Piaget (1896–1980)**	• Cognitive development theory • Developmental psychologist
6.	**Abraham Harold Maslow (1908–1970)**	• American psychologist • *Maslow's hierarchy of needs*
7.	**Carl Rogers (1902–1987)**	• Psychotherapy and counseling • Client-centered therapy
8.	**BF Skinner (1904–1990)**	• Concept of *reinforcement* and *operant conditioning*
9.	**Eugen Bleuler (1857–1939)**	• Coined the term 'schizophrenia.' • 4 'A's and secondary symptoms
10.	**Emil Kraepelin (1856–1926)**	• *Dementia precox and Manic depressive psychosis (MDP)* • Psychiatric methodology
11.	**Harry Stack Sullivan (1892–1949)**	• The Interpersonal Theory of Psychiatry
12.	**Kurt Schneider (1887–1967)**	• **F**irst **R**ank **S**ymptoms of **S**chizophrenia
13.	**John Bowlby (1907–1990)**	• Attachment theory and Grief theory
14.	**John F Cade (1912–1980)**	• Discovered (in 1948) the effects of *lithium carbonate* as a mood stabilizer
15.	**Joseph Wolpe (1915–1997)**	• Behavior therapy: Systematic desensitization
16.	**Aaron T Beck**	• Cognitive therapy
17.	**Julius Wagner-Jauregg (1857–1940)**	• Malarial therapy in General Paresis of Insane
18.	**Ugo Cerletti (1877–1963)**	• Discovered the method of electroconvulsive therapy (ECT)
19.	**Arvid Carlsson (1923–)**	• Swedish scientist, in 1957 he demonstrated that ***dopamine*** was a neurotransmitter in the brain which is implicated in psychosis

Contd...

Contd...

20.	**Egas Moniz (1874–1955)**	• Founder of psychosurgery and cerebral angiography. • Nobel Prize in 1949
21.	**Maxwell Jones**	• Therapeutic Community
22.	**Karl Jaspers**	• Phenomenology
23.	**Karl Leonhard**	• Cycloid psychosis (later MDP)
24.	**Jacob Moreno**	• Psychodrama
25.	**Kubler Ross (1926–2004)**	• Stages of grief
26.	**Leo Kanner (1894–1981)**	• Childhood Autism
28.	**Ivan Pavlov (1849–1936)**	• Classical Conditioning
29.	**Clifford Beers (1876–1943)**	• The founder of the American mental hygiene movement. • *A Mind That Found Itself* (1908), an autobiographical is an account of his hospitalization
30.	**Philippe Pinel (1745–1826)**	• French physician known for humane psychological approach care of psychiatric patients and 'moral therapy'
31.	**William Tuke (1732–1822)**	• English businessman, philanthropist • He started the York Retreat in 1796 for humane care of people with mental disorders
32.	**John Conolly (1830)**	• Removed restraints at the Hanwell Asylum
33	**William Cullen**	• Coined the term 'neurosis'
34.	**Hildegard Peplau (1909–1999)**	• Interpersonal Theory of Nursing
35.	**Linda Richards (1841–1930)**	• First psychiatric nurse, who set up nurse-training schools in several hospitals for mentally ill patients
36.	**Alois Alzheimer (1864–1915)**	• *Alzheimer's disease*
37.	**Franz Mesmer (1734–1815)**	• *Mesmerism*
38.	**William Battie (1758)**	• The first text book on psychiatric conditions—*Treatise on Madness*
39.	**Kahlbaum (1874)**	• Described *catatonia*
40.	**Hecker**	• Described *hebephrenia*
41.	**Jean-Etienne Esquirol (1772–1840)**	• Coined the term *hallucination*
42.	**Georges Gilles de la Tourette**	• *Tourette's disorder (tics and compulsive coprolalia).*
43.	**Benjamin Rush (1745–1813)**	• Father of American Psychiatry • Emblem of American Association of Psychiatry bears his portrait.

Contd...

Contd...

44.	**David T Wong (1940)**	• Discovered *fluoxetine*
45.	**Herbert Y Meltzer (1932)**	• *Clozapine*
46.	**Carl Wernick (1848–1950)**	• Aphasia, language
47.	**Korbian Broadman (1868–1918)**	• Cytoarchitecture—definition of the cerebral cortex into 52 distinct regions
48.	**Sergei Korsakoff (1853–1900)**	• *Korsakoff's psychosis*
49.	**Jean Martin Charcot (1825–1893)**	• Explained *hysteria* as a condition
50.	**Carl Gustav Jung (1875)**	• Introversion and extroversion
51.	**Hans Berger (1873–1941)**	• Electroencephalography (EEG)
52.	**Jacob Kasanin**	• Schizoaffective disorders

Evolution (History) of Psychiatric Nursing Practices

- Fourth century AD, during the period of *Emperor Ashoka*, hospitals started with 15 beds for mentally ill with two male and two female nurses. In 1964–65 Psychiatric nursing was included in curriculum.
- For the first time in India, 11 British nurses along with one matron were brought from the UK to work in the mental hospital at Ranchi in the 1930s.
- Short training courses of three to six months were conducted in Ranchi in 1921, which were recognized by the Royal Medical Psychological Association.
- During 1948–50 four nurses were sent to the UK by Goverment of India for mental health nursing diploma.
- From 1943, the Chennai Government organized a three months' psychiatric nursing course (subsequently stopped in 1964), for male nursing students at the Mental Hospital, Chennai (in lieu of midwifery).
- During 1954 Nur Manzil Medical Health centre, Lucknow gave psychiatric nursing orientation course of 4–6 weeks duration.
- Goverment of India decided to start training psychiatric nurses during 1953–54 and started the first organized course at All India Institute of Mental Health (presently NIMHANS).
- In 1964–1965, the Indian Nursing Council (INC) made it a requirement to integrate psychiatric nursing in the nursing diploma and degree courses.
- In 1967, a separate Psychiatric Nursing Committee was formed in the Trained Nurses Association of India.
- Diploma in Psychiatric Nursing is conducted in three institutions in India.
- Master of Psychiatric Nursing (MPN) program is conducted in many institutions.
- Doctoral program in psychiatric nursing (PhD) at NIMHANS, Bangalore.

PREVALENCE AND INCIDENCE OF MENTAL HEALTH PROBLEMS AND DISORDERS

World

WHO estimated that globally over 450 million people suffer from mental disorders. Currently mental and behavioral disorders account for about 12 percent of the global burden of diseases. This is likely to increase 15 percent by 2020.

World Health Organization Global Study

The World Health Organization is currently undertaking a global survey of 26 countries in all regions of the world, based on ICD and DSM criteria.

The first published figures on the 14 country surveys completed to date indicate that, of those disorders assessed, anxiety disorders are the most common in all countries. (Prevalence rate 2.4 to 18.2%) and mood disorders next most common (12-month prevalence of 0.8 to 9.6%), while substance disorders (0.1–6.4%) and impulse-control disorders (0.0–6.8%) were consistently less prevalent.

India

In 2000 a review of epidemiological studies estimated that the prevalence of mental disorders in India was 70 per 1000 in rural and 73 per 1000 in the urban population. In 1999, a study stated that the prevalence of mental disorders in child and adolescent population was 9.4 percent. Similarly, another study from Bangalore in 2005 documented the burden of mental disorders to be 12.5 percent. The study also showed that there were no significant differences among prevalence rates of mental disorders in urban middle class, slum and rural areas with annual incidence of 18 per 1000 population.

The prevalence of mental disorders among 0-3 yr old children was 13.8 percent, most commonly due to breath holding spells, pica, behavior disorder, expressive language disorder and mental retardation.

The prevalence rate in the 4–16 year old children was 12.0 percent mainly due to enuresis, specific phobia, hyperkinetic disorders, stuttering and oppositional defiant disorder. Compared with the general population, industrial workers were more predisposed to mental disorders.

In 2002, the prevalence rate of mental disorders in the Indian industrial population was estimated to be 14 to 37 percent.

Prevalence of Suicide

- National crime record International Journal of Scientific and Research Publications, Volume 3, Issue 2, February 2013, India reported, 27.7 percent increase in recorded number of suicides between 1995 and 2005 with suicide rate of 10.5 per million.
- A study conducted in rural areas of south India, in 2010 reported 37% of those who died by suicide had a mental disorder. The two most common reasons were alcohol dependence (16%) and adjustment disorders (15%).

Statistics

Mental disorders diagnosed and treated in the six states is given in Table: 1.1 and 1.2

Table 1.1: Prevalence of 'psychosis' in 6 states

State	Need (% diagnosed)	Covered (% Treated)
Assam	1.0	39.1
Karnataka	0.7	85.2
Maharashtra	2.2	48.7
Rajasthan	3.6	36.2
Uttar Pradesh	2.7	45.5
West Bengal	1.8	66.5

The treated cases were in the urban areas (61.7% vs 47.5%); higher, The rate of treatment was lower in the rural population.

Table 1.2: Prevalence of 'depression ' in 6 states

State	Need (% diagnosed)	Covered (% treated)
Assam	3.2	32.3
Karnataka	9.2	13.0
Maharashtra	27.3	9.6
Rajasthan	7.3	29.7
Uttar Pradesh	7.4	8.2
West Bengal	11.7	17.8

Though the prevalence rates of depression are higher than psychoses, the rates treated are far lower, pointing to the limited awareness in the community. The rate of treatment was lower in the rural population.

Box 1.6: Existing mental health services in India and prevalence of mental disorders

- 70 million mentally ill in the country out of 1 billion populations.
- 20,000 beds in 42 mental hospitals.
- 2000 to 3000 beds for psychiatric patients in general and teaching hospitals.
- At the most 10% alone receive active psychiatric assistance or help.
- Point prevalence is that 10 to 20/1000 populations are affected by serious mental disorder.
- 20 to 30 million people may require mental health care.
- 1 bed available for psychiatric patient per 32,500 populations.
- 10% of the patients require urgent mental health care.
- Roughly 2,50,000 new psychiatric cases with serious mental disorders manifesting each year.

Uneven Distribution

In relation to above box 1.6, diagram represents need and availability of mental health services in which need exceeds the services.

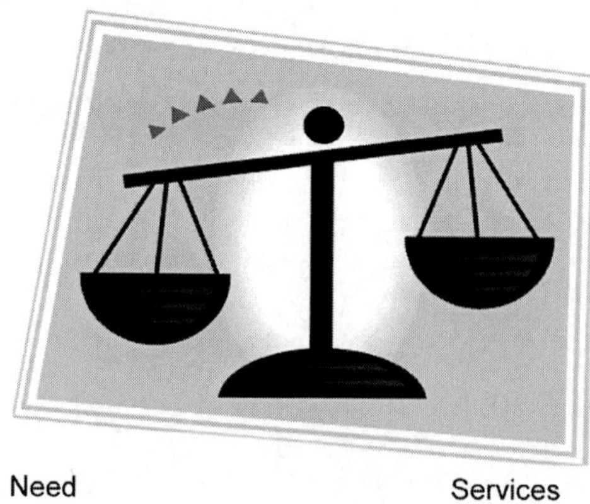

Fig. 1.1: Uneven distribution of mental health need and services

Box 1.7: Man power distribution in mental health field

Psychiatrists (4,000)
Psychologists (200)
Psychiatric social workers (2,000)
Psychiatric nurses (400)

MENTAL HEALTH ACT

The Mental Health Act, which was drafted by the parliament in 1987, was executed into effect in all the states and union territories of India in 1993. This act replaces the Indian Lunacy Act of 1912, which had earlier replaced the Indian Lunatic Asylum Act of 1858. After the independence, The Indian Psychiatric Society was established in the year 1947 and the Mental Health Act was passed in the year 1987.

The main purpose of Mental Health Act 1987 was to consolidate and amend law relating to treatment and care of mentally ill persons and for better provision with respect to property and affairs of mentally ill persons. According to this act some previously used terms were replaced such as nursing home or asylum to a psychiatric hospital, lunatic to mentally ill person and a criminal lunatic to a mentally ill prisoner.
(Refer chapter 14 for detail explanation of Mental Health Act.)

NATIONAL MENTAL HEALTH POLICY *VIS-À-VIS* NATIONAL HEALTH POLICY

National Mental Health Policy

The National Mental Health Policy outlines the prioritized agenda for extending within a pragmatic time-frame basic mental health care facilities to all sections of the population across the country by the year 2020. The tactical vehicle for implementing the said policy will be the refocused National Mental Health Programme, initially formulated in 1982, with five key areas:

1. The District Mental Health Programme (DMHP), redesigned around a Nodal Institution which in most instances will be the Zonal Medical College.

2. Strengthening the Medical Colleges with a view to develop psychiatric manpower (HRD), improve psychiatric treatment facilities at the secondary level and to promote the development of general hospital psychiatry in order to reduce and eventually to eliminate a large extent the need for big mental hospitals with a huge proportion of long-stay patients.
3. Streamlining and modernization of Mental Hospitals to transform them from the present mainly custodial mode to tertiary care centers of excellence with a dynamic social orientation for providing leadership to research and development (R and D) in the field of community mental health.
4. Strengthening of Central and State Mental Health Authorities in order that they may effectively fulfill their role of monitoring ongoing Mental Health Programmes, determining priorities at the ventral/state level and promoting intersectoral collaboration and linkages with other national programmes.
5. Research and training aimed at building up an extensive database of epidemiological information relating to mental disorders and their course/outcome, therapeutic needs of the community, development of better and more cost-effective intervention models, promotion of intersectoral research and providing the necessary inputs/conceptual framework for health and policy planning.

Prioritized Goals

Subject to availability of resources the following time-frame is visualized for attainment in a phased manner for above mentioned policies:

10th Five Year Plan (2002–2007)

- District Mental Health Programme (DMHP) will be extended to one district attached to each of the 100-Medical College in Country, thereby covering 100-Districts by the end of the plan period including the 27-districts where DMHP is already in place, thus making a total of 100- districts across the Country.
- Strengthening of Medical Colleges with allocation of ₹ 50.00 lakhs each to 100-Medical Colleges preferably located in backward areas for upgrading the departments of psychiatry with the aim of instituting post graduate training courses leading to MD (Psychiatry).
- Streamlining and modernization of Mental Hospitals with the aim of reduction in chronicity through intensive therapeutic intervention using non-conventional antipsychotic medications, promoting care of chronically mentally ill patients in the community using outreach maintenance.
- Strengthening of Central and State Mental Health Authorities by facilitating the establishment of permanent secretariats and related machinery and networking of the state authorities with that at the national level to ensure effective coordination in all areas of activity.
- Research and training by sponsoring relevant community based research projects and building up an extensive database which will form the basis for development of intervention models and policy planning.

11th Five year Plan (2007–2012)

The district mental health programme will be extended to other 100-districts while consolidating the same in the 100-districts covered at the end of the 10th plan. Psychiatry Department of the remaining Medical Colleges will be upgraded and the infrastructure created during the previous plan will be reinforced. Qualitative as well as quantitative improvements will be introduced in the areas of research, training and International Electrotechnical Commission (IEC), with more focused attention on epidemiological catchments area surveys on a larger scale.

12th Five Year Plan (2012–2019)

The district mental health programme will be extended to the remaining 161-districts and the gains made in the previous plans will be consolidated, upgradation of the remaining 39-Medical College Psychiatry Departments will be undertaken and 20-Mental Hospitals will be taken up for disinvestments/reconstruction.

Non-viable mental hospitals will be closed down or merged with general hospitals to create general hospital psychiatry units (GHPUs). Central and State Mental Health Authorities will be further reinforced and technologically more sophisticated long-term research projects will be initiated in selected institutions while continuing support to community based research. IEC activities will be augmented to cover all sections of the population across the whole country.

Box 1.8: Strategies of MHP

The National Mental Health Policy is aimed at doing 'the greatest good to the largest number' through five interdependent and mutually synergistic strategies, to be implemented in a phased manner over the next two decades:

1. Extension of basic mental health care facilities to the primary level.
2. Strengthening of psychiatric training in Medical Colleges at the undergraduate as well as postgraduate level.
3. Modernization and rationalization of mental hospitals to develop them into tertiary care centres of excellence.
4. Empowerment of Central and State Mental Health Authorities for effective monitoring, regulation and planning of mental health care delivery systems.
5. Promoting research in frontier areas to evolve better and more cost-effective therapeutic interventions as well as to generate seminal inputs for future planning.

National Health Policy

The Ministry of Health and Family Welfare, Government of India, evolved a National Health Policy in 1983 and 2002.

- The policy lays stress on preventive, promotive, public health and rehabilitation aspects of health care.
- The policy stresses the need of establishing comprehensive primary health care services to reach the population in the remote area of the country.

Aims

- A greater awareness of health problems and means to solve them.
- Supply of safe drinking water and basic sanitation.
- Reduction of existing imbalance in health services by concentrating on the rural health infrastructure.

- Establishment of dynamic health management information system to support health planning.
- Provision of legislative support to health protection and promotion.
- Research into alternative methods of healthcare delivery and low cost health technologies.
- Greater coordination of different systems of medicine.

Objectives

- To achieve an acceptable standard of good health amongst the general population of the country.
- To increase access to the decentralized public health system by establishing new infrastructure in deficient areas, and by upgrading the infrastructure in the existing institutions.
- To ensuring a more equitable access to health services across the social and geographical expanse of the country.
- To increase the aggregate public health investment through a substantially increased contribution by the Central Government.
- To strengthen the capacity of the public health administration at the State level to render effective service delivery.
- To enhance the contribution of the private sector in providing health services for the population group which can afford to pay for services.
- To rationalize use of drugs within the allopathic system.
- To increase access to tried and tested systems of traditional medicine.

Box 1.9: National mental health policy *vs* national health policy

Mental health policy	Health policy
The National Mental Health Policy outlines the prioritized agenda for extending within a pragmatic time-frame basic mental health care facilities to all sections of the population across the country by the year 2020. The tactical vehicle for implementing the said policy will be the refocused National Mental Health Programme, initially formulated in 1982, with five key areas: • The District Mental Health Programme (DMHP), redesigned around a Nodal Institution which in most instances will be the Zonal Medical College. • Strengthening the Medical Colleges with a view to develop psychiatric manpower (HRD), improve psychiatric treatment facilities at the secondary level and to promote the development of general hospital psychiatry in order to reduce and eventually to eliminate to a large extent the need for big mental hospitals with a huge proportion of long-stay patients.	The Ministry of Health and Family Welfare, Government of India, evolved a National Health Policy in 1983 and 2002. • The policy lays stress on preventive, promotive, public health and rehabilitation aspects of health care. • The policy stresses the need of establishing comprehensive primary health care services to reach the population in the remote area of the country. **Aims:** • A greater awareness of health problems and means to solve them. • Supply of safe drinking water and basic sanitation. • Reduction of existing imbalance in health services by concentrating on the rural health infrastructure. • Establishment of dynamic health management information system to support health planning

Contd...

Contd...

Mental health policy	Health policy
• Streamlining and modernization of Mental Hospitals to transform them from the present mainly custodial mode to tertiary care centers of excellence with a dynamic social orientation for providing leadership to research and development (R–D) in the field of community mental health. • Strengthening of Central and State Mental Health Authorities in order that they may effectively fulfill their role of monitoring ongoing Mental Health Programmes, and promoting intersectoral collaboration and linkages with other national programmes. • Research and training aimed at building up an extensive database of epidemiological information relating to mental disorders and their course/ outcome. ***Five strategies of mental health policy:*** • Extension of basic mental health care facilities to the primary level. • Strengthening of psychiatric training in Medical Colleges at the undergraduate as well as postgraduate level. • Modernization and rationalization of mental hospitals. • Empowerment of Central and State Mental Health Authorities for effective monitoring, regulation and planning of mental health care delivery systems. • Promoting research.	• Provision of legislative support to health protection and promotion. • Research into alternative methods health care delivery and low cost health technologies. • Greater coordination of different systems of medicine. **Objectives:** • To achieve an acceptable standard of good health amongst the general population of the country. • To increase access to the decentralized public health system by establishing new infrastructure in deficient areas, and by upgrading the infrastructure in the existing institutions. • To ensuring a more equitable access to health services across the social and geographical expanse of the country. • To increase the aggregate public health investment through a substantially increased contribution by the Central Government. • To strengthen the capacity of the public health administration at the State level to render effective service delivery. • To enhance the contribution of the private sector in providing health services for the population group which can afford to pay for services. • To rationalize use of drugs within the allopathic system. • To increase access to tried and tested systems of traditional medicine.

NATIONAL MENTAL HEALTH PROGRAMME

The Government of India launched the National Mental Health Programme (NMHP) in 1982, keeping in view the heavy burden of mental illness in the community, and the absolute inadequacy of mental health care infrastructure in the country to deal with it.

NMHP has three Components

1. Treatment of Mentally ill.
2. Rehabilitation.
3. Prevention and promotion of positive mental health.

Objectives

- To ensure availability and accessibility of minimum mental health care for all in the foreseeable future, particularly to the most vulnerable and underprivileged sections of population.
- To encourage application of mental health knowledge in general health care.
- To promote community participation in the mental health services development.

(Refer chapter 15 for detail explanation of mental health programme)

MENTAL HEALTH TEAM

A Multidisciplinary/Interdisciplinary Approach

Team work is important in any setting so as in a mental health setting. In mental health care setting, different professionals act hand in hand to help the patient with an overall objective of patient wellness.

For the promotion of a therapeutic environment, members of various discipline coordinate their activity. Four health care professionals constitute the core mental health disciplines: ***Psychiatric nursing, psychiatry, clinical psychology and psychiatric social work.***

Teamwork is a coordinated and dedicated effort of each and every member of the team toward achievement of a vested interest, target or goal of the team as an entity. It becomes more significant in a mental health setting where the contribution of all the members is extremely vital for a comprehensive care of the mentally ill client.

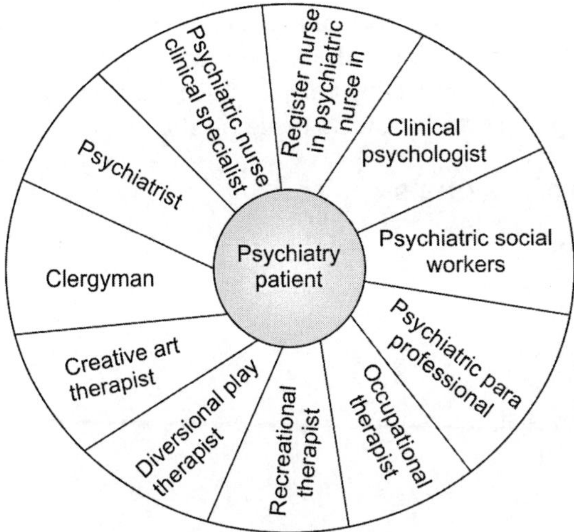

Fig. 1.2: Mental health team members

Psychiatrist

The psychiatrist is a doctor with a postgraduation in psychiatry with 2 to 3 years of residential training. He is responsible for diagnosis, treatment and prevention of mental disorders, prescribe medicines and somatic therapies and function as a leader of the mental health team.

Psychiatric Nurse Clinical Specialist

The psychiatric nurse clinical specialist should have a master degree in nursing, preferably with postgraduate research work.

She/he participates actively in primary, secondary and tertiary prevention of mental disorder and provides individual, group and the family psychotherapy in a hospital and community setting. She/he also takes the responsibility of teaching, administration and research, etc. in a mental health setting. She/he takes up the role of a leader and can practice independently.

Registered Nurse in a Psychiatric Unit

The registered nurse undergoes a General Nursing and Midwifery program or BSc Nursing/PB BSc Nursing program with added qualification such as diploma in psychiatric nursing, and should have registration with state nursing council.

She/he is skilled in caring for the mentally ill, gives holistic care by assessing the patient's mental, social, physical, psychological and spiritual needs and applies psychiatric nursing process.

Clinical Psychologist

The clinical psychologist holds a Doctoral degree in clinical psychology and is registered with clinical psychologist's association. He/she conducts psychological tests, interprets and evaluates the finding of these tests and implements a program of behavior modification.

Psychiatric Social Worker

The psychiatric social worker is a graduate in social work and postgraduate in psychiatric social work. He/She assesses the individual, the family and community support system, helps in discharge planning, counseling for job placement and is aware of the state laws and legal rights of the patient and protects these rights.

Psychiatric Para-professionals

- Psychiatric nursing aids
- ECT technicians
- Auxiliary personnel
- Occupational therapist
- Recreational therapist
- Diversion play therapist
- Creative art therapist
- Clergyman.

NATURE AND SCOPE OF MENTAL HEALTH NURSING

The scope of mental health nursing is not restricted within the confines of the bed-side nursing care. A mental health nurse needs to be skilled and clinically competent, sensitive to the social environment, the advocacy of the needs of the patient's and their families as well as beware of the legal and ethical dilemmas.

Philosophical Beliefs in Nursing Practice [Nature of Mental Health Nursing]

- Individual has intrinsic worth and dignity and respect.
- Each person foundation as a holistic being, who acts, interacts with and reacts to the environment as a universal person.
- All behavior of the individual is meaningful. It arises out from personal needs and goals and can be understood only by the person's internal frame of reference and within the context in which it occurs.
- Behavior consists of perceptions, thought, feelings, and actions.
- Individual vary in their coping capacities, which depend on genetic, environmental influence, nature and degree of stress, and available resources. All individual have the potential for both health and illness.

- The goal of nursing care is to promote wellness, maximize functioning, and enhance self-actualization of clients.
- An interpersonal relationship will produce change and growth within the individual.
- The psychiatric nurse adopts knowledge from the psychosocial and biophysical sciences and theories of the personality and the human behavior.

Scope of Mental Health Nursing

The areas concerned for the psychiatric mental health nurse include a wide range of actual or potential mental health problem.

A mental health nurse needs to be skilled and clinically competent, sensitive to the social environment, the advocacy needs of the clients and their families as well as be aware of the legal and ethical dilemma.

Components of Scope of Mental Health Nursing

There are six components involved in the Nurse patient partnership or the Nurse patient relationship:

1. Clinical competence.
2. Patient family advocacy.
3. Fiscal responsibility.
4. Interdisciplinary collaboration.
5. Social accountability.
6. Legal ethical parameters.

Apart from the six components there are other different areas that include the following:

- **Current issues and trends** in care involving in health care, economic issues, changes in illness orientation, changes in care delivery system, information technology, consumer empowerment, deinstitutionalization, physician shortage and gaps in service, demographic changes, and changes in patient needs.
- **Educational programs** for the psychiatric nurse from Diploma to Doctorate and also various short-term training program.
- **Standards nursing practice** is a beginning step toward of quality of nursing care and standards are provided in all the health team members therefore they improve the quality of care in mentally ill patients.
- **Development of code of ethics** to take up independent roles in all therapy and protect the rights and act as patient advocate.
- **Legal aspects** in Psychiatric Nursing.
- Promotion of **research in Mental Health Nursing** aids in the innovative findings in the both theories and research.
- **Cost effective nursing care** to identify the cost involved in the training of the nurse and the quality care output.
- **Focus of care** on certain target groups like elderly, children, women, mentally retarded and chronic mentally ill.
- **Role of nurse in contemporary mental health** care that involve both the extended role and the other areas of working.

ROLES AND FUNCTIONS OF MENTAL HEALTH NURSE

Role in Contemporary Mental Health Care

- Community mental health nurse.
- Psychiatric home care nurse.
- Forensic psychiatric nurse.
- Psychiatric consultation liaison nurse.
- Case manager.
- Gero psychiatric nurse.
- Parish nurse.
- Tele *health/Tele* nurse.
- Psychiatric Nurse Educator.
- Nurse Manager.

Role of Nurse in Various Settings

Role in Mental Hospital

- Patient care.
- Education and supervision.
- Ward management.
- Interpersonal Process Recording (IPR) and communication.
- Role in other therapies like,
  - *Chemotherapy*
  - *Family therapy*
  - *ECT and Physical therapy.*

Role of Nurse in Community Mental Health

- Consultative role
- Clinical role
- Therapeutic role
- Researcher
- Trainer
- Administrator
- Domiciliary care.

Factor Affecting the Level of Nursing Practice

- Increased consumer.
- Awareness of community in early detection and treatment of mental illness.
- Availability of multidisciplinary team approach.
- Reorganization of physical structure of the hospital.
- Change in method of treatment.
- Increased priority on rehabilitation of the patient.
- Expansion of psychiatric services within general hospital.
- Emphasis of mental health services in national health policy.

Box 1.10: Qualities of a psychiatric nurse

- Self-awareness
- Self-acceptance
- Accepting the patient
- Being sincerely interested in patient care
- Being available
- Empathizing with the patient
- Reliability
- Professionalism
- Accountability
- The ability to think critically.

Concepts of Normal and Abnormal Behavior

Concept of Normal Behavior

People having average amount of intelligence, personality, stability, and social adaptability are considered as normal.

Do You Know?

Word normal derived from ***latin*** word ***norma*** means ***rule***. To follow rule or pattern or standards.

Box 1.11: Normal behavior

Definition: When the individual is able to function adequately and performs his daily living activities efficiently and feel satisfied with his life style called as normal behavior.

Concept of Abnormal Behavior

Abnormality refers to maladjustment to one's society and culture which surrounds him. It is the deviating from the normal in an unfavorable and pathological way. In other words, it deals with the unusual behavior of man. The unusual or maladapted behavior of many persons which do not fit into our common forms of behavior is known as abnormal behavior.

Box 1.12: Abnormal behavior

Definition: Disturbances seen in behavior which manifests in cognitive domain (thinking, memory) affective domain (emotion and feeling) and conative domain (psychomotor activity).

A close analysis of various types of abnormal behavior indicates that abnormal behavior circumscribes a wide range of maladaptive reactions like *psychoneuroses, psychoses, delinquents, sexually deviants, and drug addicts, etc.* The abnormal deviants who are about 10 percent of the general population are classified into four main categories:

1. Psychoneurotic
2. Psychotic
3. Mentally defective
4. Antisocial.

Thus, abnormality and normality can only be defined in terms of conformity to the will and welfare of the group and in the capacity for self-management.

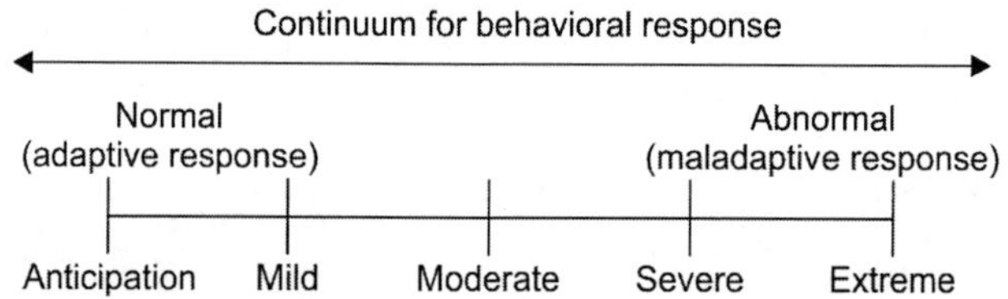

Box 1.13: Characteristics

Normal behavior	Abnormal behavior
• A perception of reality. • A positive attitude toward one's self, acceptance of weakness and pride in strengths. • Capacity for withstanding anxiety and stress. • Adequate in work, play and leisure willingness to use problem solving approaches in life process. • Capacity to adapt oneself to current situation.	• Change in person's thinking process, memory, perception and judgment. • Work efficiency will be reduced. • Forgetfulness. • Unhappiness. • Unable to cope, worried, anxious disturbance in daily routine activities. • No respect will be given to others or self. • Lack of gratification. • Lack of self-confidence.

CONCEPT OF NORMAL BEHAVIOR AND ABNORMAL BEHAVIOR EXPLAINED THROUGH MODELS

Defining the concepts of normal and abnormal behavior is found to be difficult. Several models have been put forward in order to explain the concept of normal and abnormal behavior.

Medical Model

Medical model describes mental illness as a result of organic pathology. According to this model, abnormality is characterized by the disturbances in thought, emotions and behavior.

Statistical Model

Statistically normal mental health falls within two Standard Deviations (SDs) of the normal distribution curve. Therefore mental illness falls outside two Standard Deviations of the normal distribution curve.

Utopian Model

Utopian model regards normal mental health as an individual's ability to blend various mental faculties so that he can function at optimum level.

Process Model

Normal behavior is the result of interacting system. This model focuses the need for developmental changes in the attainment of mature adult functioning.

Social Model

Normality is defined in context with social norms prescribed by the culture. When there is a deviation from the social norms, it is considered as an abnormal behavior.

Behavioral Model

Behavior that is adaptive and socially acceptable is considered as normal. Abnormal behavior is a set of faulty behaviors acquired through learning.

There is no clear demarcation between Normality and Abnormality because no individual is static and their behavior or nature varies and the continuum also will be deviated but it is depicted on the basis of the general derivation systematically processing.

2 Principles and Concepts of Mental Health Nursing

CONCEPTS OF MENTAL HEALTH NURSING

Psychiatric mental health nursing, it is a core mental health profession in nursing field. Psychiatric mental health nurses provide comprehensive, patient-centred mental health and psychiatric care and outcome evaluation in a variety of settings across the entire continuum of care.

Why should Nurse Understand the Concepts of Mental Health Nursing?

- The nurse can expect to use mental health nursing principles in a variety of health care settings.
- Basic mental health concepts are useful in understanding a patient's behavioral responses to disease and dysfunction.
- Behavior is the manner in which a person performs any or all of the activities of daily living.
- Mental health is one's ability to cope-up with and adjust to the recurrent stresses of everyday living.

Box 2.1: Mental health

'An adjustment of human beings to the world and to each other with a maximum of effectiveness and happiness'.

—*Karl Menninger (1947)*

Box 2.2: Mental health nursing

'It is a specialized area of nursing practice employing theories of human behavior, as a science and the purposeful use of self as art in the diagnosis and treatment of human responses to actual or potential mental health problems.'

—*American Nurses Association (1994)*

Interventions include the continuous and comprehensive primary mental health care services necessary for the improvement of optimal mental health, the prevention of mental illness, rehabilitation from mental disorders, and health maintenance.

SIGNS AND SYMPTOMS OF MENTAL ILLNESS (TERMINOLOGIES USED)

Signs and symptoms of mental illness are common in patients of all kinds; therefore, students require sound knowledge of these symptoms and signs. In psychiatric clinical practice, diagnosis is not made on a single symptom or signs, but on the pattern of several clinical features.

Box 2.3: Symptoms and signs of psychiatric disorder

- Abnormalities of behavior and movements.
- Abnormalities of mood and emotion.
- Abnormalities of speech.
- Abnormalities of thinking.
- Abnormalities of perception.
- Abnormalities of awareness of self and others.
- Abnormalities of consciousness.
- Abnormalities of attention and concentration.
- Abnormalities of memory.
- Abnormality of judgment.
- Abnormality of insight.
- Abnormality of sleep, eating and sex.

Abnormalities of Behavior and Movements

- ***Aggression:*** Verbal or physical hostile behavior, with rage and anger.
- ***Akathisia:*** Inability to keep sitting still, due to compelling subjective feeling of restlessness (patient is fully aware of restlessness).
- ***Catatonic excitement:*** Marked agitation, impulsivity and aggression without external provocation.
- ***Catatonic stupor:*** It is characterized by extremely slowed motor activity, to the point of being motionless and seeming unawareness of the environment.
- ***Compulsions:*** Compelling repeated irrational actions associated with obsessions. For example, repeated hand washing.
- ***Dyskinesia:*** Restless movement of group of muscles (face, neck, hands).
- ***Dystonia:*** Painful severe muscle spasm.
- ***Echopraxia:*** Imitative repetition of movement of somebody.
- ***Mannerism:*** Odd goal-directed movements, e.g. repeated hand movement resembling a military salute.
- ***Psychomotor agitation:*** Restlessness with psychological tension. (patient is not fully aware of restlessness).
- ***Stereotypies:*** Purposeless repetitive involuntary movements, e.g. foot tapping, thigh rocking.
- ***Stupor:*** A state in which a person does not react to the surroundings (mute, immobile and unresponsive).
- ***Tics:*** Sudden repeated involuntary muscle twisting, e.g. repeated blinking, grimacing.
- ***Torticollis:*** Contraction of neck muscles.
- ***Waxy flexibility*:** Patient's limbs may be moved like wax, holding position for long period of time before returning to previous position (patient obeys to remain in abnormal position for long time even it is too difficult).

Abnormalities of Mood and Emotion

- ***Alexithymia*:** Inability or difficulty in expressing one's own emotions.
- ***Anxiety:*** Feeling of apprehension accompanied by autonomic symptoms caused by anticipation of danger.
- ***Anhedonia:*** Lack of pleasure in acts which are normally pleasurable.
- ***Apathy:*** Lack of emotion, interest or concern, associated with detachment.
- ***Ambivalent mood:*** Coexistence of two opposing emotional tones towards same object in the same person at same time.

- ***Depressed mood:*** Feeling of sadness, pessimism and a sense of loneliness.
- ***Dysphoria:*** Mixture feelings of sadness and apprehension.
- ***Elevated mood:*** A mood more cheerful than usual.
- ***Elation:*** Feeling of elevated mood with optimism and self-satisfaction.
- ***Euphoria:*** Intense elation with feeling of grandeur.
- ***Expansive mood:*** Expression of euphoria with an overestimation of self-importance.
- ***Fear:*** Anxiety caused by realistic consciously recognized danger.
- ***Flat affect:*** Absence of emotional expression.
- ***Grief:*** Sadness appropriate to a real loss (e.g. death of a relative).
- ***Grandiosity***: Feeling and thinking of great importance (in identity or ability).
- ***Guilt:*** Unpleasant emotion secondary to doing what is perceived as wrong.
- ***Inappropriate affect:*** Disharmony between emotions and the idea, thought, or speech, accompanying it.
- ***Irritable mood:*** Easily annoyed and provoked to anger.
- ***Labile affect:*** Rapid, abrupt changes in emotions in the same setting, unrelated to external stimuli.
- ***LaBelle indifference:*** Inappropriate denial of expected affect and lack of concern about physical disability (seen in conversion disorders).
- ***Panic:*** Acute, self-limiting, episodic intense attack of anxiety associated with overwhelming dread and autonomic symptoms.
- ***Perplexity:*** Anxious mood with bewilderment.
- ***Phobia:*** Irrational exaggerated fear and avoidance of a specific object, situation or activity.
- ***Shame:*** Unpleasant emotion secondary to failure to live up to self-expectation.

Abnormalities of Speech

- ***Circumstanciality:*** Over inclusion of details delaying reaching the desired goal.
- ***Clang associations (rhyming):*** Association of word similar in sound but not in meaning (e.g. deep, keep, sleep).
- ***Dysarthria:*** Difficulty in articulation and speech production.
- ***Echolalia:*** Imitation of words or phrases made by others.
- ***Elective mutism:*** Refusal to speak in certain circumstances.
- ***Motor aphasia:*** Impairment in the ability to formulate fluent speech due to lesion affecting Broca's (motor) area.
- ***Mutism:*** Inability to speak.
- ***Poverty of speech:*** Restricted amount of speech.
- ***Pressure of speech***: Rapid, uninterrupted speech that is increased in amount.
- ***Stuttering (stammering):*** Frequent repetition or prolongation of sound or syllable, leading to markedly impaired speech fluency.
- ***Punning:*** Playing upon words, by using a word of more than one meaning (e.g. ant, aunt).
- ***Word salad:*** Incoherent mixture of words and phrases.

Abnormalities of Thinking

A. Abnormal Stream of Thoughts

- *Poverty of thoughts:* Few, slow, unvaried thoughts associated with poverty of speech.
- *Pressure of thoughts:* Rapid abundant varying thoughts associated with pressure of speech and flight of ideas.

Thought block: Sudden cessation of thought flow with complete emptying of the mind not caused by an external influence.

B. Abnormal Thought Link (*Also called formal thought disorders)*

- *Flight of ideas:* Successive rapidly shifting of incomplete ideas but with an understandable link.
- *Loosening of associations:* Lack of logic connection between thoughts.
- *Thought perseveration:* Repeating the same sequence of thoughts persistently and inappropriately.

C. Abnormal Thought Content

- *Overvalued ideas:* Strongly held false ideas but shakeable (e.g. personal conviction that vitiligo is a contagious disease).
- *Obsessions:* Repetitive ideas, images, feelings or urges insistently entering person's mind despite resistance. They are unwanted, distressful and recognized as senseless and irrational. Obsessions are frequently followed by compelling actions (compulsions). (Box 2.4)

Box 2.4: Common obsessional content

- Dirt/contamination/cleaning
- Orderliness/symmetry
- Doubts/checking/counting
- Aggressive impulses/inappropriate acts:
  - **Ruminations:** obsessional thoughts
  - **Rituals:** Certain repeated compulsions.

- *Delusions:* Unshakable false beliefs out of keeping with the person's cultural background, not arrived at through logic thinking and not amenable to reasoning.

Box 2.5: Common delusional contents

- **Persecutory (paranoid) delusion:** Delusion of being persecuted (cheated, mistreated, harassed, etc.)
- **Grandiose delusion:** Delusion of exaggerated self-importance, power or identity.
- **Delusion of reference:** Delusion that some events and others' behavior refer to oneself.
- **Delusion of jealousy:** Delusion that a loved person (wife/husband) is unfaithful (infidelity delusion).
- **Erotomanic delusion:** Delusion that someone, (usually inaccessible, high social class person) is deeply in love with the patient.
- **Nihilistic delusion:** Delusion of nonexistence of self, part of the body, belongings, others or the world.
- **Delusion of self-accusation:** Delusion that a patient has done something sinful, with excessive feeling of remorse and guilt.

Contd...

Contd...

- **Delusion of influence:** Delusion that person's thoughts, actions, or feelings are controlled by outside forces.
- **Passivity phenomena:** Person reports being made feel, made think or made act.

D. Thought Alienation

- ***Thought insertion:*** Delusion that some of person's thoughts being put into the mind by an external force (other people, certain agency).
- ***Thought withdrawal:*** Delusion that some of person's thoughts being taken out of the mind.
- ***Thought broadcasting:*** Derived from *'Idea of Reference'*: misattribution of events as referring to oneself. Delusion that others can read or hear the person's thoughts, as they are broadcast over the air, radio or some other unusual way.

Box 2.6: Delusions can be either

Mood-congruent Delusion	Mood-incongruent delusion
Mood-congruent delusion means when patient's **delusional** content has **association** to **mood.** **For example:** *In depressed mood:* delusion of self-accusation. - *In elevated mood:* Grandiose delusion.	Mood-incongruent Delusions means when patient's **delusional content** has **no association** to **mood.** **For example:** patient with elevated mood has delusion of thought insertion.

Box 2.7: Delusions can be either

Systematized delusion	Bizarre delusion
Delusion united by a single event or theme, e.g. delusion of jealousy.	Totally odd and strange delusional belief, e.g. delusion that person's acts are controlled by stars.

Abnormalities of Perception

- ***Illusions:*** Misperceptions or misinterpretations of real external sensory stimuli, e.g. shadows may be misperceived as frightening figures.
- ***Hallucinations:*** Perception in the absence of real external stimuli; experienced as true perception coming from the external word (not within the mind), e.g. hearing a voice of someone when actually nobody is speaking within the hearing distance.

Box 2.8: Types and sub-types of hallucination

- Auditory hallucinations (hearing voices, sound, noise in the absence of auditory stimuli).
- **Second-person hallucinations:** Voice speaking to the person addressing him as 'you'.
- **Third-person hallucinations:** Voice talking about the person as 'he' or 'she'.
- **Thought echo:** Hearing one's own thoughts spoken aloud.
- Visual hallucinations (images/sights).
- Olfactory hallucinations (smell/odor).
- Gustatory hallucinations (taste).
- Tactile hallucinations (touch).
- Somatic hallucinations (visceral and other internal sensations).
- **Hypnagogic hallucinations:** Hallucinations when falling asleep.
- **Hypnopompic hallucinations:** Hallucinations when waking from sleep.
- **Pseudo-hallucinations:** Sensory deceptions perceived as emanating from within the mind.

Abnormalities of Awareness of Self and Others

- *Depersonalization:* The experience of altered self-awareness; being unreal, strange or detached.
- *Derealization:* The experience of changed reality; environment is unreal or changed.
- *Fugue*: Assuming a new identity with amnesia for the old identity often involves travel or wandering to new environment.

Abnormalities of Conciousness

- *Drowsiness:* Diminished awareness with inclination to sleep.
- *Somnolence:* Severe abnormal drowsiness.
- *Disorientation:* Disturbance of orientation in time, place, or person.
- *Confusion:* Muddled thinking with disorientation and disturbance of consciousness.
- *Clouding of consciousness:* Drowsiness with impaired attention and reaction to stimuli.
- *Delirium*: Disorientation with disturbed memory, perception, emotion, thinking and behavior.
- *Coma*: Profound degree of unconsciousness.

Abnormalities of Attention and Concentration

- *Distractibility*: A state in which attention is easily drawn to irrelevant external stimuli.
- *Inattention:* Inability to focus attention on a stimulus.
- *Selective inattention*: Choosing not to focus attention on unwanted stimuli.
- *Hypervigilance:* Excessive attention concentration; continually watching or on guard.

Abnormalities of Memory

- *Amnesia:* Inability to recall past information and experiences.
- *Hypermnesia:* Exaggerated degree of retention and recall.
- *Confabulation*: Unintentional filling of memory gaps by imagined experiences.
- *Déjà vu:* False feeling of familiarity; illusion of visual recognition in which a new situation is incorrectly regarded as a repetition of a previous memory.
- *Jamais vu:* Unfamiliarity with a real situation that a person has experienced before.
- *Deja pense:* Illusion that a new thought is recognized as a thought previously felt.

Box 2.9: Types of amnesia

- **Anterograde amnesia:** Amnesia for events occurring after a point in time.
- **Retrograde amnesia:** Amnesia for events occurring before a point of time.
- **Memory blackout:** Amnesia experienced by alcoholics for events during drinking bouts.
- **Dissociative (hysterical) amnesia:** Unconscious forgetting of painful memories.

Abnormality of Insight

What is insight?

The capacity to gain an accurate and deep understanding of someone or something.

Levels of Impaired Insight—rated based on grades:

Grade I: Complete lack of insight (denial of illness).

Grade II: Diminished insight.

Grade III: Being aware of abnormal experiences but denying being mentally ill.

Grade IV: Being aware of mental illness but attributing it to an imagined external force (e.g. persecutors).

Grade V: Being aware of mental illness but denying the need of psychiatric treatment.

Grade VI: Being aware of mental illness and the need of psychiatric treatment but actually not motivated to be treated. (intellectual but not actual insight).

Abnormalities of Sleep

- *Insomnia:* Diminished or lack of sleep.
- *Hypersomnia:* Excessive prolonged sleep.
- *Parasomnia:* Disturbed behavior during sleep. Common are:
  - **Nightmare:** A terrifying dream in which the dreamer experiences feelings of helplessness and extreme anxiety.
  - **Night terrors:** Sudden awakening from Non-REM (repid eye movement) sleep with autonomic arousal (person may scream).
  - **Somnambulism (sleepwalking):** While still asleep a patient walks with open eyes but with poor concentration and appears unresponsive.
  - **Sleep talking:** Talking few words or sentences during sleep.
  - **Sleep paralysis:** Inability to perform voluntary movements during the transition between wakefulness and sleep; person is conscious but cannot move.
  - **Sleep related bruxism:** Tooth grinding occurring during sleep.

Abnormalities of Eating

- *Anorexia*: Loss of, or decrease in appetite.
- *Hyperphagia*: Increase in appetite and intake of food.
- *Bulimia:* Episodes of uncontrolled excessive eating with insatiable hunger (binge eating).
- *Pica*: Craving and eating of non-food substances, such as clay and paint.
- *Psychogenic vomiting*: Repeated episodic vomiting without a medical cause; occurs commonly after meals and without nausea.

Abnormalities of Sex

- *Diminished libido:* Decreased sexual interest, drive and performance.
- *Impotence:* Inability to maintain erection enough for completion of satisfactory coitus.
- *Premature ejaculation:* Ejaculation before person's wish.
- *Vaginimus*: Involuntary painful contraction of vaginal introitus in response to attempts at penetration, that interferes with intercourse.
- *Dyspareunia:* Persistent or recurrent genital pain during, before or after intercourse.

CLASSIFICATION OF MENTAL (PSYCHIATRIC) DISORDERS

There are two most important modern psychiatric classifications basically given by two organizations. They are:

i. *International Classification of Diseases and Related Health Problems* **(ICD-10)** given by ***WHO***.

ii. *Diagnostic and Statistical Manual of Mental Disorder, 4th Edition, Text Revision* **(DSM-IV-TR)** published by ***The American Psychiatric Association (APA).***

I. International Statistical Classification of Diseases and Related Health Problems (ICD-10).

This system was developed by the World Health Organization (WHO). Mental disorders were first included in its 6th edition (ICD-6) in 1948. The latest version is ICD-10, introduced in 1992.

The chapter 'F' classifies psychiatric disorder as mental and behavioral disorder and codes them on an alphanumeric system from F00 to F99. The main categories in ICD-10 are as follows:

F00–F09	Organic, including symptomatic and mental disorders
F00	Dementia in Alzheimer's disease
F01	Vascular dementia
F02	Dementia in other diseases classified elsewhere
F03	Unspecified dementia
F04	Organic amnesic syndrome, not induced by alcohol and other psychoactive substances
F05	Delirium, not induced by alcohol and other psychoactive substances
F06	Other mental disorders due to brain damage and dysfunction, and physical disease
F07	Personality and behavioral disorders due to brain disease, damage and dysfunction
F09	Unspecified organic or symptomatic mental disorder
F10–F19	**Mental and behavioral disorders due to psychoactive substances used**
F10	Mental and behavioral disorders due to use of alcohol
F11	Mental and behavioral disorders due to use of opioids
F12	Mental and behavioral disorders due to use of cannabinoids
F13	Mental and behavioral disorders due to use of sedatives or hypnotics
F14	Mental and behavioral disorders due to use of cocaine
F15	Mental and behavioral disorders due to use of other stimulants, including caffeine
F16	Mental and behavioral disorders due to use of hallucinogens
F17	Mental and behavioral disorders due to use of tobacco
F18	Mental and behavioral disorders due to use to volatile solvents
F19	Mental and behavioral disorders due to multiple drug use and use of other psychoactive substances
F20–F29	**Schizophrenia, schizotypal and delusional disorders**
F20	Schizophrenia
F21	Schizotypal disorder
F22	Persistent delusional disorders
F23	Acute and transient psychotic disorders

Contd...

Contd...

F24	Induced delusional disorder
F25	Schizoaffective disorders
F28	Other nonorganic psychotic disorders
F29	Unspecified nonorganic psychosis
F30–F39	**Mood (affective) disorders**
F30	Manic episode
F31	Bipolar affective disorder
F32	Depressive episode
F33	Recurrent depressive disorder
F34	Persistent mood (affective) disorders
F38	Other mood (affective) disorders
F39	Unspecified mood (affective) disorder
F40–F48	**Neurotic, stress-related and somatoform disorders**
F40	Phobic anxiety disorders
F41	Other anxiety disorders
F42	Obsessive-compulsive disorder
F43	Reaction to severe stress, and adjustment disorders
F44	Dissociative (conversion) disorders
F45	Somatoform disorders
F48	Other neurotic disorders
F50–F59	**Behavioral syndromes associated with physiological disturbances and physical factors**
F50	Eating disorders
F51	Nonorganic sleep disorders
F52	Sexual dysfunction, not caused by organic disorder or disease
F53	Mental and behavioral disorders associated with the puerperium, not elsewhere classified
F54	Psychological and behavioral factors associated with disorders or diseases classified elsewhere
F55	Abuse of non-dependence-producing substances
F59	Unspecified behavioral syndromes associated with physiological disturbances and physical factors
F60–F69	**Disorders of adult personality and behavior**
F60	Specific personality disorders
F61	Mixed and other personality disorders
F62	Enduring personality changes, not attributable to brain damage and disease
F63	Habit and impulse disorders
F64	Gender identity disorders
F65	Disorders of sexual preference
F66	Psychological and behavioral disorders associated with sexual development and orientation

Contd...

Contd...

F68	Other disorders of adult personality and behavior
F69	Unspecified disorder of adult personality and behavior
F70–F79	**Mental retardation**
F70	Mild mental retardation
F71	Moderate mental retardation
F72	Severe mental retardation
F73	Profound mental retardation
F78	Other mental retardation
F79	Unspecified mental retardation
F80–F89	**Disorders of psychological development**
F80	Specific developmental disorders of speech and language
F81	Specific developmental disorders of scholastic skills
F82	Specific developmental disorder of motor function
F83	Mixed specific developmental disorder
F84	Pervasive developmental disorders
F88	Other disorders of psychological development
F89	Unspecified disorder of psychological development
F90–F98	**Behavioral and emotional disorders with onset usually occurring in childhood and adolescence**
F90	Hyperkinetic disorder
F91	Conduct disorders
F92	Mixed disorders of conduct and emotions
F93	Emotional disorders with onset specific to childhood
F94	Disorders of social functioning with onset specific to childhood and adolescence
F95	Tic disorders
F98	Other behavioral and emotional disorders with onset usually occurring in childhood and adolescence
F99	Unspecified mental disorder
F99	Mental disorder, not otherwise specified.

II. Diagnostic and Statistical Manual of Mental Disorder, 4th Edition, Text Revision (DSM-IV-TR)

This system was developed by The American Psychiatric Association (APA). The first edition (DSM–1) was published in 1952 as an alternative to ICD–6 which had been widely criticized. It is now in its fourth edition DSM-IV which was introduced in 1994, and reviewed (DSM–4 Text Revision) in 2000. Although designed for use in the United States, it is used in other countries, especially for research purposes. Categories are as follows:

Box 2.10: The main categories of disorders in DSM–IV

- Disorders usually first diagnosed in infancy, childhood, or adolescence
- Delirium, dementia and amnestic, and other cognitive disorders
- Mental disorders due to a general medical condition
- Substance-related disorders
- Schizophrenia and other psychotic disorders
- Mood disorders
- Anxiety disorders
- Somatoform disorders
- Factitious disorders
- Dissociative disorders
- Sexual and gender identity disorders
- Eating disorders
- Impulse-control disorders
- Adjustment disorders

Multiaxial Classification

DSM –IV is a multiaxial system that evaluates patients along several variables and contains five axes:

Box 2.11: Multiaxial classification

Axis I: It consists of clinical disorders and other conditions that may be a focus of clinical attention.

Axis II: It consists of personality disorders and/or mental retardation.

Axis III: It lists any physical disease relevant to mental disorder.

Axis IV: It is used to code the psychosocial and environmental problems that significantly contribute to the development or exacerbation of the current disorder.

Axis V: It is a global assessment of functioning scale.

Only the first three axes are used commonly in everyday clinical practice, and can be recorded without assigning them to separate axes.

Other Classification of Mental Disorders

Although this classification is no longer used in the official current systems of classification, in everyday clinical practice these terms are still used widely; hence, it is of practical value to know this distinction.

III. Organic Versus Functional Classification

Organic disorders are disorders with definite underlying neuropathology (e.g. delirium, dementia), whereas functional disorders are psychiatric disorders without structural brain disease (e.g. schizophrenia, mood disorders).

Box 2.12: Psychiatric disorders

Organic	Functional
• ***Global:*** – *Acute:* Delirium; *Chronic:* Dementia • ***Focal:*** – Amnestic syndrome – Complex partial seizures – Frontal lobe syndrome – Others	• Schizophrenia • Mood disorders • Schizoaffective disorders • Delusional disorders • Anxiety disorders • Adjustment disorders • Others.

IV. Neurosis Versus Psychosis Classification

Box 2.13: Psychiatric illness or mental disorders

Psychosis	Neurosis
Mental disorders in which the patient is unable to distinguish between subjective experience and reality, as evidenced by delusions, hallucinations lack of insight. ***Examples:*** Schizophrenia, Mood disorders, delirium, and delusional disorders.	Generally, less severe forms of psychiatry disorders in which the patient is able to distinguish between subjective experience and reality (no lack of insight, delusions or hallucinations). ***Examples:*** Anxiety, panic and phobic disorders.

REVIEW OF PERSONALITY DEVELOPMENT AND DEFENCE MECHANISM

The personality development can be described as a process in which one can refine and polish one's own persona building the best possible image. In large social sense, the meaning of personality development include the sum total of human happiness by fostering self-awareness and self-esteem, by developing talents, by facilitation. This is achieved through social and professional interaction and by contributing to the expression and realization of hopes, wishes and ambitions.

What is personality?

The combination of character, behavioral temperamental, emotional and mental traits these are unique to each specific individual.

Definition

The *DSM-IV-TR* defines *personality* as 'enduring patterns of perceiving, relating to, and thinking about the environment and oneself that are exhibited in a wide range of social and personal contexts'.

Personality is the total quality of an individual's behavior as it is shown in his habits of thinking, attitude, interests, manner of acting and personal philosophy of life.

The above concept is clearly understood through various theories of personality development.

Theories of Personality Development

Developmental stages are identified by age. Behaviors can then be evaluated for age-appropriateness. Ideally, an individual successfully fulfils all the tasks associated with one stage before moving on to the next stage (at the appropriate age). The environment may also influence one's developmental pattern.

There are a number of approaches for studying the human personality development. There are several theories of personality development which have been developed by various psychologists to explain personality difference.

Table 2.1: Classification and review of each theories of personality development

S. No.	Theories of personality development	Theories contributed by
1.	Psychoanalytic theory	Sigmund Freud (1961)
2.	Interpersonal theory	Sullivan (1953)
3.	Theories of psychosocial development	Erik Erikson (1959)
4.	Theory of object relations	Mohler
5.	Humanistic approach (Theory of self-actualization)	Maslow

1. Psychoanalytic Theory (Psycho-Sexual Theaory)

Sigmund freud given a personality based theory in the form of *psychoanalytical theory,* can be conceptualized according to the *structure* and *dynamics* of the personality, topography of the mind and stages of personality development.

- **Structure of the personality:** Freud organized the structure of the personality into the three major component: (Fig 2.1)

1. **ID:** The ID is the locus of instinctual drives ***'the pleasure principle'***, present at birth, it endows infant with the instinctual drives and seek to satisfy need and achieves immediate gratification.
2. **The ego:** Also called the rational self (works on ***'reality principle'***). It begins to develop between the ages of 4 and 6 months. The primary function of the ego is to maintain harmony among the external world, the id and the superego.
3. **Superego:** Referred as, ***perfection principle.*** The superego which develops between ages of 3 and 6 years, internalizes the value and moral set forth by primary care givers. The superego is important in the socialization of the individual because it assist in controlling the id.

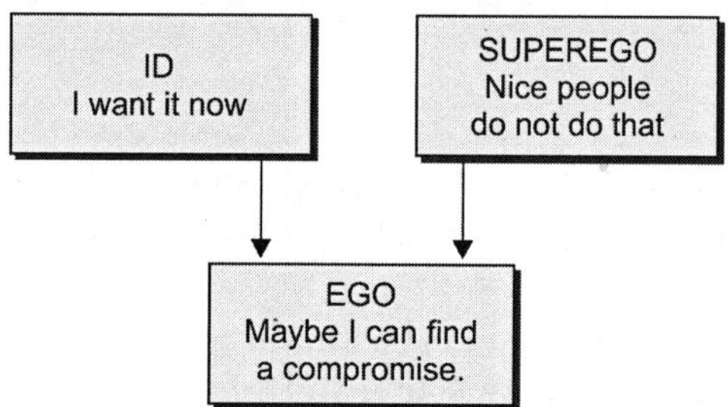

Fig. 2.1: Example of ID, ego and superego

- **Topography of the mind:** Sigmund freud classified all mental contents and operations into three categories are as follows:

1. **The conscious mind:** Events and experience that are easily remembered and retrieved are considered to be within the *conscious mind.* It is the smallest of all three categories and thought to be under the control of ego.

   For example, Telephone numbers, birthday of self, friends and special holiday days, etc.

2. **The preconscious mind:** All memories that may have been forgotten or not in present awareness but with little mental effort it can be brought into *consciousness.*
   For example Telephone numbers or addresses one known but little used and feelings associated with significant life events.
3. **The unconscious mind:** It includes all memories that one is unable to bring conscious awareness even with mental effort but can be retrieved through therapies. It is the largest of three topographical levels and consists of *unpleasant* memories that have been *repressed* (Fig.2.2)

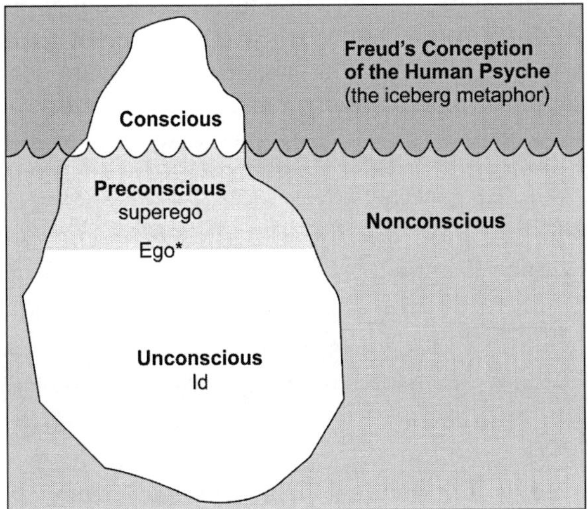

Fig. 2.2: Freud's topography of mind: The iceberg metaphor

Note: Ego is freefloating in all three levels

- **Dynamics of the personality:** Freud believed that *psychic energy* is the force required for mental functioning. Originating in the id, it instinctually fulfils basic physiological needs. Freud called the psych energy or the drive is to fulfil basic physiological needs such as hunger, thirst, the libido (sex).
  As the child matures, psychic energy is diverted from *id* to form *ego* and from *ego* to form *superego.*
- **Freud stages of personality development:** Sigmund Freud described formation of the personality through five stages of *psychosexual development*.
  1. ***Oral stage (birth to 18 months):*** During the oral stage, the behavior is directed by id, and the goal is immediate gratification needs, the focus of energy is the mouth with the behaviors that include, sucking, chewing, and biting.
  2. ***Anal stage (18 months to 3 years):*** The major tasks in the anal stage are gaining independence and control with particularly focus on the excretory function; *toilet training* is the main task to achieve during this stage.
  3. ***Phallic stage (3–6 years):*** In this stage, the focus of energy shifts to the genital area. Discovery of differences between genders results in a heightened interest in the sexuality of self and others. Freud proposed that the development of the ***Oedipus complex (males)* or *Electra complex (females)*** occurred during this stage of development.

What is Oedipus complex (males) and Electra complex (females)?

Child's unconscious desire to eliminate the parent of the same sex and to possess the parent of the opposite sex for himself or herself.

4. ***Latency stage (6–12 years):*** During this stage, focus change from *egocentrism* to more interest in *group activities, learning, socialization* with the peer group members. Sexuality is not absent during this period but remains obscure and imperceptible to others. The preference is *homosexual;* children of this age show a distinct preference of same sex relationship, even rejecting members of the opposite sex.
5. ***Genital stage (13–20 years):*** In this stage, maturation of genital organs results in a reawakening of the libidinal drive. The focus is on relationship with the members of the opposite sex and preparations for selecting a mate.

Table 2.2: Overview of Freud's stages of personality development

S.No.	Age	Stage	Development
1.	**Birth to 18 months**	Oral	Relief from anxiety through oral gratification of needs
2.	**18 months to 3 years**	Anal	Learning independence and control—excretion focusing
3.	**3–6 years**	Phallic	Identification with same sex—sexual identity (parent)
4.	**6–12 years**	Latency	Sexuality repressed—focus with same sex relationship
5.	**13–20 years**	Genitalia	Relationship with opposite sex members—friend

2. Interpersonal Theory

Sullivan (1953) believed that individual behaviors and personality development are the direct result of the interpersonal relationship. Before the development of his own theoretical framework, Sullivan traced the concepts of Freud, later he changed the form of his work from the interpersonal view of Freud to one with more interpersonal flavor in which human behavior could be observed in social interactions with others.

Sullivan's Stages of Personality Development

1. **Infancy (Birth to 18 months):** During the beginning stage, the image developmental task for the child is the gratification of needs. This is accomplished through activity associated with the mouth, such as crying, noising and thumb sucking.
2. **Child hood (18 months to 6 years):** At ages 18 months to 6 years, the child learns that interference with fulfilment of personal wishes and desires may result in delayed gratification, lead to parental approval. Tools of this stage included the mouth, language experimentation, manipulation, and identification.
3. **Juvenile (6—9 years):** The major task of the juvenile stage is the formation of satisfactory relationship with peer groups. This is accomplished through the use of competition, and cooperation, compromises.
4. **Preadolescence (9—12 years):** The tasks at the preadolescence stage focus on developing relationships with person of the same sex. One's ability to collaborate with and show love and affection for another person begins at this stage.
5. **Early adolescence (12–14 years):** During this period, the child is struggling with developing a sense of identity that is separate and independent from the parents. This major task is formation of satisfactory relationship with members of the opposite sex.

Sullivan saw the emergence of lust in response to biological changes as a major force occurring during the period.

6. **Late adolescence (14–21 years):** The late adolescent period is characterized by tasks associated with the attempt to achieve interdependence within the society and the formation of a lasting, intimate relationship with selected members of the opposite sex. The genital organs are the major development focuses of this stage.

Table 2.3: Overview of Sullivan's stages of personality development

S.No.	Age	Stage	Major development tasks
1.	**Birth to 18 months**	Infancy	Relief from anxiety through oral gratification of needs
2.	**18 months to 6 years**	Childhood	Learning to experience or delay in personal gratification without undue anxiety
3.	**6–9 years**	Juvenile	Learning to form satisfactory peer relationships
4.	**9–12 years**	Preadole-scence	Learning to form satisfactory relationship with persons of same sex, initiating feelings of affection for another person.
5.	**12–14 years**	Early adolescence	Learning to form satisfactory relationship with persons of the opposite sex, developing sense of identity
6.	**14–21 years**	Late adolescence	Establishing self-identity, experiencing, satisfying relationships, working to develop a lasting intimate opposite sex relationships.

3. Theories of Psychosocial Development

Erik Erikson's (1959) theory of psychosocial development has eight distinct stages. Like Freud, Erikson assumes that a crisis occurs at each stage of development. These crises are of a psychosocial nature because they involve psychological needs of the individual.

According to the theory, successful completion of each stage results in a healthy personality. Failure to successfully complete a stage can result in a reduced ability to complete further stages and therefore a more unhealthy personality.

Erik Erikson's Psychosocial Stages of Personality Development

1. Trust mistrust: Is the world a safe place or is it full of unpredictable events and accidents waiting to happen?

During this stage, the infant is uncertain about the world in which they live. To resolve these feelings of uncertainty, the infant looks towards their primary caregiver for stability and consistency of care. If the care the infant receives is consistent and reliable, they will develop a sense of trust and they will be able to feel secure even when threatened. If the care has been harsh, unpredictable and unreliable, then the infant will develop a sense of mistrust.

Success in this stage will lead to the virtue of **hope.** Failing to acquire the virtue of hope will lead to the development of fear.

2. Autonomy shame and doubt: Between the ages of 18 months and 3 years, children begin to assert their independence, by walking away from their mother, picking toy to play, making choices about what they like to eat, etc.

If children in this stage are encouraged and supported in their increased independence, they become more confident and secure in their own ability to survive in the world.

If children are criticized, overly controlled, or not given the opportunity, they begin to feel lack self-esteem, and feel a sense of *shame or doubt* in their own abilities.

Success in this stage will lead to the virtue of **will.**

3. Initiative guilt: During this period, the primary feature involves the child regularly interacting with other children at school. Central to this stage is play, as it provides children with the opportunity to explore their interpersonal skills through initiating activities.

If given opportunity, children develop a sense of initiative, and feel secure in their ability to lead others and make decisions.

If criticized during this stage, children develop a sense of guilt.

A healthy balance between initiative and guilt is important. Success in this stage will lead to the virtue of **purpose.**

4. Industry inferiority: Children are at the stage (aged 5–12 years) where they will be learning to read and write, to do sums, to do things on their own. Teachers begin to take an important role in the child's life as they teach the child specific skills.

The child now feels the need to win approval by demonstrating specific competencies that are valued by society, and begin to develop a sense of pride in their accomplishments.

If children are encouraged and reinforced for their initiative, they begin to feel industrious. If this initiative is not encouraged, if it is restricted by parents or teacher, then the child begins to feel inferior, doubting his own abilities and therefore may not reach his or her potential.

Success in this stage will lead to the virtue of **competence**.

5. Identity role confusion: During adolescence, (aged 12–18 years), the transition from childhood to adulthood is most important. Children are becoming more independent, and begin to look at the future in terms of career, relationships, families, etc. The individual wants to belong to a society and fit in.

During this period, they explore possibilities and begin to form their own identity based upon the outcome of their explorations. Failure to establish a sense of identity within society ('I don't know what I want to be when I grow up') can lead to role confusion. Role confusion involves the individual not being sure about themselves or their place in society.

Success in this stage will lead to the virtue of **fidelity**.

(Fidelity involves being able to commit one's self to others on the basis of accepting others.)

6. Intimacy isolation: Occurring in young adulthood (aged 18–40 years) and successful completion of this stage can lead to comfortable relationships, safety, and care within a relationship. Avoiding intimacy and relationships can lead to isolation, loneliness, and sometimes depression.

Success in this stage will lead to the virtue of **love**.

7. Generativity stagnation: During middle adulthood (aged 40–65 years), individual establish careers, settle down within a relationship and give back to society through raising children, being productive at work. By failing to achieve these objectives, person become stagnant and feels unproductive.

Success in this stage will lead to the virtue of **care**.

8. Ego integrity despair: As person grow older (65+ years) and become senior citizen, productivity will slow down, and explore life as a retired person. During this time, person contemplate accomplishments and develop integrity if he sees himself leading a successful life.

If he sees lives as unproductive, then he become dissatisfied with life and develops despair, often leading to depression and hopelessness.

Success in this stage will lead to the virtue of **wisdom**.

Table 2.4: Overview of psychosocial stages of personality development

S. No	Stages	Issue	Description of task
1	0–18 months (infant)	Trust mistrust	Developed through consistent love and support
2	1–3 years (toddler)	Autonomy shame and doubt	Independence fostered by support and encouragement
3	3–6 years (Pre-school)	Initiative guilt	Developed by exploring and accepting challenges
4	6–12 years (School age)	Industry inferiority	Mastery comes from success and recognition
5	12–18 years (puberty)	Identity role confusion	Exploration of different paths to attain a healthy identity
6	18–40 years (Young adulthood)	Intimacy isolation	Form positive, close relationships with others
7	40–65 years (Late adulthood)	Generativity stagnation	Transmitting something positive to the next generation
8	65 years and above	Integrity despair	Life review and retrospective evaluation of one's past.

4. Theory of Object Relations

Object relation is a theory of the human personality developed by Mahler, reflects the mother-infant bond. The theory holds that the infant's experience in relationship with the mother or primary caregiver is the primary determinant of personality formation and that the infant's need for attachment is the motivating factor in the development of the infantile self.

She describes this process as progressing through three major phases. Phase III further divided into 4 sub phase.

- **Phase I: Autistic phase (birth to one month)** In the autistic phase, also called normal autisms, the infant exist in a half-sleeping half-walking state and does not perceive the existence of other people or an external environment. The fulfilment of basic needs for survival and comfort is the main focus.

- **Phase II: Symbolic phase (1–5 month)** Symbiosis is a type of psychic fusion of mother and child. The child views the self as an extension of mother, but with a developing awareness that it is she who fulfils his or her every need.
- **Phase III: Separation-Individuation (5–36 Months)** This third phase represents what Mohler calls the psychological birth of the child. Separation is defined as the physical and psychological attachment of a sense of personal distinction from the mothering figure.

  Four sub phases through which the child evolves in his or her profession from symbolic extension of the mothering figure to a distinct and separate being are as follows:
  - **Sub phase I: Differentiation (5–10 months)** The differentiation phase begins with the childs initial physical movements away from the mothering figure.
  - **Sub phase II: Practicing (1–16 months)** With advanced locomotors functioning, the child experience feelings of exhilaration from increased independence. He or she is now able to move away from and return to the mothering figure.
  - **Sub phase III: Rapprochement (16–24 months)** This third sub phase, rapprochement, is extremely critical to the childs healthy ego developments. During this time, the child becomes increasingly aware of his or her separation from the mothering figure, in which the sense of for bidden and omnipotence diminishes.

    The child now recognize the mother or a separate individual wishes to re-establish closeness with her but shuns total re engulfment of the symbolic stage. The need is for the mothering figure to be available to provide 'emotional refuelling or demand.
  - **Sub phase IV: Consolidation (24–36 Months)** With achievement of the consolidation sub phase a definite individually and sense of separation of self-care established. Objects are represented as whole with child having the ability to integrate both 'good and bad'.

    A degree of object constancy is established as the child is able to internalize a sustained image of the mothering figure are enduring and loving, while maintaining the perception of her or separate person in the outside world.

5. Humanistic Approach

Maslow's humanistic theory of personality states that 'people achieve their full potential by moving from basic needs to self-actualization'.

Maslow has set up a hierarchy of five levels of basic needs (Fig 2.3). Beyond these needs, higher levels of needs exist. These include needs for understanding, aesthetic appreciation and purely spiritual needs. In the levels of the five basic needs, the person does not feel the second need until the demands of the first have been satisfied, nor the third until the second has been satisfied, and so on. Maslow's basic needs are as follows:

- **Physiological needs**: These are biological needs. They consist of needs for oxygen, food and water. They are the strongest needs because if a person were deprived of all needs, the physiological ones would come first in the person's search for satisfaction.
- **Safety needs**: When all physiological needs are satisfied and are no longer controlling thoughts and behaviors, the need for security can become active.

- **Need of love, affection and belongingness**: When the need for safety and for physiological well-being are satisfied, the next class of needs for love, affection and belongingness can emerge. Maslow states that people seek to overcome feelings of loneliness and alienation. This involves both giving and receiving love, affection and the sense of belonging.
- **Need for esteem**: When the first three classes of needs are satisfied, the need for esteem can become dominant. These involve need for both self-esteem and for the esteem, a person gets from others.

  Humans have a need for a stable, firmly based, high level of self-respect, and respect from others. When these needs are satisfied, the person feels self-confident and valuable as a person in the world.

Need for self-actualization: When all of above needs are satisfied, then only need is to achieve self-actualization. Maslow describes self-actualization as a person's need to be and do that which the person was 'born to do.' A musician must make music, an artist must paint, and a poet must write.

The hierarchic theory is often represented as a pyramid which is given below.

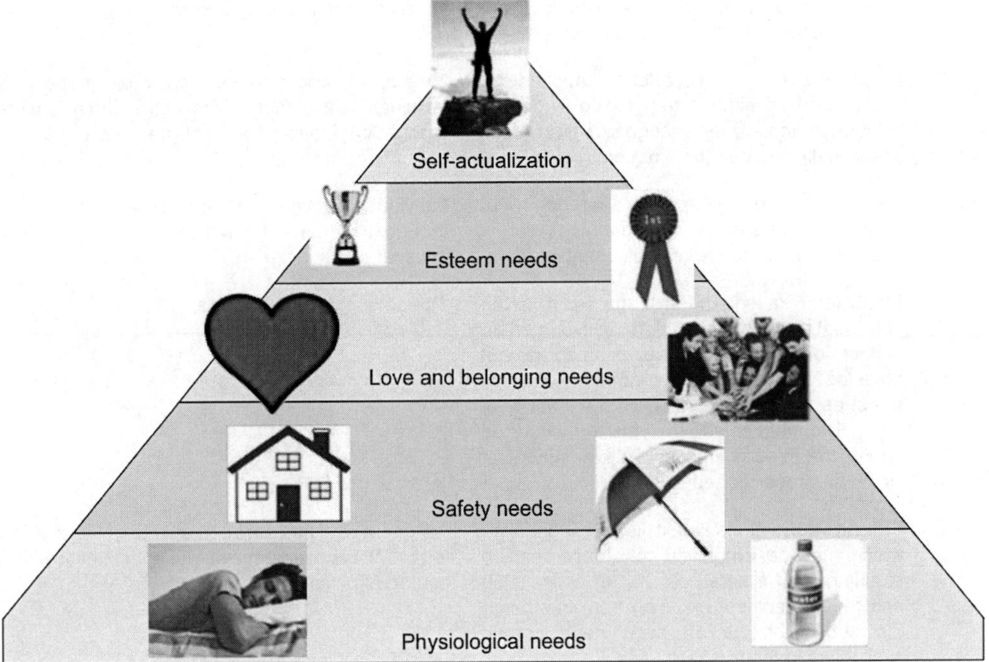

Fig. 2.3: Pyramidal representation of Maslow's hierarchy of need

Defense Mechanisms

Sigmund Freud stated the structure of personality as *id, ego* and *superego.* There is always danger of having conflict among the id, the superego and the external reality situation. Main function of ego is to control the situation and make course of action, which is compatible with reality situation not to frustrating the id and superego.

Mental mechanisms are also referred to as ego defense mechanisms or coping mechanism. These mental mechanisms function to protect the ego from overwhelming anxiety, for the most part; they operate on an unconscious level. They are the patterns of adjustment through which an individual relieves or decreases anxiety caused by an uncomfortable situation that threatens self-esteem.

Definition

Defense mechanisms as the automatic psychological process protecting the individual against anxiety and from the awareness of internal or external dangers or stressors.

Box 2.14: Classifications of defence mechanism and their descriptions with examples

S.No	Classification	Example
A.	**Defense Mechanisms Originating in Oral Phase:**	
1.	**Compensation:** *Compensation* is a mechanism by which one's weaknesses are compensated by excelling in some other area.	A handicapped boy who is unable to participate in sports compensates by becoming a great scholar.
2.	**Displacement:** In this defense mechanism, an emotional feeling is transferred to person or objects who are less dangerous than those who initially aroused the emotion.	A student, who has received a low grade in a terminal examination, can't show anger on the teacher but blows up at her sister when she asks about her grade
3.	**Denial:** In denial, the individual does not accept the existence of something that is disturbing or existence of unpleasant realities.	Individual continue to smoke cigarettes even though they have been told of the health risk involved.
4.	**Fixation:** Fixation refers to the point in the individual's development at which certain aspects of the emotional development do not advance. The reasons are not clear but this arrest appears to develop from the inability of the individual to solve problems that occurred during the specific phase of development at which progress ceased or stopped.	Thumb sucking in adult age.
5	**Substitution:** Substitution is a mechanism which may be employed to reduce tension resulting from frustration. To get satisfaction and reduce tension, resulting from frustration the substitutive action must have certain similarities to the frustrated one.	A student who has not been able to get admission to the MBBS course may try to substitute it with a course of physiotherapy.
B.	**Defense Mechanisms Originating in Habit Training Period:**	
1.	**Conversion:** Conversion is exactly what it says strong emotional conflicts are expressed as or converted into physical symptoms.	A boy does not want to go school, he frightened to communicate with his parents who are very strict, unconsciously adopts the mechanism of conversion develops weakness and pain in the leg and cannot walk. Parents suggest not to go to school and resolving the conflict temporarily.

Contd...

Contd...

S.No	Classification	Example
2.	**Identification:** Identification is a useful defense mechanism which plays an important part in the development of child's personality. The person has unconscious assumption of similarity between himself and the person whom he admires.	After hospitalization for a minor surgery, a girl decides to become a nurse because she developed an admiration for the nurse who looked after her.
3.	**Introjection:** In introjections, individual unconsciously takes the qualities, values and characteristics of significant persons and incorporate in one's personality.	For instance, a woman who likes to live in a simple way introjects in her the sophisticated way, of living like her husband.
4.	**Reaction Formation:** In this, unacceptable real feelings are repressed and acceptable opposite feelings are expressed. This is an important device for the development of character.	For instance, a woman who actually dislikes her mother-in-law hides her feelings by being always very nice to her.
5.	**Transference:** In transference, the image of one person is unconsciously identified with that of another.	A patient who is fond of his daughter finds the nurse of the same age and height as his daughter. So, he transfers his positive emotions to the nurse as his daughter.
6.	**Suppression:** Suppression is a device where a conscious effort is made by the individual to dismiss the impulses, feelings and thoughts that are unpleasant to the pre conscious mind. So, unacceptable feelings and thoughts are consciously kept out of awareness.	A young woman who is depressed about a pending divorce proceeding tells the nurse, 'I just don't want to talk about the divorce. There is nothing I can do about it anyway'.
7.	**Sublimation:** Sublimation is a positive mechanism in which unwanted primitive impulses or feeling are diverted to some socially-accepted channels.	A teenage boy with strong competitive and aggressive drives becomes the star football player in his high school team.
C.	**Defense Mechanisms Originating in Later Period of Childhood:**	
1.	**Repression:** The hostile feelings are pushed into the unconscious mind. It is the basic or primary defense and protects us from anxiety but they are still present in the unconscious mind.	A man is jealous of his good friend's success but is unaware of his feelings of jealousy.
2.	**Regression:** Regression is a mechanism of going from the present pattern to the past level of behavior. The individual returns to patterns of behavior that were successful in earlier stages of development.	Tears and temper tantrums in adults, which is child like behavior, are sometimes very effective in overcoming stressful situations. A person who is depressed may withdraw to his or her room, curl up in a fetal position on the bed, and sleep for long periods.
3.	**Rationalization:** This is the mechanism by which unacceptable behavior, feeling, ideas or motives are justified logically with acceptable reasons or explanations.	The woman who overspends to buy a dress explains its purchase to her husband herself that the dress was on sale and she may not get it so cheap afterwards. (A phrase 'grapes are sour' is another example or rationalization).

Contd...

Contd...

S.No	Classification	Example
D.	**Defense Mechanisms Originating in Latency Phase:**	
1.	**Projection:** It is a defense mechanism by which one attributes to others, one's own unacceptable or unwanted thoughts and/or emotions.	A young soldier who has an extreme fear of participating in military combat tells his sergeant that the others in his unit are 'a bunch of cowards'.

Box 2.15: Defense mechansim classification according to behavioral type

Narcissistic	Immature	Neurotic	Mature
Denial	Acting-out	Displacement	Altruism
Projection	Regression	Dissociation	Humor
Distortion	Passive-aggressive	Reaction formation	Sublimation
Splitting	Schizoid fantasy	Repression	Anticipation
	Somatization	Isolation	Suppression
	Introjections	Rationalization	Asceticism
	Hypochondriasis	Sexualization	
	Blocking	Intellectualization	

Maladaptive behavior of individual and group: stress and crisis-it is explained detail in Chapter-13).

ETIOLOGY: BIOPSYCHOSOCIAL FACTORS

Diagnosing mental illness is not like diagnosing other chronic diseases. Heart disease is identified with the help of blood tests and electrocardiograms. Diabetes is diagnosed by measuring blood glucose levels. But classifying mental illness is a more subjective endeavor. No blood test exists for depression; no X-ray can identify a child at risk of developing bipolar disorder.

Although, the exact cause of most mental illnesses is not known, it is becoming clear through research that many of these conditions are caused by a combination of biological, psychological, and environmental factors.

Biological Factors

Some mental illnesses have been linked to abnormal functioning of nerve cell circuits or pathways that connect particular brain regions. Nerve cells within these brain circuits communicate through chemicals called *neurotransmitters.*

Any abnormal firing of these neurotransmitters causes a range of mental disorders in an individual. In addition, defects in or injury to certain areas of the brain have also been linked to some mental conditions.

Other biological factors that may be involved in the development of mental illness include:

- **Genetics (heredity):** Mental illnesses sometimes run in families, suggesting that people who have a family member with a mental illness may be somewhat more likely to develop themselves. Susceptibility is passed on in families through genes.

Experts believe many mental illnesses are linked to abnormalities in many genes rather than just one or a few and that how these genes interact with the environment is unique for every person (even identical twins). That is why a person inherits a susceptibility to a mental illness and does not necessarily develop the illness.

Mental illness itself occurs from the interaction of multiple genes and other factors such as stress, abuse, or a traumatic event which can influence, or trigger, an illness in a person who has an inherited susceptibility to it.

- **Infections:** Certain infections have been linked to brain damage and the development of mental illness or the worsening of its symptoms. For example, a condition known as Paediatric Autoimmune Neuropsychiatric Disorder (PANDA) associated with the Streptococcus bacteria has been linked to the development of obsessive-compulsive disorder and other mental illnesses in children.
- **Brain defects or injury:** Defects in or injury to certain areas of the brain have also been linked to some mental illnesses.
- **Prenatal damage**: Some evidence suggests that a disruption of early fetal brain development or trauma that occurs at the time of birth. For example, loss of oxygen to the brain may be a factor in the development of certain conditions, such as autism.
- **Substance abuse:** Long-term substance abuse, in particular, has been linked to anxiety, depression, and paranoia.
- **Other factors:** Poor nutrition and exposure to toxins, such as lead, may play a role in the development of mental illnesses.

Psychological Factors

- Severe psychological trauma suffered as a child, such as emotional, physical, or sexual abuse
- An important early loss, such as the loss of a parent
- Neglect
- Poor ability to relate to others.

Social Factors

Certain stressors can trigger an illness in a person who is susceptible to mental illness. These stressors include:

- Death or divorce
- A dysfunctional family life
- Feelings of inadequacy, low self-esteem, anxiety, anger, or loneliness
- Changing jobs or schools
- Social or cultural expectations (For example, a society that associates beauty with thinness can be a factor in the development of eating disorders)
- Substance abuse by the person or the person's parent.

What Science does know?

Mental illnesses have several dimensions that are helpful to review:

- **BIO** → Biology–Refers to the structure of the brain, chemicals in the brain, genes inherited from parents, etc. Science is gaining more knowledge about the large influence of biology on the risk for acquiring a mental illness.

- **PSYCHO** → Psychology–refers to personality, personal beliefs, thoughts, experiences, etc.
- **SOCIAL** → Sociology–Refers to environmental stress (e.g. trauma of war, assault), cultural factors, discrimination, etc.

  Therefore, treatment needs to be aimed at all three of these areas:

1. **BIO:** Medication, nutrition, general physical health.
2. **PSYCHO:** Education [SAFE (Support and family education) Program], psychotherapy, coping skills.
3. **SOCIAL:** Environmental management, stigma of mental illness, advocacy.

Psychopathology of Mental Disorders

Review of structure and function of brain, limbic system and abnormal neurotransmission.

Box 2.16: Read and understand this before you study about Brain!!!

'The human brain, it has been said, is the most complexly organized structure in the universe and to appreciate this you just have to look at some numbers. The brain is made up of one hundred billion nerve cells or 'neurons' which is the basic structural and functional units of the nervous system. Each neuron makes something like a thousand to ten thousand contacts with other neurons and these points of contact are called *synapses* where exchange of information occurs. And based on this information, someone has calculated that the number of possible permutations and combinations of brain activity, in other words the numbers of brain states that 'exceeds the number of elementary particles in the known universe.'

—VS Ramachandran

The above words are said by VS Ramachandran, from the book 'The Tell Tale Brain' is the expression of infinite concept about brain that gives us a clear cut idea that brain is more complexly arranged organ in our body.

He also expresses more ideas about brain cells which is very interesting to listen in his own word that he says, 'How can a three-pound mass of jelly that you can hold in your palm, it can imagine angels, contemplate the meaning of infinity, and even question its own place in the cosmos? It can also think about its own ability to think and wonder about its own ability to wonder. With the arrival of humans, it has been said, the universe has suddenly become conscious of itself. This truly, the greatest mystery of all.'

The above paragraph explains about, 100 billion brain cells have the ability to think about its thinking capacity and it can wonder about its ability to wonder. This gives us a clear cut picture about importance of brain and brain cells which controls our body. But any abnormal firing of group of neurons can cause a wide range of mental illness. So, the concept of studying normal and abnormal structure and functions of brain is necessary which explained as below.

Overview

Nothing in the world can compare with the human brain. This mysterious three-pound organ controls all necessary functions of the body, receives and interprets information from the outside world.

The brain receives information through five senses: sight, smell, touch, taste, and hearing–often many at one time. It assembles the messages in a way that has meaning for us, and can store that information in our memory. The brain controls our thoughts, memory and speech, movement of the arms and legs, and the function of many organs within our body. It also determines how we respond to stressful situations (such as taking a test, losing a job, or suffering an illness) by regulating heart and breathing rate.

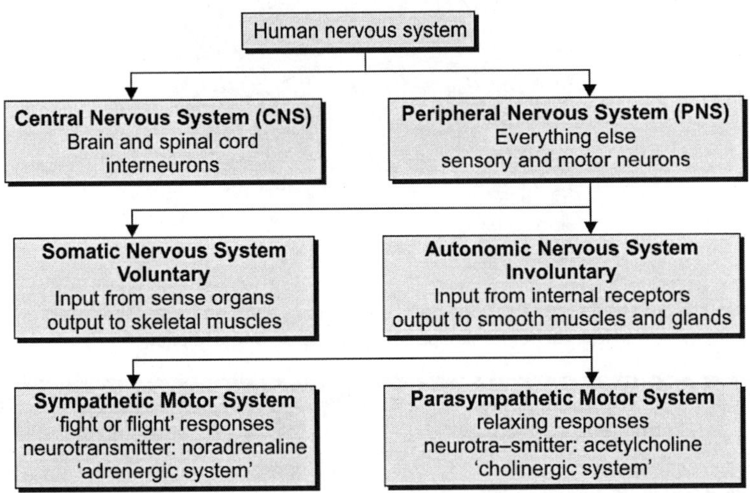

Fig. 2.4: Components of nervous system

NERVOUS SYSTEM

The nervous system is divided into central and peripheral systems. The central nervous system (CNS) is composed of the brain and spinal cord. The peripheral nervous system (PNS) is composed of spinal nerves that branch from the spinal cord and cranial nerves that branch from the brain which explained in schematic diagram (Fig. 2.4)

Brain

The brain is composed of the ***cerebrum, cerebellum, and brainstem*** (Fig. 2.5).

- ***Cerebrum:*** It is the largest part of the brain and is composed of right and left hemispheres. It performs higher functions like interpreting touch, vision and hearing, as well as speech, reasoning, emotions, learning, and fine control of movement.
- ***Cerebellum:*** It is located under the cerebrum. Its function is to coordinate muscle movements, maintain posture, and balance.
- ***Brainstem:*** It includes the midbrain, pons, and medulla. It acts as a relay center connecting the cerebrum and cerebellum to the spinal cord. It performs many automatic functions such as breathing, heart rate, body temperature, wake and sleep cycles, digestion, sneezing, coughing, vomiting, and swallowing. Ten of the twelve cranial nerves originate in the brainstem.

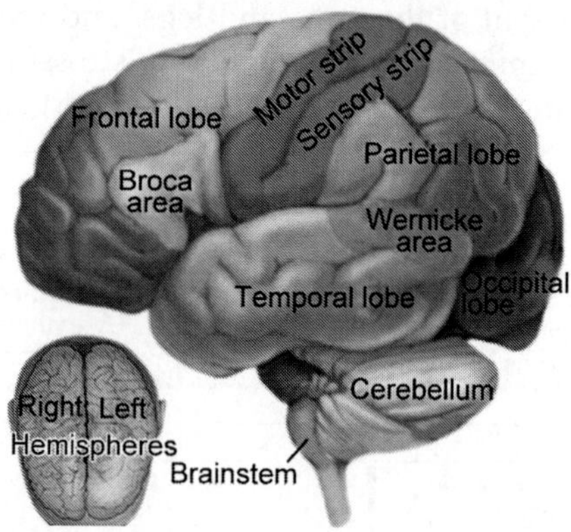

Fig. 2.5: Diagram showing parts of brain: brainstem, cerebellum, and cerebrum. The cerebrum is divided into four lobes: frontal, parietal, temporal, and occipital.

Box 2.17: Lobes of Cerebrum and its functional areas

Frontal lobe	Parietal lobe
• Personality, behavior, emotions • Judgment, planning, problem solving • **Speech:** speaking and writing (Boca's area) • Body movement (motor strip) • Intelligence, concentration, self-awareness	• Interprets language, words • Sense of touch, pain, temperature (sensory strip) • Interprets signals from vision, hearing, motor, sensory and memory • Spatial and visual perception
Occipital lobe	**Temporal lobe**
• Interprets vision (color, light, movement).	• Understanding language (Wernicke's area) • Memory • Hearing • Sequencing and organization.

Gray and White Matter

The surface of the cerebrum has a folded appearance called the *cortex*. The cortex contains about 70% of the 100 billion nerve cells. The nerve cells body color the cortex gray-brown, giving it its name–gray matter (Fig. 2.6). Beneath the cortex are long connecting fibers between neurons, called *axons*, which make up the white matter.

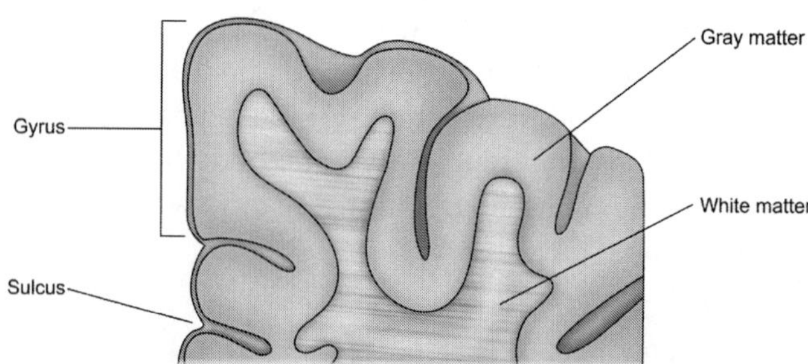

Fig. 2.6: The surface of the cerebrum is called cortex (gray matter), which are interconnected to other brain areas by axons (white matter). The cortex has a folded appearance

The folding of the cortex increases the brain's surface area allowing more neurons to fit inside the skull and enabling higher functions. Each fold is called a ***gyrus***, and each groove between folds is called a ***sulcus***.

Right Brain – Left Brain

The right and left hemispheres of the brain are joined by a bundle of fibers called the ***corpus callosum*** that delivers messages from one side to the other. Each hemisphere controls the opposite side of the body.

Functions

In general, the left hemisphere controls speech, comprehension, arithmetic, and writing. The right hemisphere controls creativity, spatial ability, artistic, and musical skills.

Lobes of the Brain

The cerebral hemispheres have distinct fissures, which divide the brain into four lobes:

- Frontal
- Temporal
- Parietal
- Occipital

Messages within the brain are carried along pathways. Messages can travel from one ***gyrus*** to another, from one lobe to another and to structures found deep in the brain (**e.g. thalamus, hypothalamus).**

Deep Structures (Fig. 2.7)

- **Hypothalamus:** It is located in the floor of the third ventricle and is the master control of the autonomic system. It plays a role in controlling behaviors such as hunger, thirst, sleep, and sexual response. It also regulates body temperature, blood pressure, emotions, and secretion of hormones.

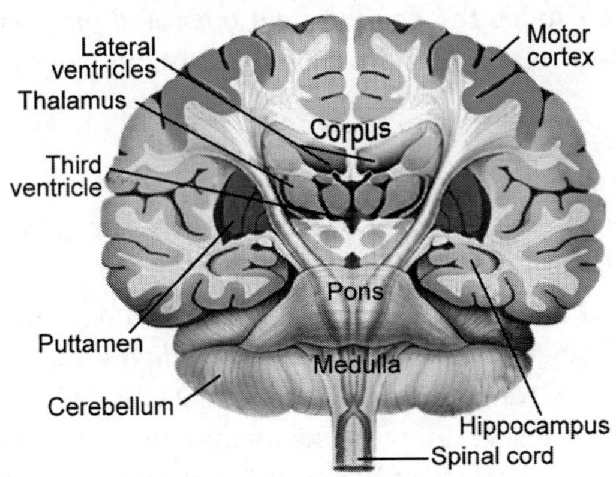

Fig. 2.7: Deep structures of brain

- **Pituitary gland:** It lies in a small pocket of bone at the skull base called the *sella turcica*. The pituitary gland is connected to the hypothalamus of the brain by the pituitary stalk known as the '*master gland*,' it controls other endocrine glands in the body. It secretes hormones that control sexual development, promote bone and muscle growth, respond to stress, and fight disease.
  - **Limbic system:** It is the center of our emotions, learning, and memory. This system includes the cingulate gyri, hypothalamus, amygdala (emotional reactions) and hippocampus (memory) (Fig. 2.8).

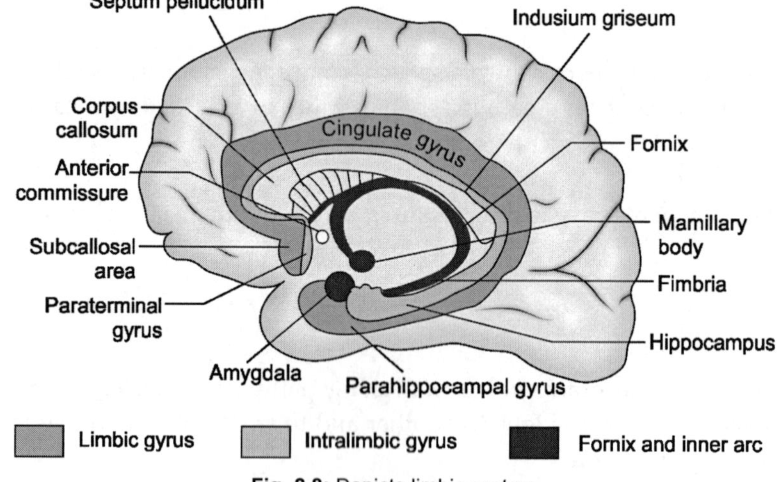

Fig. 2.8: Depicts limbic system

  - **Pineal gland:** It is located behind the third ventricle. It helps in regulate the body's internal clock and circadian rhythms by secreting melatonin. It has some role in sexual development.
  - **Thalamus:** Serves as a relay station for almost all information that comes and goes to the cortex. It plays a role in pain sensation, attention, alertness and memory.
  - **Basal ganglia:** Includes the ***caudate, putamen and globus pallidus.*** These nuclei work with the cerebellum to coordinate fine motions, such as fingertip movements.

Cranial Nerves

The brain communicates with the body through the spinal cord and 12 pairs of cranial nerves (Fig. 2.9). Ten of the twelve pairs of cranial nerves originate in the brainstem. The cranial nerves for smell and vision, originate in the cerebrum.

Meninges: The brain and spinal cord are covered and protected by three layers of tissue called *meninges*. They are: ***dura, arachnoid and pia mater.***

1. **The dura mater:** It is a strong, thick membrane that closely lines the inside of the skull.
2. **The arachnoid mater**: It is a thin, web-like membrane that covers the entire brain.
3. **The pia mater**: Hugs the surface of the brain following its folds and grooves.

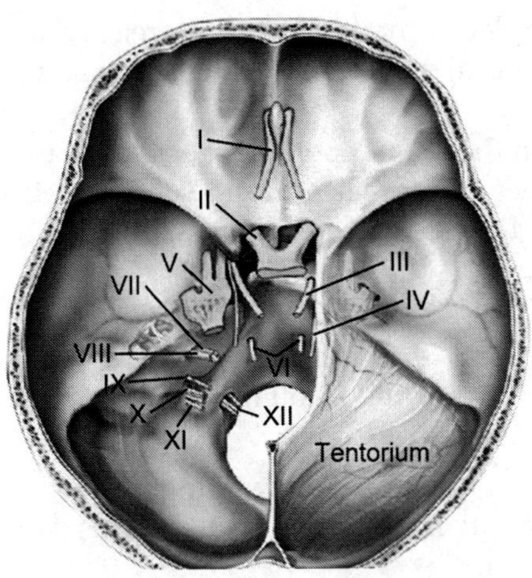

Fig. 2.9: Location of 12 cranial nerves

Table 2.5: List of cranial nerves

S.No	Cranial nerves	Functions
I	Olfactory	Smell
II	Optic	Sight
III	Oculomotor	Movement of eyes and pupil
IV	Trochlear	Movement of eyes
V	Trigeminal	Facial sensation
VI	Abducens	Movement of eyes
VII	Facial	Movement of face and salivation
VIII	Vestibulocochlear	Hearing and balance
IX	Glossopharyngeal	Taste, swallow
X	Vagus	Heart rate, digestion
XI	Accessory	Movement of head
XII	Hypoglossal	Movement of tongue

Ventricles and Cerebrospinal Fluid

The brain has hollow fluid-filled cavities called *ventricles*. Inside the ventricles is a ribbon-like structure called the *choroid plexus* that makes clear colorless cerebrospinal fluid (CSF).

There are two ventricles deep within the cerebral hemispheres called the *lateral ventricles*. They both connects with the third ventricle through a separate opening called the *foramen of Monro*. The third ventricle connects with the fourth ventricle through a long narrow tube called the *aqueduct of Sylvius*. From the fourth ventricle, CSF flows into the subarachnoid space where it bathes and cushions the brain.

Normal and Abnormal Brain Functions

Aphasia is a disturbance of language affecting production, reading or writing, due to brain injury—like stroke or trauma. The type of aphasia depends on the affected brain area:

- **Broca's area:** Lies in the left frontal lobe. If this area is damaged, leads to difficulty in moving the tongue or facial muscles to produce the sounds of speech called *Broca's aphasia.*
- **Wernicke's area:** Lies in the left temporal lobe. Damage to this area causes Wernicke's aphasia. The individual may speak in long sentences that have no meaning, add unnecessary words, and even create new words.

Memory

Memory is a complex process that includes three phases: encoding (deciding what information is important), storing, and recalling. Different areas of the brain are involved in memory depending on the type of memory:

- **Short-term memory**: It is also called working memory, it stores information for about 1 minute and capacity is limited to about 7 items. For example, dialling a phone number someone just told.
- **Long-term memory:** It is processed in the hippocampus of the temporal lobe and is activated when to memorize something for a longer time.

Nerve Cells (Brain Cells)

The brain is made up of two types of cells: Nerve cells (neurons) and glial cells.

1. **Nerve cells:** There are many sizes and shapes of neurons, but all consist of a cell body, dendrites and an axon. The neuron conveys information through electrical and chemical signals.

Neurons transmit their energy, or 'talk', to each other across a tiny gap called a *synapse* (Fig. 2.10). A neuron has many arms called *dendrites,* which act like antennae picking up messages from other nerve cells. These messages are passed to the cell body, which determines if the message should be passed along. Important messages are passed to the end of the axon where sacs containing neurotransmitters; open into the synapse.

Neurotransmitters

Definition

Neurotransmitters are chemicals located and released in the *brain* to allow an impulse from one nerve cell to pass to another nerve cell.

Neurotransmitters are chemicals that transmit messages from one nerve cell (neuron) to another. The nerve impulse travels from the first nerve cell through the axon—a single smooth body arising from the nerve cell—to the axon terminal and the synaptic knobs.

Each synaptic knob communicates with a dendrite or cell body of another neuron, and the synaptic knobs contain neurovesicles that store and release neurotransmitters. For the impulse to continue traveling across the synapse to reach the next cell, the synaptic knobs release the neurotransmitter into that space, and the next nerve cell is stimulated to pick up the impulse and continue it.

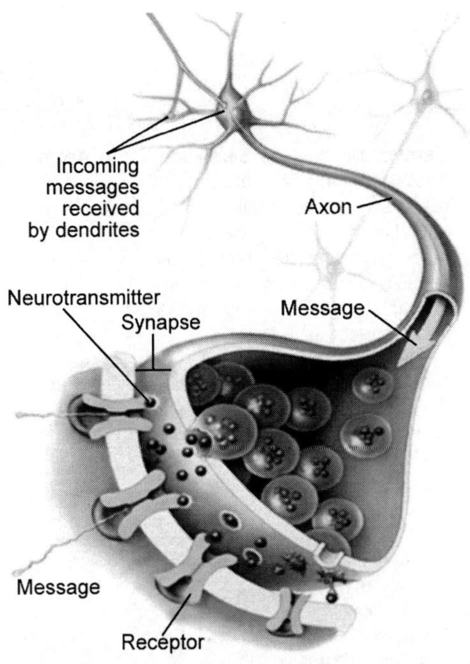

Fig. 2.10: Nerve cell consists of cell body, dendrites and axon

Box 2.18: Neurotransmitters and its implication in psychiatric illness

<table>
<tr><th rowspan="2">Group</th><th rowspan="2">Name</th><th rowspan="2">Site of secretion</th><th rowspan="2">Function</th><th colspan="2">Psychiatric implications</th></tr>
<tr><th>Increased</th><th>Decreased</th></tr>
<tr><td rowspan="2">Amino acids</td><td>GABA</td><td>Cerebral cortex, cerebellum, basal ganglia, retina and spinal cord</td><td>Slow down the body activity</td><td rowspan="2">Huntington's disease, temporal lobe epilepsy, spinal cerebellar degenerations</td><td rowspan="2">Huntington' s disease, anxiety disease, schizophrenia, and various forms of epilepsy</td></tr>
<tr><td>Glycine</td><td>Forebrain, brainstem, spinal cord and retina</td><td>Recurrent inhibition of motor neurons</td></tr>
<tr><td>Cholinergics</td><td>Acetylcholine</td><td>Cerebral cortex, basal ganglia, hippocampus and limbic structure</td><td>Sleep, arousal, pain perception, movement, memory</td><td>Depression</td><td>Alzheimer's, Huntington's and Parkinson's disease</td></tr>
<tr><td>Monoamines</td><td>Norepinephrine</td><td>Sympathetic postsynaptic nerve terminals; CNS: Thalamus, hypothalamus, limbic system, hippocampus, cerebellum, cerebral cortex</td><td>Mood, cognition, perception, locomotion, cardiovascular functioning, and sleep and arousal</td><td>Depression</td><td>Mania, anxiety states, schizophrenia</td></tr>
</table>

Contd...

Contd...

Group	Name	Site of secretion	Function	Psychiatric implications	
				Increased	Decreased
	Serotonin	Cerebellum, basal ganglia, retina and spinal cord, hippocampus and limbic structure, GI tract, lungs and platelets	Sleep and arousal, libido, appetite, mood, pain aggression, perception,	Anxiety states	Depression
Neuro-peptides	Endorphins and enkephalins	Hypothalamus, thalamus, limbic structure, mid brain and brainstem.	Modulation of pain and reduced peristalsis	Modulation of dopamine activity by opioid peptides may indicate some link to the symptoms of schizophrenia	
	Substance p	Hypothalamus, limbic structure, brainstem, thalamus and spinal cord also found in GI tract and salivary gland	Pain regulation	Depression	Huntington's disease and Alzheimer's disease.

Abbreviations: GABA- gamma-aminobutyric acid; CNS- Central nervous system; GI track- Gastrointestinal tract.

PRINCIPLES OF MENTAL HEALTH NURSING

Principles are formulated based on the concept that every individual has an intrinsic worth and dignity, potentialities and capabilities. Principles form the guidelines which will help the client to meet his emotional needs and also bring about desirable changes in his behaviors. The following are the principles of psychiatric nursing:

- Accept the patient exactly as she is
- Self-understanding is used as a therapeutic tool
- Consistency is used to contribute to the patient's security
- Reassurance to be given in acceptable and realistic manner
- Patient behavior can be changed through emotional experience not by rational interpretation
- Avoid unnecessary increase in patient's anxiety
- Observe objectively to understand and interpret the patient behavior
- Maintain realistic i.e professional relationship
- Verbal and physical force must be avoided if possible
- Nursing care centered on patient as a person not on control of symptoms
- Routine procedures explained at patient's level of understanding
- Positive reinforcement to be used wherever is possible

- Structured activity schedule as a part of psychiatric nursing
- Many procedures are modified but basic principle remain unaltered

Detail Description of Principles of Psychiatric Nursing

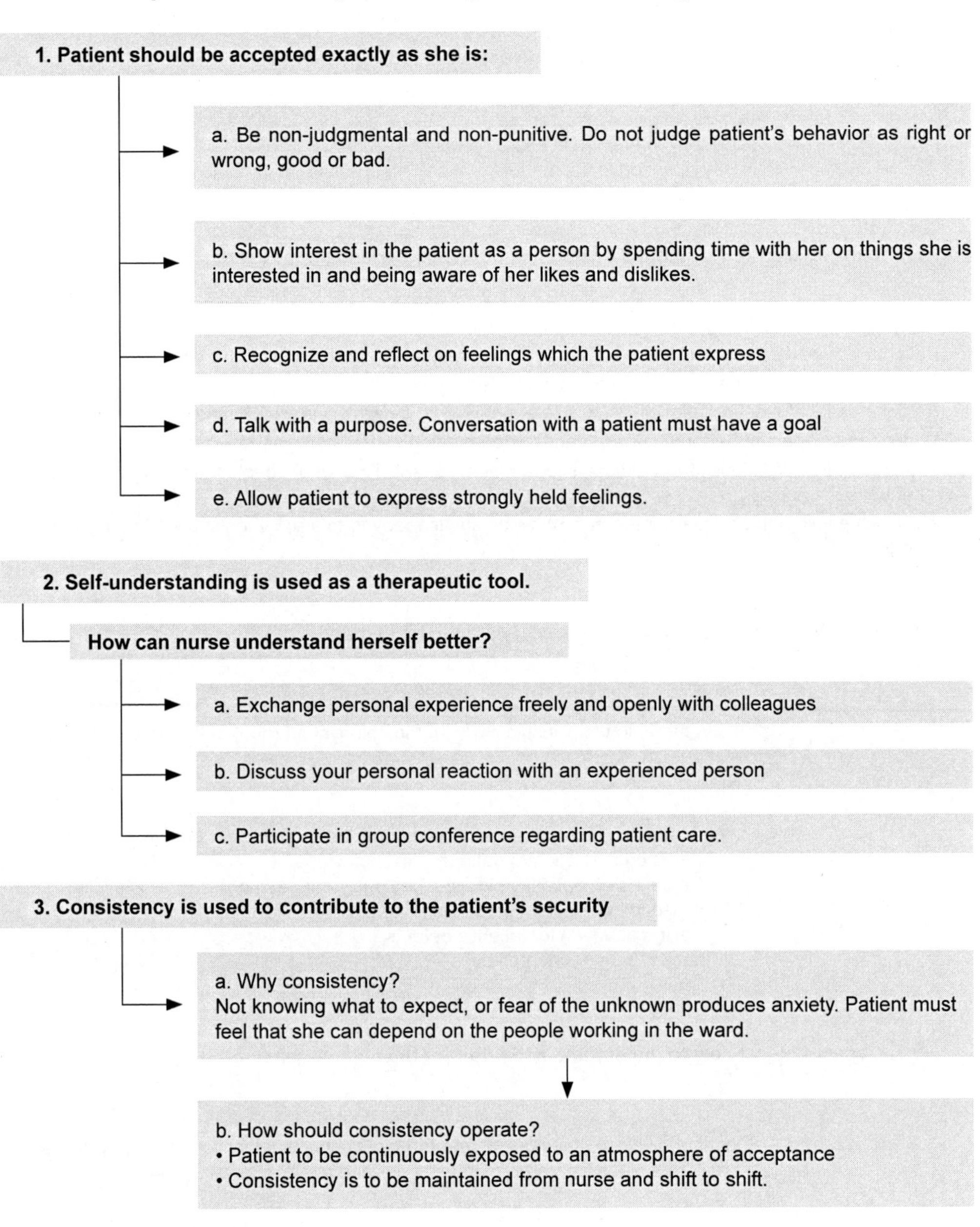

4. Reassurance to be given in a suitable and acceptable manner.

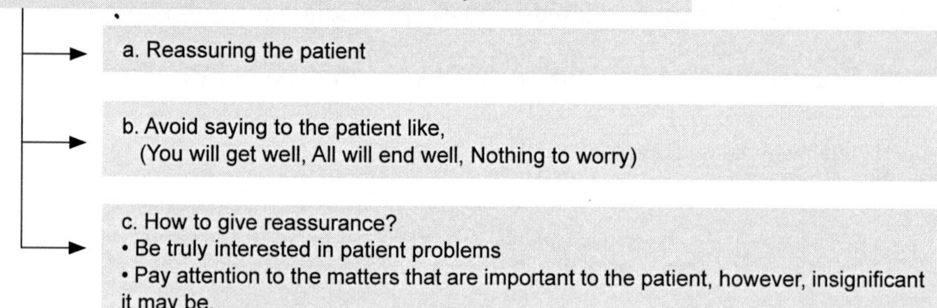

5. Patient's behavior is changed through emotional experience not by rational interpretation.

- Major focus is on feeling aspect, not on intellectual aspect
- Patients' defensive behavior against anxiety producing stress is based on strong emotional needs
- The more beliefs are challenged, the more the patient becomes defensive
- Help the patient to feel emotionally secure to enable her to develop and understands her behavior
- Understanding cannot be forced. Insight and understanding of one's own behavior is painful
- Interpretation is only done when patient is ready for it, i.e. secure enough to tolerate and able to apply it to alter her behavior
- Attitude are also not identified for the patient, when she is ready to tolerate, then she will identify them herself.

6. Unnecessary increase in patient's anxiety should be avoided.

a. What is anxiety?
It is a threat to biological integrity of the self-system (ego) of the person.

b. What factors, situation, topics or approaches can increase anxiety?
- Direct contradiction of patient's psychotic ideas
- Demands on patient which she obviously cannot meet
- Indiscriminate use of professional terms
- Calling attention to patient's defects
- Lack of proper orientation.

7. Observe objectively to understand and interpret the patient behavior

Continuous close observations are the most important function of the psychiatric nurse. This helps to interpret the behavior and avoid untoward incidences.

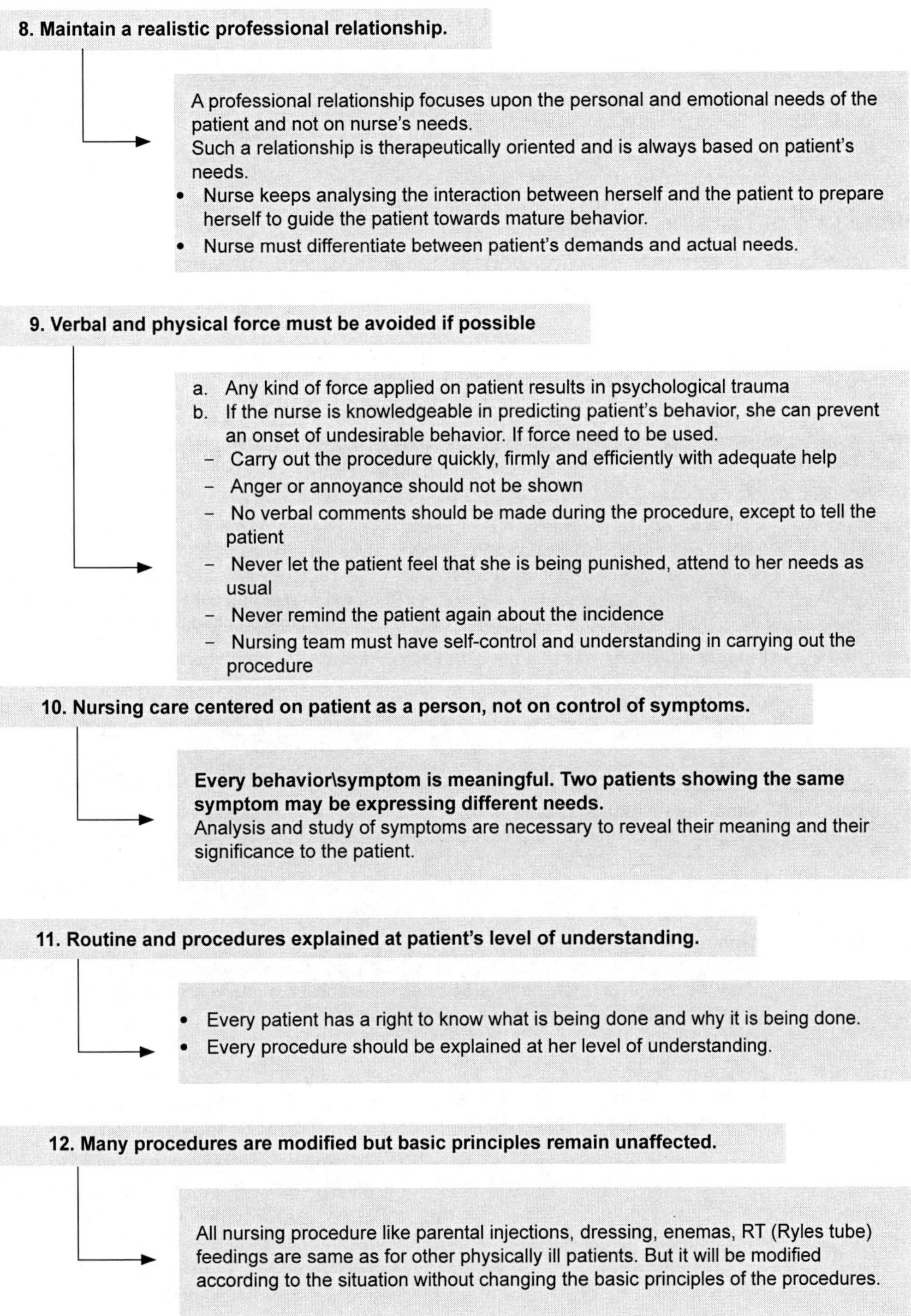

8. Maintain a realistic professional relationship.

A professional relationship focuses upon the personal and emotional needs of the patient and not on nurse's needs.
Such a relationship is therapeutically oriented and is always based on patient's needs.

- Nurse keeps analysing the interaction between herself and the patient to prepare herself to guide the patient towards mature behavior.
- Nurse must differentiate between patient's demands and actual needs.

9. Verbal and physical force must be avoided if possible

a. Any kind of force applied on patient results in psychological trauma
b. If the nurse is knowledgeable in predicting patient's behavior, she can prevent an onset of undesirable behavior. If force need to be used.

- Carry out the procedure quickly, firmly and efficiently with adequate help
- Anger or annoyance should not be shown
- No verbal comments should be made during the procedure, except to tell the patient
- Never let the patient feel that she is being punished, attend to her needs as usual
- Never remind the patient again about the incidence
- Nursing team must have self-control and understanding in carrying out the procedure

10. Nursing care centered on patient as a person, not on control of symptoms.

Every behavior\symptom is meaningful. Two patients showing the same symptom may be expressing different needs.
Analysis and study of symptoms are necessary to reveal their meaning and their significance to the patient.

11. Routine and procedures explained at patient's level of understanding.

- Every patient has a right to know what is being done and why it is being done.
- Every procedure should be explained at her level of understanding.

12. Many procedures are modified but basic principles remain unaffected.

All nursing procedure like parental injections, dressing, enemas, RT (Ryles tube) feedings are same as for other physically ill patients. But it will be modified according to the situation without changing the basic principles of the procedures.

STANDARDS OF MENTAL HEALTH NURSING PRACTICE

What is Standard?

Standards may be defined as 'a benchmark of achievement which is based on a desired level of excellence'. Standards of care (SOC's) measure the degree of excellence in nursing care and describe a competent level of nursing care.

—Dianne McMahon

Standards of Nursing Practice

The standards of nursing practice pertain to professional nursing activates that are demonstrated by the nurse through nursing process. Those involve assessment, diagnosis, outcome identification, planning, implementation and evaluation. Nursing process is a foundation of clinical decision making and empowers all significant action plan taken by Nurses in providing psychiatric mental health care to all clients.

—(American Psychiatric Nurses Association)

Box 2.19: Descriptions of each standard

Standards		Rationale
Standard 1	**Assessment:** The psychiatric mental health registered nurse collects comprehensive health data that is pertinent to patient's health or situation.	The psychiatric mental health registered nurse uses linguistically and culturally effective communication skills, interviewing, observation, record review and collection of collateral information to make sound clinical assessments.
Standard 2	**Diagnosis:** The psychiatric mental health registered nurse analyzes the assessment of data in determining diagnoses or problems including level of risk.	Through comprehensive and focused assessment and data analysis the psychiatric mental health nurse identifies patient needs related to actual or potential psychiatric disorders, mental health problems, and potential co-morbid physical illnesses.
Standard 3	**Outcomes Identification:** The psychiatric mental health registered nurse identifies expected outcomes for a plan individualized to the patient or to the situation.	Psychiatric mental health registered nurses provide nursing care to influence positive patient outcomes including the achievement of individualized mental and physical health goals.
Standard 4	**Planning:** The psychiatric mental health registered nurse develops a plan that prescribes strategies and alternatives to attain expected outcomes.	A plan of care is used systematically to guide therapeutic interventions and document progress.
Standard 5	**Implementation:** The psychiatric mental health registered nurse implements the identified plan.	Standard 5A: Coordination of care Standard 5 B: Health teaching and health promotion Standard 5 C: Milieu therapy Standard 5 D: Pharmacological, biological and complimentary Interventions Standard 5E: Prescriptive, authority and treatment Standard 5F: Psychotherapy Standard 5G: Consultation

Contd...

Contd...

Standards		Rationale
Standard 6	**Evaluation**	The psychiatric mental health registered nurse evaluates progress toward attaining expected outcomes.
Standard 7	**Quality of practice**	The psychiatric mental health registered nurse systematically enhances the quality and effectiveness of nursing practice.
Standard 8	**Education**	The psychiatric mental health registered nurse attains knowledge and competency that reflects current nursing practice.
Standard 9	**Professional practice evaluation**	The psychiatric mental health registered nurse evaluates his/her own practice in relation to the professional practice standards and guidelines, relevant statutes, rules, and regulations.
Standard 10	**Collegiality**	The psychiatric mental health registered nurse interacts with and contributes to the professional developments of peers and colleagues.
Standard 11	**Collaboration**	The psychiatric mental health registered nurse collaborates with patients, family and others in the conduct of nursing practice.
Standard 12	**Ethics**	The psychiatric mental health registered nurse integrates ethical provisions in all areas of practice.
Standard 13	**Research**	The psychiatric mental health registered nurse integrates research findings into practice.
Standard 14	**Resource utilization**	The psychiatric mental health registered nurse considers factors related to safety, effectiveness, cost, and impact on practice in the planning and delivery of nursing services.
Standard 15	**Leadership**	The psychiatric mental health registered nurse provides leadership in the professional practice setting and the profession.

CONCEPTUAL MODELS AND THE ROLE OF NURSE

Core concept of conceptual model

A conceptual model is a framework of related concepts. It address the bases for behavior in order to direct intervention.

Most mental health professionals practice within the framework of a conceptual model of psychiatric treatment. A model is a way of organizing a complex body of knowledge, such as concepts related to human behavior. They are:

- Existential model
- Psychoanalytical model
- Behavioral model
- Interpersonal model
- Medical model.

Existential Model

Ellis, Rogers

The existential model focuses on the person's experience in the here and now, with much less attention to the person's past than in other theoretical models.

View of Behavioral Deviations

Existentialist theorists believe that behavioral deviations result when the individual is out of touch with the self or the environment. This alienation is caused by self-imposed restrictions. The individual is not free to choose from among all alternative behavior. Deviant behavior frequently is a way of avoiding more socially acceptable or more responsible behavior.

The person who is self-alienated feels helpless, sad, lonely, self-criticism and lack of self-awareness prevent participation in authentic, rewarding relationships with others. Theoretically, the person has many choices in terms of behavior. However, existentialists believe that people tend to avoid being real and instead give in to the demands of others.

Existential Therapeutic Process

There are several existential therapies, all of which assume that the patient must be able to choose freely from what life has to offer. Although the approaches are somewhat different, the goal is to return the patient to an authentic awareness of being.

The existential therapeutic process focuses on the encounter is not merely the meeting of two or more people, it also involves their appreciation of the total existence of each other. Through the encounter, the patient is helped to accept and understand personal history, to live fully in the present, and to look forward to the future.

Roles of nurse and patient

Existential theorist emphasize that the therapist and the patient are equal in their common humanity. The therapist acts as a guide to the patient, who has gone astray in the search for authenticity. The therapist is direct in pointing out areas where the patient should consider changing. However, caring and warmth are also emphasized. The therapist and the patient are to be open and honest. The therapeutic experience is a model for the patient; new behaviors can be tested before risks are taken in daily life.

The patient is expected to assume and accept responsibility for behavior. Dependence on the therapist generally is not encouraged. The patient treated is an adult. Frequently, illness is de-emphasized. The patient is viewed as a person alienated from the self and others, but for whom, there is hope if the therapist is trusted and directions are followed. The patient is always active in therapy, working to meet the challenge presented by the therapist.

Psychoanalytical Model

Freud, Erickson

Psychoanalytical theory was developed by Sigmund Freud in the late nineteenth and early twentieth century's. It focused on the nature deviant behavior and proposed a new perspective on human development. Many of Freud's ideas were controversial, particularly in the Victorian society to that time. Objective observation of human behavior was a great contribution the psychoanalysts, as was the identification of a mental structure. Such concepts as id, ego, superego, and ego defense mechanism are still widely used. Most people also accept the existence of an unconscious level of mental functioning; first introduced by Freud.

Id: Personality process that wants to experience only pleasure, is impulsive and without morals.

Ego: Personality process that focuses on reality while striving to meet the needs of the id. The ego experiences anxiety and uses defense mechanism for protection.

Superego: Personality process that is concerned with right and wrong consequences. It provides the ego with an inner control to help cope with the id.

View of Behavior Deviations

Psychoanalysts trace disrupted behavior in the adult to earlier developmental stages. Each stage of development has a task that must be accomplished. If too much emphasis is placed on any stage or if unusual difficulty arises in dealing with the associated conflicts, psychological energy (libido) becomes fixated in an attempt to deal with anxiety.

Psychoanalysts believe that neurotic symptoms arise when so much energy goes into controlling the anxiety that it interferes with the individual's ability to function. They believe that everyone is neurotic to some extent. Everyone carries the burden of childhood conflicts and is influenced in adulthood by childhood experiences. Psychoanalysts in training must undergo personal analysis so that their own neurotic behavior does not hinder their objectivity as therapist.

According to psychoanalytic theory, symptoms are symbols of the original conflict. For instance, compulsive handwashing may represent the person's attempt to cleanse the self of impulses that a parent labelled unclean during the anal stage of development. However, the meaning of the behavior is hidden from the conscious awareness of the person, who usually is upset about these uncontrollable thoughts, actions, and feelings.

Psychoanalytical Therapeutic Process

Psychoanalytic uses free association and dream analysis to reconstruct the personality. Free association is the verbalization of thought as they occur without any conscious screening or censorship. Off course, there is always unconscious censorship of thought and impulses that threaten the ego.

The psychoanalyst searches for patterns in the areas that are unconsciously avoided. Conflictual areas that the patient does not discuss or recognize are identified as resistance. Analysis of the patient's dreams can provide additional insight into the nature of the resistances, since dreams symbolically communicate areas of intrapsychic conflict.

The therapist helps the patient to recognize intrapsychic conflicts by using interpretation. Interpretation involves explaining to the patient the meaning of dream symbolism and the significance of the issues that are discussed or avoided.

Strong positive transference causes the patient to want to please the therapist and to accept the patient's behavior. Strong negative transference may impede the progress of therapy as the patient actively resists the therapist's interventions. Countertransference, or the therapist's response to the patient, can also interfere with therapy if the analyst is unaware of it or unable to deal with it.

Since the therapist can temporally replace the significant other of the patient's early life experience, previously unresolved conflicts can be brought into the therapeutic situation. These conflicts can be worked through a healthier resolution. Psychoanalytical therapy is usually long term and is time consuming and expensive.

Roles of Patient and Psychoanalyst

The roles of the patient and the psychoanalyst were defined by Freud. The patient was to be an active participant, freely revealing all thoughts exactly as they occurred and describing all dreams. The patient often lies during therapy to induce relaxation, which facilitates free association.

The psychoanalyst is a shadow person. The patient is expected to reveal all private thoughts and feelings and the analyst reveals nothing personal. The analyst usually is out of the patient's sight to ensure that nonverbal responses do not influence the patient. Verbal responses are brief and noncommittal for the most part to prevent interference with the associate flow.

The therapist uses free association (letting the patient say everything that comes to mind) so that repressed material can be identified and interpreted for patient. Dream analysis helps patients uncover the meaning of dreams, which also increases awareness about present behavior. Transference that occurs in the relationship is used to encourage working through feelings that would otherwise remain unconscious.

The therapist changes this communication style when interpreting behavior. Interpretations are presented for the patient to accept or reject, but rejections suggest resistance. Likewise, frustration that the patient expresses toward the analyst is interpreted as transference. By the end of therapy, the patient should be view the analyst realistically, having worked through conflicts and dependency needs.

Behavioral Model

This model assumes that:

- All human behavior is a response to a stimulus.
- Human being can control or determine the behavior of others.

- Human personality is mere pattern of stimulus response chain.

Both adaptive and non-adaptive behaviors are learned and strengthened through reinforcement.

Therapies Based on Behavior Model

- **Assertive training:** To alleviate anxiety when the patient's anxiety is arising from interpersonal relationships. Assertiveness implies the ability to stand-up for one's own rights while not infringing on the rights of others.
- **Aversion therapy:** It refers to the use of painful stimulus usually an electrical shock, to create an aversion to a stimulus. It tries to anti-abuse therapy.
- **Token economy:** It is positive reinforcement program. One use of this system is to encourage socially acceptable behavior in chronically hospitalized patients. The person is rewarded with a token generally an eatable or a cigarette, when desirable behavior occurs. He is penalized by removal of tokens when undesirable behavior takes place.
- **Shaping:** Another behavioral reinforcement technique is used to condition the close approximations of some desired adaptive behavior.

Interpersonal Model

Sullivan, Peplau

According to Sullivan, the purpose of all behavior is to get needs met through interpersonal interactions and decrease or avoid anxiety.

Sullivan coined the term *security operation* to describe those measures that the individual employs to reduce anxiety and enhance security. Collectively, all of the security operation of an individual's uses to defend him or herself against anxiety and ensure self-esteem to make up the self-system.

View of Behavioral Deviations

Interpersonal theorists believe that behavior evolves around interpersonal relationship. While Freudian theory emphasizes a person's intrapsychic experience. Interpersonal theory emphasizes social or interpersonal experience. Sullivan, like Freud, traces a progression of psychological development. Sullivan's theory states the person bases behavior on two drives, the drive for satisfaction and the drive for security. Satisfaction refers to the basic human drives, including hunger, sleep, lust, and loneliness.

When Peplau defined nursing as an interpersonal process, she also discussed the importance of basic human needs. Needs must be met if a healthy state is to be achieved and maintained. For Peplau, the two interacting components of health are psychological demands and interpersonal conditions.

Interpersonal Therapeutic Process

The interpersonal therapist, like the psychoanalyst, explore the patient's life history. The idea is that by experiencing a healthy relationship with the therapist, the patient can learn to have more satisfying interpersonal relationships. The therapist actively encourage the development of trust by relating authentically to the patient.

Therapy is completed when the patient can establish satisfying human relationships, thereby meeting basic needs. Termination is a significant part of the relationship that must be experienced and shared by both the therapist and the patient. The patient learns that leaving a significant other involves pain but can also be an opportunity for growth.

Roles of Patient and Interpersonal Therapist

The patient-therapist dyad is viewed as a partnership in interpersonal therapy. Sullivan describes the therapist as a 'participant observer' whose role is to engage the patient, establish trust, and empathize. There is an active effort to help the patient realize that other people have to speak openly.

The therapist interact as a real person who also has beliefs, values, thoughts, and feelings. The patient's role is to share concerns with the therapist and to participate as fully as possible in the relationship. The relationship itself is meant to serve as a model of adaptive interpersonal relationships.

Interpersonal nursing roles have been identified by Peplau. These roles may be assumed by the nurse or assigned to others. The therapist helps the patient to meet the goals of therapy; need satisfaction and personal growth. Self-awareness is essential to success as an interpersonal therapist.

Medical Model

The medical model refers to psychiatric care that is based on the traditional physician-patient relationship. It focuses on the diagnosis of a mental illness, and subsequent treatment is based on this diagnosis.

Somatic treatments, including pharmacotherapy and electroconvulsive are important component of the treatment process. The interpersonal aspect of the medical model varies widely, from intensive insight-oriented intervention to brief session involving medical management of medications. Much of modern psychiatric care is dominated by the medical model. Other health professionals may be involved in interagency referrals, family assessment, and health teaching, but physicians are viewed as the leaders of the team when this model is in effect.

A positive contribution of the medical model has been the continuous exploration for causes of mental illness using the scientific process.

View of Behavioral Deviations

The medical model proposes that deviant behavior is a symptom of a CNS disorder. Currently, the exact nature of the psychological disruption is not well understood. It is thought that the psychotic disorders such as bipolar disorder, mayor depression; and schizophrenia involve an abnormality in the transmission of neural impulses. It is also thought that this difficulty occurs at the synaptic level and involves neurochemicals such as dopamine, serotonin, and norepinephrine.

Research currently is taking place so that the brain's involvement in emotional response can be better understood. Another branch of research focuses on stressors and the human response to stress.

Summarization of Conceptual Models

Model	View of behavioral deviation	Therapeutic process	Roles of patient and therapist
Psychoanalytical (S Freud, Erikson, A Freud, Klein, horney, Fromm Reichmann, Menninger)	• Based on adequate resolution of developmental conflicts • Ego defenses inadequate to control anxiety. • Symptoms result in effort to deal with anxiety.	• Uses techniques of free association and dream analysis • Identifies problem areas through interpretation of patient's resistances and transferences	• Patient verbalizes all thoughts and dreams: considers therapist's interpretations • Therapist remains remote to encourage development of transference and interprets patient's thoughts and dreams.
Interpersonal (Sullivan, Peplau)	• Anxiety arises and is experienced interpersonally • Basic fear is fear of rejection • Person needs security and satisfaction that result from positive interpersonal relationships	• Relationship between therapist and patient builds feeling of security • Therapist helps patient experience trusting relationship and gain interpersonal satisfaction	• Patient shares anxieties and feelings with therapist • Therapist uses empathy to perceive patient's feelings, and uses relationship as a corrective interpersonal experience
Existential: (Perls, Glasser, Ellis, Rogers, Frankl)	• Life is meaningful when the person can fully experience and accept the self • The self can be experienced through authentic relationships with other people	• Person aided to experience authenticity in relationships • Therapy frequently conducted in groups • Patient encouraged to accept self and to assume control of behavior	• Patient participates in meaningful experience to learn about real self • Therapist helps patient recognize value of self, clarify realities of situation, and explore feelings
Medical (Meyer, Kraepl in, Spitzer)	• Behavioral disruption result from a biological disease process • Symptoms result from a combination of psychological, genetic, environmental and social factors	• Treatment is related to diagnosis and includes somatic therapies and various interpersonal techniques • Treatment approach adjusted depending on symptomatic response	• Patient complies with prescribed therapy and reports effects of therapy to physician. • Therapist diagnoses illness and prescribes therapeutic approach.

3 Assessment of Mental Health Status

The evaluation of psychiatric clients is a multifaceted endeavor, most effectively performed by interdisciplinary team of mental health professionals. The ability to assess clients is one of the most important skills of a psychiatric nurse.

PSYCHIATRIC NURSING INTERVIEW

An interview is a conversation with a deliberate purpose that ideally is accepted by the participants. In no other branch of medicine is the history-taking interview as important as in psychiatry.

The purpose of the psychiatric nursing interview is to gather information which is necessary to understand and treat the clients.

The content and process of the interview vary according to the state of the participants and the context in which the interview takes place. The members of multidisciplinary team share the responsibility for data collection.

The content of the psychiatric nursing interview focuses on the client's biopsychosocial history and current mental status examination.

Biopsychosocial History

Psychiatric history helps to gather information about a client and helps the examiner to make diagnosis about his problem. Psychiatry has no external validating criteria, no laboratory test to confirm the diagnosis. Psychiatric history collection is having an important role in making the diagnosis of client's problem, which depends on the skills and knowledge of the examiner.

Definition

'The psychiatric history is record of patient's life and it allows the mental health team members to understand who that patient is, where the patient has come from and where patient is likely to go in future.'

Purpose

- To allow the clients and family members to express their feelings freely in their own words.
- Psychiatric history collection helps to identify the symptoms, how these symptoms are developed and the effect of these symptoms on person's life.

- Helps to identify the causes of illness.
- Helps to make easy diagnosis and management of the illness.
- To identify psychiatric emergencies.
- To provide insight into the nature of relationship with closest people.

Box 3.1: History collection overview

- Identification of data of the client
- Informant
- Presenting chief complaints
- History of present illness
- Treatment history
- Past psychiatric and medical history
- Family history
- Personal history

Identification and Demographical Details

These details includes client's name, age, sex, religion, address, socio-economic status, inpatient number, education, occupation, marital status, details of informant and relation to the patient.

Presenting Chief Complaints

Here, symptoms are written in chronological order with its duration. These details are collected from patient and if he deny then collect from relatives. Write down the details in patient's own words without changing its meaning.

Enquire about the onset of illness also; it may be acute or insidious. The progress may be steady and progressive, diminishing or reappearing periodically.

History of Present Illness

In this record, all the details of symptoms from its starting. Patient's history can be supplemented with data available from other sources. Record the data.

Treatment History

Record the details of treatment like psychopharmacological drugs, electroconvulsive therapy (ECT), psychological therapies, etc.

Past Psychiatric and Medical History

Collect the details about the past psychiatric history. If patient had any previous episode of psychiatric illness, its nature, duration, the treatment received and outcome should be recorded.

If the patient has any medical illnesses it should be included in the history. The duration of illness, its treatment, history of any accidents, hospitalizations, etc. should be recorded.

Family History

Collect the details of family like type and size of family. The presence of any psychiatric illness on the paternal or maternal side; note specifically the history of suicide, mental retardation, epilepsy or any other genetically transmitted disorders. Construct the family composition and genogram (family tree) with the collected details of the family members.

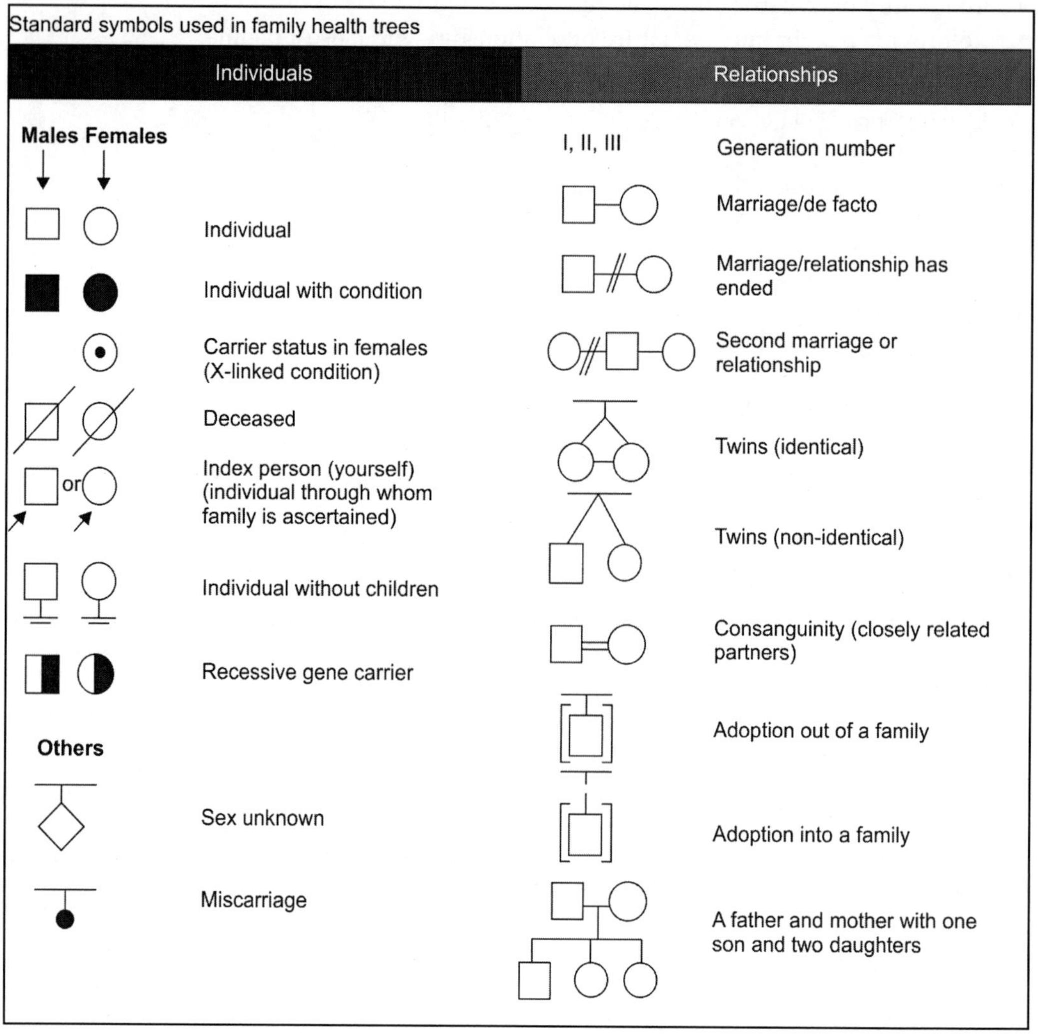

Standard symbols used in family health trees

Individuals	Relationships
Males Females	I, II, III — Generation number
Individual	Marriage/de facto
Individual with condition	Marriage/relationship has ended
Carrier status in females (X-linked condition)	Second marriage or relationship
Deceased	Twins (identical)
Index person (yourself) (individual through whom family is ascertained)	Twins (non-identical)
Individual without children	Consanguinity (closely related partners)
Recessive gene carrier	Adoption out of a family
Others	Adoption into a family
Sex unknown	A father and mother with one son and two daughters
Miscarriage	

Fig. 3.1: Common pedigree symbols

Personal History

Personal history includes the developmental, educational, occupational as well as the sexual history of the patient. *Developmental history* includes the details of pregnancy and delivery, developmental milestones, occurrence of any significant events like separation from parents, migration, etc.

The *educational history* relates to the details of levels of performance in school, relation with peers and teachers, academic achievements, etc. and in *occupational history,* collects the details of type of work, job satisfaction, frequent change in job, etc.

In *sexual history* collects the details about sexual development, attitude towards sexuality. In *marital history,* enquire about married life, relation with spouse and children.

Collect the details of *premorbid personality;* it is the personality of the individual prior to the illness. Ask about the social relationship, interests and hobbies, mood changes, habits, character, fantasies, ambition, religious view, etc. ***(See Appendix 1)***

Mental Status Examination (MSE)

Mental status examination (MSE) is a standardized format in which the clinician records the psychiatric signs and presents at the time of interview.

The MSE of psychiatric patients is analogous to the physical examination in physical medicine. It provides a format for the systematic observation and recording of information about a person's thinking, emotions, and behavior. These data combined with information from the history are the basis for formulating a differential diagnosis.

Box 3.2: Aspects of mental status examination (MSE)

Physical
- General appearance
- Motor activity and behavior

Emotional
- Mood and Affect

Cognitive
- Speech
- Attention, concentration
- Memory
- Thought
- Intelligence
- Abstract thinking
- Perception
- Insight
- Orientation
- Judgment.

General Appearance and Behavior

This is the general description of patient's behavior. This shows his sensorium, alertness, cooperativeness, mannerisms, involuntary movements, etc.

Speech

The manner of speaking and its defects are recorded under speech. Assess the rate, quantity and flow of speech. Check for the initiation. Record a sample of speech for later analysis.

Thought

Inference about the thought and its disorders are made from the speech sample or the writing sample of the patient. Disorders of form, content and possession may be present. Check for delusions, obsessive ruminations and thought alienation.

Mood and Affect

The patient should asked about his affective state. Check that his mood is appropriate or not. Is the emotional expression is blunt and colorless? Does the patient has any suicidal ideas?

Perception

Observe for any type of perceptual abnormalities like illusions and hallucinations. If hallucination is present, find out which type of hallucination and patients reaction.

Attention and Concentration

Assess the patient's ability to attend and maintain attention during the allocated task.

How is his concentration? Can his attention be easily aroused and sustained? Is he distractible?

Some simple tests can be administered. Ask the client to name the days of week or names of months forwards and backwards. He may be asked to subtract 7 or 3 from 100 (100, 93, 86, 79, etc) up to 1.

Orientation

Check whether the patient is oriented to time, place and persons. A defect in orientation reflects cognitive disorders. Orientation involves the ability to tell correctly the time of day, date, week, month, where he is and how he came and correct identification of people around him.

Memory

In which the immediate, recent and remote memory should be tested. *Immediate memory* can be tested by asking to repeat the digits or letters presented to him. *Recent memory* can be tested by asking some events of past 24 hours. *Remote memory* can be tested by asking the details of his past life, schooling, etc.

Intelligence

Patient's educational level, vocabulary, abstract thinking and reasoning give an idea about his intellectual capacity.

Insight and Judgment

Awareness of illness and readiness for taking treatment reflects the insight of the patient. Judgment refers the patient's plans for his future. ***(See Appendix 2)***

INVESTIGATIONS

After taking psychiatric interview and mental status examination, it is important for the mental health care professionals to know about some of the medical investigations and neuro imaging techniques. These investigations are carried out based on the diagnostic and etiological possibilities.

These tests may perform as a part of routine examination, to identify the drug concentrations in blood (e.g. lithium), before starting the administration of some psychiatric drugs, in case of side effects of drug and prior to ECT. Some of the common investigations are given in the box below.

Box 3.3: Common investigations performed

Name of tests	Type of tests
Complete hemogram	Total and differential count, ESR, hemoglobin
Renal function tests (RFTs)	Blood urea, serum creatinine
Urinalysis	Routine examination
Liver function tests (LFTs)	SGOT, SGPT, serum alkaline, phosphatse, bilirubin level
Thyroid function tests (TFTs)	T_3,T_4,TSH
Blood sugar	Fasting and post prandial blood sugar
Serum electrolytes	Level of sodium, potassium, calcium and chlorides
Serum lithium	Patient with the treatment of lithium salts
X-ray skull, ECG	Prior to ECT.

Abbreviations: ECG—Electrocardiagram; ESR–Erythrocyte sedimentation rate; SGOT—Serum glutamic oxaloacetic transaminase; SGPT—Serum glutamic pyruvic transaminase; T3—Triiodothronine; T4—Thyroxine; TSH—Thyroid stimulating harmone; ECT—Electroconvulsive therapy

NEUROIMAGING TECHNIQUES

Brain function can be identified by using various imaging techniques which helps in determining the normal and abnormal activities of brain and also helps in identifying various anatomical differences in various psychiatric disorders. Various neuroimaging techniques are given in the box.

Box 3.4: Common neuroimaging techniques used

Name of test	Procedure	Indications
Electroencephalo graphy (EEG)	Graphical representation of brain waves with the help of electrodes	Dementia, seizures, other degenerative disorders
Computed tomography (CT) scan	Study of brain structures by the radiographic, three dimensional images obtained through computer	Structural changes in schizophrenia, bipolar disorders, dementia, delirium, seizures
Magnetic resonance image (MRI)	Brain activity and functions are notified by placing head in the magnetic field which induces brain to emit radiowaves	Structural and functional changes in brain, any ischemic changes (transient ischemic attack)
Brain electrical activity mapping (BEAM)	A computed tomographic technique is used to display the EEG recording of the brain electrical activity by using flash light, or sudden sound	To assess the brain activity and function
Positron emission tomography (PET)	A radioactive substance is injected in the brain which shows bright spots on the scan taken up by different tissues	To study the brain structure and physiology like neurotransmitter activity

Contd...

Contd...

Name of test	Procedure	Indications
Single positron emission computed tomography (SPECT)	It is similar to PET, more stable substances than PET are used to visualize the blood flow pattern in the brain	To detect cerebrovascular accident (CVA) and brain tumor.

Neurological Examination

The neuro assessment is a key component in the care of the neurological patient. Nurses working in psychiatric department need to have knowledge and skill in performing a neurological assessment.

Purpose

- To rule out nervous system dysfunction
- To establish a baseline for mental status
- To monitor the progress of disease
- To determine the type of therapy.

Components of Neurological Assessment

Following are the components of neurological examination:

- Patient history
- Level of consciousness
- Mental status examination
- Cranial nerve testing
- Motor function
- Sensory function
- Cerebellar function.

Patient History

A thorough history is the most important part of neurological examination and must be performed before any other procedures unless impossible. History can be collected from patient or from a reliable informant.

Level of Consciousness

Consciousness is the most sensitive indicator of neurological change. Consciousness can be defined as a state of general awareness of oneself and the environment. Consciousness is difficult to measure directly but it is estimated by observing how patients respond to certain stimuli.

Assessing the level of consciousness is an important part of neurological examination.

There are various terms used to describe altered level of consciousness like alert, lethargy, stuporous, semicomatose, comatose, etc.

Glasgow Coma Scale (GCS) is one of the common measure to assess the level of consciousness which quantifies the level of consciousness from 3 to 15, a score of 15 indicates best level and a score of 3 indicates the least level of consciousness.

Box 3.5: Glasgow Coma Scale (GCS)

Eye opening	Verbal response	Motor response	Score
		Obeys commands	6
	Oriented	Localizes pain	5
Spontaneous	Confused	Flexion withdrawal	4
To speech	Inappropriate words	Abnormal flexion	3
To pain	Incomprehensible sounds	Extension	2
None	None	None	1
Total best score of 15.			

Mental Status Examination

The client's higher cognitive functioning can be assessed by examining orientation, attention, concentration, memory, judgment and abstract thinking. The details of MSE has been already discussed in this chapter earlier.

Cranial Nerve Examination

The cranial nerves arise directly from the central nervous system (CNS). Most often, a neurological problem is detected through the assessment of these nerves. There are 12 pairs of cranial nerves, and the cranial nerve assessment tests are summarized in the box below.

Box 3.6: Assessment of cranial nerve functioning

Nerve	Function	Assessment
I. Olfactory	Smell	Instruct the patient to close the eyes, occlude one nostril and ask to identify the odor. Repeat for the opposite nostril. (Familiar substances such as coffee, lemon, peppermint, etc. are used).
II. Optic	Vision	Gross assessment of visual field is carried out in the following manner. Instruct the patient to close one eye. The examiner closes his/her opposite eye then positions her fingers off to the side at eye level at the same distance between the patient and herself. The examiner's moving finger is then brought into the main boundaries of the visual field. The patient states when the moving finger is seen. This exercise is repeated with the opposite eye.
		Fundoscopic examination: The retina, retinal arteries, veins of optic nerve are visualized through an ophthalmoscope. Increased intracranial pressure is indicated when the vein is congested of the optic nerve head is swollen .

Contd...

Contd...

Nerve	Function	Assessment
III. Oculomotor	Eyelid elevation, EOM (extraocular movements), pupil size and reactivity	Instruct the patient to fix his eyes on an object. Shine the beam of torch directly into each pupil. Note the size, shape of reaction of the pupils to the light stimulus. The pupil size should be noted before and after the light is directed into the eye.
IV. Trochlear	EOM—turns eye downward and laterally	To assess ocular movements ask the patient to follow an object moved systematically in various directions up, down to the right, and to the left. Note for diplopia, limited eye movements of the presence or absence of nystagmus.
V. Trigeminal	Facial sensation and jaw movements	The patient is asked to close his eyes while a wisp of cotton is passed gently over various parts of the face. The patient is asked to identify where the cotton is applied each time. The motor component is evaluated by telling the patient to open his / her mouth wide of hold tightly. The examiner then attempts to close the patient's mouth using hands.
VI. Abducens	EOM—turns eye laterally	Same as like occulomotor and trigeminal nerve test.
VII. Facial	Facial expression, taste, corneal reflex, eyelid and lip closure	The patient is asked to identify the taste of sugar after which a sip of water is given. The same procedure is followed using a salty, sour and bitter substance. Motor function is tested by having the patient wrinkle forehead, smile, showing teeth and wrinkling eyes. Asymmetrical movement or facial drooping is to be noted.
VIII. Vestibulocochlear	Hearing, equilibrium	Tested by using a ticking watch one to two inches away from the patient's ear or using a tuning fork, hearing in both the lift and right ears should be compared. The Weber test and Rinne test may be done to differentiate between conduction deafness of nerve deafness.
IX. Glosso-pharyngeal	Swallowing, gag reflex, taste	• Instruct the patient to open mouth and say 'ah'. The soft palate of uvula elevate in the midline normally. If there is paralysis, uvula deviates to the side.
X. Vagus	Swallowing, gag reflex, phonation	• Use the tip of a tongue depressor, very gently stimulate the back of the pharynx nose, any asymmetrical contractions of the palate, uvula and pharynx. • Test for swallowing reflex by asking the patient to drink clear fluid to note the reaction.

Contd...

Contd...

Nerve	Function	Assessment
XI. Spinal accessory	Shoulder movement, head rotation	• Assess the *trapezius muscle* function by instructing the patient to raise both shoulder of hold tightly while the examiner applies resistance to both shoulders using hands. • Evaluate the *sternocliedomastoid muscle* function by asking the patient to turn his/ her head against resistance applied by the examiner's hands.
XII. Hypoglossal	Tongue movement, speech articulation	Ask the patient to protrude tongue normally, protrudes in the midline. To assess the tongue strength, instruct the patient to move her tongue to the right or to the left.

Assessment of Motor Function

When assessing motor function from a neurological perspective, the assessment should focus on arm and leg movement. Consider the following:

- Muscle size
- Muscle tone
- Muscle strength
- Involuntary movements
- Posture, gait.

When assessing apply maximum force to the extremity while the patient pushes against the observer's fixed resistance. Use following abbreviations when referring to each extremity:

D – Distal
P – Proximal
RUE – Right Upper Extremity
RLE – Right Lower Extremity
LUE – Left Upper Extremity
LLE – Left Lower Extremity.

Box 3.7: Motor power grading

Grade	Description
5/5	Full range of motion against gravity with extreme resistance
4/5	Full range of motion against gravity with some resistance
3/5	Full range of motion against gravity with no resistance
2/5	Full range of motion with gravity eliminated
1/5	Slight contraction visible
0/5	No movement.

Assessment of Sensory Function

When assessing sensory function remember that there are three main pathways for sensation and they should be compared bilaterally:

1. Pain and temperature sensation
2. Position sense (*proprioception*)
3. Light touch.

- Touch is assessed by passing a wisp of cotton gently touch various areas on the body, asking the patient to identify the area.
- To assess the pain, gently touch various parts of the body with a sterile needle and request the patient to identify where the sensation is felt.
- Temperature response is evaluated by touching the patient with test tubes filled with warm water and cracked ice alternatively. The patient is asked to distinguish between hot and cold.
- Sense of position is evaluated by instructing the patient to close eyes; the examiner grasp the patients index finger at the last joint from the side of gently raises or lowers it. The patient is asked whether the index finger is positioned up or down. This exercise is repeated using the patient's great toe.

Assessment of Cerebellar Functions

The cerebellum is responsible for muscle coordination and balance on the same side. To test cerebellar function, use the following tests:

- ***Finger to finger test***: The patient is asked to place index finger on the nurse's index finger. This is repeated in succession on both sides.
- ***Finger to nose test***: The patient is asked to extend his/her finger touch the tip of his/her nose several times in rapid succession. This is done with eyes opened eyes closed also.
- ***Patting test***: The patient is asked to hold his/her hands and arms above his/her thighs with palms positioned downward and slap his/her thighs simultaneously. The same is repeated several times in rapid succession with palms positioned upwards also.
- ***Romberg test***: The patient is instructed to stand with feet together, closed eyes and arms at the sides for 10 seconds. The Romberg test is considered positive only if there is actual loss of balance.
- ***Tandem walking test***: The patient is asked to stand in the normal erect, standing position to walk on a straight line. Note any *lurching*, unsteadiness or broadening of gait.

PSYCHOLOGICAL TESTS

Psychological tests are ideally conducted by a clinical psychologist who has been trained in the administration, scoring and interpretation of these tests. This will aid the psychiatrist in diagnosis the disorder. The psychiatric nurse should have knowledge on all these tests, this will enable her to clarify the doubts of the client and family members.

The common psychological tests used are:

Intelligence tests:

- Stanford-Binet test
- Wechsler's adult intelligence test (WAIS)

- Wechsler's children intelligence test
- Binet kamat test (BKT)
- Bhatia battery test.

Personality test:

- Thematic apperception test (TAT)
- Minnesota multiphasic personality inventory (MMPI)
- 16 PF (16 Personality factor) test
- Draw a person test (DAPT)
- Sentence completion test
- Bender-Gestalt test.

Rating Scales

- Brief psychiatric rating scale (BPRS)
- Scale of assessment of negative symptoms (SANS)
- Scale of assessment of positive symptoms (SAPS)
- Hamilton's anxiety rating scale (HARS)
- Hamilton's depression rating scale (HDRS)
- Yale-Brown obsessive compulsive scale (Y-BOCS).

Role of Nurse in Psychological Tests

The psychiatric nurse should have knowledge about all the above psychological tests. This will enable her to clarify the patients and relatives doubts regarding the psychological tests they have to undergo.

Nurses should have good rapport with the patient of family members. Hence, the patients and relatives are more comfortable approaching the nurse for any clarifications.

The nurse should reassure the patient about the safety of the tests of confidentiality of the observations of the psychologist.

The nurse observes the patient's behavior and the changes, which occur once therapy is commenced. She observes and records the changes in the patient's chart. Better observation is possible by the nurse since the patient is under her care for 24 hours, where as the other team members interact with patient for a limited period of time.

A nurse who is *knowledgeable* and skilled is an empowered nurse who is able to function as per with other team member also.

Box 3.8: Mini-mental status examination (MMSE)

A. Orientation	Score
• What is your age? • What is your occupation? • What day is it today? • Where are you now? • In which ward are you staying? • Which is your native place? • What is the name of this study?	10

Contd...

Contd...

• What is time now? • Which is the current season of the year? • Since how many days are you staying here?	
B. Registration	
Name three objects: One second to say each. Then ask the patient all three after you have said them. Give one point for each correct answer. Repeat them until he learns all the three. Count the trials and record number of trials.	**3**
C. Attention and concentration	
Begin with 100 and count backwards by 7 (stop after 5 answers). Alternatively spell 'WORLD' backwards.	**5**
D. Recall	**3**
Ask for three objects repeated above. Give one point for each other.	
E. Language	
• Show a pencil and a watch, and ask subject to name them.	**2**
• Repeat the following; 'No ifs, 'ands', or 'buts'.	**1**
• A three stage command: 'Take a paper in your right hand; fold it in half, and put in on floor'.	**3**
• Read and obey the following (show subject the written them)	**1**
Close your eyes Write a sentence. Copy a design (For example, complex polygon) 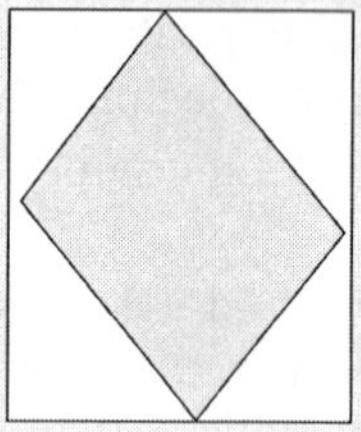	**1** **1**

4 Therapeutic Communication and Nurse-Patient Relationship

THERAPEUTIC COMMUNICATION

Introduction

Communication is the basic element of human interactions that allows people to establish, maintain and improve contacts with others. It is the transmission and receiving information, feelings and or attitudes with the overall purpose of having understood producing a response.

Communication is much more than an understanding of the spoken or written language. It includes symbols, gestures, and illustrations that accompany either the spoken or the written word.

Nursing is a communicative intervention and is founded on effective communication.

Do you know?

Communication is derived from the Latin word *communis* which means '*to share*', that is, sharing of ideas, concepts, feelings and emotions.

Key Terms

***Therapeutic communication*:** It is a process in which the nurse consciously influences a client or helps the client to a better understanding through verbal or nonverbal communication.

***Interpersonal relationship*:** The nurse-client relationship is a dynamic partnership that defines, directs, and evaluates treatment outcomes.

***Therapeutic Relationship*:** An interaction between two people (usually a caregiver and a care receiver) in which input from both participants contributes to a climate of healing, growth promotion, and/or illness prevention.

***Nurse-patient relationship*:** It is an interpersonal process between a professional nurse and a client that helps the client to foster and promote growth of personality, to help the client improve in construction and productive way of living.

Definition

'Communication is a process of sharing thoughts, feelings, facts, and other information, includes verbal and nonverbal behavior'.
— Sue C Delaune

'Communication is the process of exchanging information and the process of generating and transmitting meanings between two or more individuals.
— Carol Taylor

'Communication is a means of persuasion to influence the other so that the desired effect is achieved'.
— Aristotle

Nurse-patient Relationship

It is a mutual learning experience and a corrective emotional experience for the patient. The nurse uses personal attributes and specified clinical techniques in working with the patient to bring about behavioral change.

Nurse-patient relationship is an interaction process in which the nurse fulfil her role by using her professional knowledge.

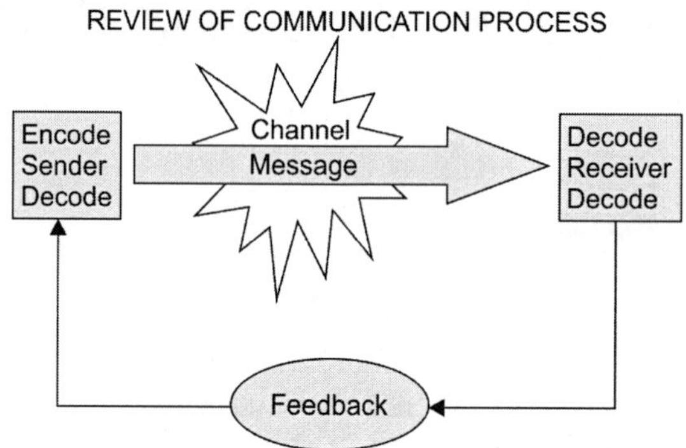

Fig 4.1: The communication process

The Elements of Communication Process

For the process of communication to be complete, it is essential that the basic elements of communication be identified. These elements are:

- *Sender/Encoder/Speaker*
- *Receiver/Decoder/Listener*
- *Message*
- *Medium*
- *Feedback*

Sender/Encoder/Speaker

The person who initiates the communication process is normally referred to as the sender.

Receiver/Decoder/Listener

The receiver is simply the person receiving the message, making sense of it, or to understand meaning of message. The receiver is also a communicator.

Message

The message is the encoded idea transmitted by the sender. The formulation of the message is very important, for an incorrect choice of words and expressions can turn the receiver hostile or make him lose interest. At this stage, the sender has to be extremely cautious.

Channel

Another important element of communication is the channel or medium in which the message being taken to receiver. It could be oral, written or nonverbal. The sender has to compose the message according to the medium of communication. Prior to the composition of the message, the medium/channel should be decided.

Feedback

Feedback is the most important component of communication. Effective communication takes place only if the receiver gives a feedback to the sender after the message has been communicated. Here, the receiver becomes again sender after respond to sender. So, communication is a continuous cyclic process.

TYPES OR FORMS OF COMMUNICATION

Basically, there are two forms in which the process of communication takes place.

Verbal	Nonverbal
Speaking **Writing**	Using through: Physical appearance and dress, touch, cues, vocal qualities, gestures, position, facial expression.

Verbal Communication

Verbal communication involves the arrangement of words in a structured and meaningful manner, adhering to the rules of grammar. The message is then conveyed to the audience in either spoken or written form.

Nonverbal Communication

Nonverbal communication is a form of communication that does not involve the use of words. It rather uses gestures, cues, vocal qualities, spatial relationships, etc. to convey a message. It is commonly used to express emotions like respect, love, dislike, unpleasantness, etc. It reflects the communicator's true feelings.

Nonverbal communication enhances the effectiveness of the message as gestures and body language, are registered easier and quicker with the audience than verbal communication.

Therapeutic Communication

The concept of 'therapeutic communication' refers to the process in which the nurse consciously influences a client or helps the client to a better understanding through verbal or nonverbal communication.

Therapeutic communication involves the use of specific strategies or techniques that encourage the patient to express feelings and ideas and that convey acceptance and respect.

Box 4.1: Difference between communication and therapeutic communication

Communication	Therapeutic communication
Communication is a process of sharing thoughts, feelings, facts, and other information, between two or more people through verbal and nonverbal behavior.	Therapeutic communication is defined as the face to face process of interacting that focuses on physical emotional wellbeing of a patient. Nurse use therapeutic communication techniques to provide support and information to the patient.

Techniques of Therapeutic Communication

Therapeutic nurse-client interaction requires warmth, trust, empathy and mutual respect. Client also should believe that the nurse cares, understands and concerned about his or her problem. To make this successful, the nurse must adopt certain therapeutic communication techniques as follows.

Table 4.1: Therapeutic communication techniques

S.No.	Techniques	Example
1.	**Active listening:** To listen actively is to be attentive to what client is saying, both verbally and nonverbally. (Several nonverbal behaviors have been designed to facilitate attentive listening).	(Mnemonics—SOLER) **S** – **S**it squarely facing the client **O** – **O**bserve an open posture **L** – **L**ean forward toward the client **E** – **E**stablish eye contact **R** – **R**elax.
2.	**Accepting:** Convey positive regard	'Yes' I follow what you said.
3.	**Giving recognition:** Acknowledging, indicating awareness	'I notice you combed your hair'.
4.	**Offering self:** Making oneself available	'Can I sit with you and talk for sometime'.
5.	**Broad opening:** The nurse allows the client to explore feelings and life problems on vast basis. The nurse communicates to patient that she is interested in him and his problems.	'Is there something you'd like to talk about?'
6.	**Offering general leads:** General leads, like broad opening statements, leave the direction of the conversation to the patient. This can be accomplished verbally or nonverbally, but nodding or through facial expressions, which demonstrate attentiveness and concern.	During the conversation, general leads, such as 'yes' or simply the 'uh hum' will usually encourage the patient to continue. Some additional samples of general leads are: 'I see' 'And then....', 'go on'
7.	**Reflecting:** In reflecting, all or part of the patient's statement is repeated to encourage him to go on. Letting him hear all of what he has said, or part of what he has said may lead him to more fully consider and expand upon his remark.	If he says, 'Everyone here ignores me' the nurse might reply, 'ignores you?'
8.	**Restating:** Lets client know whether an expressed statement has or has not been understood by nurse.	**Client:** 'I can not sleep. I stay awake all night'. **Nurse:** You have difficulty in sleeping.
9.	**Using silence:** In certain circumstances, attentive silence may be preferable. This allows the nurse to temporarily slow the pace of the conversation and gives the patient an opportunity to think about his problem, then speak further about his feelings. Also, silence allows the nurse to observe the patient for nonverbal clues and to assemble her own thoughts.	After several minutes of silence, the nurse can help the patient to resume verbal activity with statements such as, 'You were saying that ...' or 'What were you thinking?'

Contd...

Contd...

S.No.	Techniques	Example
10.	**Making observations:** Here, the nurse shares with the patient her observations regarding behavior of a patient.	'You appear tense' 'I notice you are biting your lips' (verbalize what is observed or perceived)
11.	**Giving information:** Nurse can do much to establish an atmosphere of helpfulness and trust in her relationship with the patient.	My name is.... i am a student nurse
12.	**Clarifying:** If the nurse has not understood the meaning of what the patient has said, she clarifies immediately.	She can use phrases such as 'I'm not sure I follow...' or 'Are you using this word to mean...' to request that the patient make his meaning clear to her.
13.	**Exploring:** Delving further into a subject, idea, experience, or relationship. The nurse should recognize when to delve further—she should refrain from probing or prying.	'Tell me more about that', 'Would you describe it more fully?' and 'What kind of work?' are examples exploring topics which the patient has brought up for discussion.
14.	**Focusing:** Taking notice of a single idea or even a single word and concentrate on that to identify definite problem.	'You said something earlier that i want you to go back to'
15.	**Presenting reality:** Clarifying misconceptions that client may be expressing. When it is obvious that the patient is misinterpreting reality, the nurse can indicate that which is real.	'I see no one else in the room', 'That sound was a car backfiring, 'and 'Your mother is not here; I'm a nurse.' [This technique is highly useful with geriatric patients, who are confused, and psychiatric patients showing high anxiety and patients who are confused due to alcohol or drugs such as Lysergic acid diethylamide(LSD).]
16.	**Voicing doubt:** Express uncertainty as to the reality of the patient's perceptions.	'Isn't that unusual?' 'Really?' 'That's hard to believe.' (Such expression permits the patient to become aware that others do not necessarily perceive events in the same way or draw the same conclusions that he does).
17.	**Suggesting collaboration:** Offering to share, to strive, to work together with the patient for his benefit.	'Perhaps you and I can discuss and discover what produces your anxiety (pain, frustration, etc.)
18.	**Validating:** When the nurse feels that the patient's need has been met, she should validate her impression with him to confirm patient need has been completely met.	'Do you feel relaxed?' or 'Are you feeling better now?'

Blocks to Therapeutic Communication (Nontherapeutic Techniques)

These are few methods in therapeutic communication should not be adopted, because it may leads to failure of an effective communication and causes ineffective interpersonal relationship between nurse and patient.

1. **Using reassuring clichés:** When a patient who has expressed apprehension is told, 'Everything will be alright'. 'You don't need to worry,' he is likely to feel that the nurse is not interested in his problem and thus will refrain from discussing it further.
2. **Giving advice:** 'What you should do is...'Why don't you...' By telling the patient what he should do, the nurse imposes her own opinions and solutions on client, rather than helping him to explore his ideas so that he can arrive at his own conclusions.
3. **Giving approval:** 'That's the right attitude' or 'That's the thing to do.' Although conceivably a useful response when the nurse wishes to motivate or encourage a patient, giving approval can sometimes create a block.
4. **Requesting and explanation:** 'Why did you do that?' 'Why are you here?' 'Why are you upset?' are examples of questions which some patients find difficult. Patients who cannot answer 'why' questions frequently invent answers. The nurse should avoid asking 'why' questions except when asking simple, direct questions pertaining to patient care, e.g. 'Why are you going to the bathroom?'
5. **Agreeing with the patient:** 'I agree with you,' or 'you must be right.' 'When the nurse introduces her own opinions or values into the conversation, it can prevent the patient from expressing himself freely.
6. **Disagreeing with the patient:** 'You're wrong', 'That's not true,' 'No, it isn't.' By contradicting the patient, the nurse indicates to him that what he has said has not been accepted. Because the nurse's judgment may cause him to feel threatened he may refrain from expressing himself further on the subject, or he may become defensive or angry.
7. **Making stereotyped comments:** 'How are you feeling?' 'Isn't it a beautiful day?' 'It's for your own good,' 'You'll be home in no time.' By using social clichés or trite phrases, the nurse may lead the patient to reply in a like manner, thus keeping the conversation at a superficial level.
8. **Changing the subject:** Client: 'I 'would like to die'. Nurse: 'Don't you have visitors this weekend?' or 'by the way...' or 'That reminds me...' Generally, the nurse changes the subject to avoid discussing a topic which makes her uncomfortable (consciously or unconsciously) or to initiate discussion of a topic which she is more interested. In either case, client blocks communication.

Clinical Alert: *Communication and the comatose client:*
Use caution when 'just talking' in the room of a comatose client. Research and clinical practice indicate that some comatose clients may be able to hear and process spoken language. Talk to unconscious clients rather than about them.

NURSE-PATIENT RELATIONSHIP

Introduction

Admission to the mental health care system can be the frightening experience. Clients bring with them a variety of thoughts and feelings about mental hospitals. The nurse is the primary individual to establish an effective relationship with client and meet the care needs of the client. To establish an effective relationship with clients and to meet their needs the nurse must have an understanding of the nurse-client relationship.

What is nurse-patient relationship?

In simple meaning, it is the therapeutic interaction between the nurse and patient for the purpose of meeting unique needs of patient.

The nurse-patient relationship (NPR), therapeutic relations, one–to–one relations, interpersonal relationship (IPR)

All above names are alternatively used which gives same meaning.

Types of Relationships

Every human being is unique. Individuals will bring their own background, beliefs and personalities. There are three possible types of relationships.

1. Social relationship
2. Intimate relationship
3. Therapeutic relationship.

Social Relationship

Man is social being and he cannot live above, so it is most common kind between individuals in everyday life. Both individuals are equally involves in this relationship and are concerned with meeting their own needs through the relationship. There is no predetermined goal or focus in the relationship and continuation of relationship is not determined at the onset. For example, colleagues, neighbors, etc.

Intimate Relationship

An intimate relationship is a relationship between two individuals committed to one another, caring for and respecting each other or love each other.

According to Erickson, the ability to develop an opposite sex relation depends on completing developmental tasks. This relationship forms the basis for marriage and other partner-type relationships.

Therapeutic Relationship

In a therapeutic relationship, the nurse and client work together toward the goal of assisting the client to regain the inner resources to meet the challenges and facilitate growth. (relationship only made for therapeutic purpose, to meet unique needs of patient)

The interaction is purposefully established, maintained and carried out with the anticipated outcome of helping the client gain new coping and adaptation skills.

Box 4.2: Difference between social and therapeutic relationship

	Therapeutic relationship	Social relationship
Technique objective	It is planned; helping the patient	It just happens with mutual interests; Having fun together or satisfying need of each other
Time duration	Planned for specific time and place Time is limited duration depends on goal achievement	It may be planned, unplanned by chance of two people meet

Contd...

Contd...

	Therapeutic relationship	Social relationship
Accountability	Nurse focus on goal during relationship	It is shared, both are responsible
Acceptance	Nurse accepts the client as here and now without judgment or interest	It is based on shared values and beliefs.
Termination	It is important part of relationship it is planned	May exist life long. May terminate gradually by shifting away to another place.

ETHICS AND RESPONSIBILITY IN RELATIONSHIP

What is ethics?

An ethics is a standard of behavior or a belief valued by an individual or group.

Why it is necessary?

- Ethics are guiding codes
- Ethics provides a framework for decision-making
- Professional nurse should follow these professional standards as they deliver health care. It can increase both the quality of the care one gives and the satisfaction the nurse receives from her practice.

Ethics and responsibilities of psychiatric nurse carrying out IPR based on the laws and spirit of humanity are as follows:

- Psychiatric nurses respect fundamental human rights of the patient by protecting individual rights and dignity.
- Psychiatric nurses strive to obtain the consent of the patient to take part in medical treatment through clear and open communication.
- Psychiatric nurses strive to minimize therapeutic restraints including seclusion.
- Psychiatric nurses are bound to secrecy concerning private matters learned through one's duties.
- Psychiatric nurses participate in continuing education in order to maintain high quality nursing as professionals.
- Psychiatric nurses strive to persistently improve effective nursing practice.
- Psychiatric nurses strive to meet the reliance and expectation of society with professional expertise and skills.
- Psychiatric nurses strive for the proliferation of mental health welfare based on the expectations of the people in the community.
- Psychiatric nurses make policy proposals as professionals in nursing for the overall improvement of the nursing standard.

The concept of responsible ethical choice, therefore, involves a dynamic decision making process for the nurse. It incorporates one's values, judgments, and actual choice. Related to the nurse's sense of ethics is the need to assume responsibility for his or her own behavior. This involves knowing one's limitation and being accountable for them.

Johari Window

A **Johari window** is a cognitive psychological tool created by Joseph Luft and Harry Inghamin, 1955 in the United States (US), used to help people to better understand their interpersonal communi-cation and relationships.

The Johari Window is a communication model that can be used to improve understanding between individuals and increase self-awareness.

Two Key Ideas Behind the Tool

- Individuals can build trust between themselves by disclosing information about them.
- They can learn about themselves and come to terms with personal issues with the help of feedback from others.
- Using the Johari model, each person is represented by their own four quadrant, or four-pane window. Each of these contains and represents personal information—feelings, motivation—about the person, and shows whether the information is known or not known by themselves or other people.

The Four Quadrants are:

- **Quadrant 1: Open area**: What is known by the person about him/herself and is also known by others.
- **Quadrant 2: Blind area, or 'blind spot':** What is unknown by the person about him/herself but which others know. This can be simple information, or can involve deep issues (for example, feelings of inadequacy, incompetence, unworthiness, rejection) which are difficult for individuals to face directly, and yet can be seen by others.
- **Quadrant 3: Hidden or avoided area**: What the person knows about him/herself that others do not.
- **Quadrant 4: Unknown area**: What is unknown by the person about him/herself and is also unknown by others.

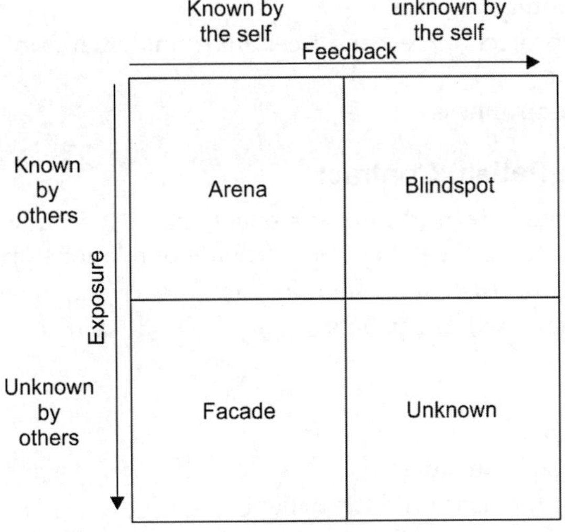

Fig. 4.2: Quadrants of Johari window

Principles of Johari Window technique

- A change in anyone quadrant; affects the all other quadrant
- If smaller the first quadrant it poorer the communication
- Interpersonal learning.

Definition of Nurse-client Relationship

'A meaningful ongoing communication with the client in an atmosphere of mutual respect and trust where by close helping relationship will be established which allows the nurse and the client to work collaboratively'.

—Wanda, K Mohr, 2006

Goals of Nurse Patient Relationship

- To help the patient to cope with the present problems
- To help the patient to understand his problems
- To assists the patient to identify emerging problems realistically
- To help the patient to find out a new alternative for his or her problem
- To help the client to communicate
- To help the patient to socialize

Purposes of Therapeutic Nurse-Patient Relation:

- It is a therapeutic goal-directed relationship between the nurse and the patient
- To bring insight and behavioral changes
- To develop mutual growth between two individuals
- To promote self-realization, self-acceptance and an increased genuine self-respect, self-identify and personal integration
- It is the central medicine through which all psychiatric care is provided to care the mental illness
- To identify appropriate nursing approaches
- To achieve developmental goals
- Provide comfort, protection, rest and freedom from demands of their usual home and work environment
- To nurture the clients illness

Elements of Nurse Patient Contract

In the introductory phase of nurse-patient relationship, the nurse and the patient first meet. As the nurse relates to the patient in this phase of relationship, the tasks are to:

- Establish a climate of trust, understanding, acceptance and open communication
- Formulate a contract with the patient

Elements of Contract

1. Name of individuals
2. Role of the nurse and the patient
3. Responsibilities of the nurse and the patient
4. Expectations of the nurse and the patient

5. Purpose of the relationship
6. Meeting location
7. Time of meetings
8. Conditions for termination
9. Confidentiality

Box 4.3: Process of formulating a contract

Step I	The contract begins with the introduction of the nurse and patient, exchange of names.
Step II	Explanation of roles. This includes the responsibilities.
Step III	Expectations of the patient and the nurse.
Step IV	Description of what nurse can and cannot do.
Step V	Discussion of the purpose of the relationship, in which the nurse emphasis that the focus of it will be the patient, his life experiences, and areas of conflict.
Step VI	Where the meetings are held? When and how often will they occur?
Step VII	How long will each be and how long will the series of meetings be?
Step VIII	The conditions of termination should be reviewed and may include a specified length of time, attainment of mutual goals or the discharge of the patient from hospital.
Step IX	The issue of confidentiality is an important one to discuss with the patient at this time. Confidentiality does not imply secrecy or the exclusive permission of information. Rather, it involves the disclosure of certain information to another specifically authorized person.

Methods of Contracting

Establishing a contract is a mutual process in which the patient participates as fully as possible. Looms describes a formal treatment contract as an openly negotiated, clearly stated set of mutual expectations that indicate what the nurse and the patient expect of each other regarding the patient health care.

Box 4.4: Loomis-model of levels of change contracts

Level I: Care contracts: Involves provision of physically and emotional safety
Level II: Social contracts: Deals primarily with behaviors and situations that can be brought under patient's conscious control.
Level III: Relationship contracts: Focuses on the repetitive or cyclical nature of patient problems as shown in their day-to-day relationships.
Level IV: Structural change and intensive psychotherapy: The emphasis here is on reworking the entire pathological structure as well as the here-and-now relationship process.

Box 4.5: Principles of therapeutic nurse-patient relationship

- Treat the client as an individual
- Accept the client as he obliques she is
- Aware the total needs of the client

Contd...

Contd...

- Emotional and involvement is essential
- Set approximate limits and goals
- Encourage the client feelings
- Therapeutic understanding (empathy in nature)
- Engage in active listening
- Realistic approach
- Establish trust and rapport.

Factors Determining Effective Nurse-Client Relationship

In nurse-patient relationship, each interaction is unique because the patient and the nurse are having their even beliefs, values, attitudes and behaviors. Some factors which can help her to develop an effective relationship are:

Self-awareness

It is an important aspect by which a nurse must identify herself/himself. Self-awareness includes self-concept, beliefs and values and life experiences.

If a nurse has a positive self-concept about herself, she will be confident of caring for her patients.

Attitude towards Patient

Nurse must develop an attitude of acceptance of the patient, tolerance of his or her disturbed behavior and helping the patient.

Rapport

It is defined as a 'relationship of mental sympathy and understanding especially between patient and therapist'. The essential qualities for developing rapport are warmth, genuineness, and empathizing ability.

Empathy

An emotional linkage between two or more people through which feelings are communicated; involves trying to imagine what it must be like to be in another person's situation. For example: Nurse: 'This must make you feel sad.'

Respect

Respect should be given in the form of nonpossessive warmth or unconditional positive regards without criticism and ridicule.

Self-disclosure

Self-disclosure is subjectively true, personal experiences about the self and is intentionally revealed to another person. The nurse may choose to share experiences or feelings that are similar to those of the client and may emphasize both the similarities and differences. This kind of self-disclosure is indicative of the closeness of the nurse-patient relationship and involves a particular kind of respect for the client.

Genuineness

It implies that the nurse is an open, honest, sincere person who is actively involved in the relationship. Genuineness means the nurse should be sincere in her relationship with clients and should not think one thing and expressing something else. This is essential because the nurse cannot expect from patient, if they lack these qualities in them.

Phases of Nurse-Patient Relationship

'Nurse-patient relationship is a series of planned purposeful interactions between a nurse and a patient'. —*Travelbee*

This definition explains that the interactions are planned and there are a series of interactions; that means the therapeutic relationship goes through various stages or phases. It is very difficult to put a statement in the beginning and end of each stage because the stages overlap. **But for the purpose of understanding the nurse-patient relationship can be described in four phases:**

1. Pre-interaction phase
2. Introductory or orientation phase
3. Working phase
4. Termination phase.

Pre-interaction Phase

Definition: Pre-interaction means a phase which a nurse goes through before the actual interaction with the patient. This phase begins when the nurse is assigned a patient to develop therapeutic relationship with him till she goes to him for interaction.

—Bimla Kapoor (2007).

This phase begins when the nurse is assigned to initiate a therapeutic relationship and this includes obtaining information about the patient from charts, significant others or health team members.

In this phase, the nurse starts with initial assessment, she evaluate her own feeling, explore fantasies, fears and ambivalence, strengths and limitations and she plan her first meeting.

Activities

The nurse plans how interaction can be established with client, what is to be achieved from this interaction and how to help patient.

Tasks of Pre-interaction Phase:

* The nurse explorer fears and anxiety
* Sets objectives for the interaction phase
* Takes help of the clinical supervisor or co-workers to overcome fears.

Introductory or Orientation Phase

Definition

Introductory or orientation phase begins when the nurse goes to the patient, introduces herself and gets introduction about patient. The nurse and the patient who are strangers meet for the first time and become acquaintances. The orientation phase ends when the nurse and the patient begin to accept each other as a unique human being.

Tasks of Introductory or Orientation Phase

Significant tasks of the orientation phase are establishment of contact, making agreement or pact and talking to him.

- **Establishment of contact**: The nurse/student nurse locates her patient. She makes an observation of who is patient and how is dressed up. Nurse introduces to the patient and asks the patient where they can sit and talk.
- **Pact:** Pact is initial encounter. The nurse makes an agreement or pact with the patient to help him towards social recovery. Nurse begins to explore onsets by telling her name, her status ad experience, name of college of nursing, the length and purpose of her stay and where she will be available. Nurse also on focus about time of termination. Nurse finds out that by which name patient would like to be called.

  During this phase, the nurse starts looking at the patient as a unique individual along with his or her environment.
- **Talking with the patient**: While talking with the patient the nurse shows trust in her behavior. Here, nurse asks 'What is your problem?' The patient gives his history and asks the nurse 'Hope you know about me now'.
  - The nurse also discusses confidentiality of information shared by patient. She clearly informs the patient that progress in therapy will be reported to team members by maintaining confidentially of specific information. Trusting relationship is also maintained by keeping up to the time.

Barriers to Orientation Phase

* Establishment, an agreement or pact is a barrier in nurse-patient relationship felt by many nurse personnel. Patient may think the nurse is here only for a few weeks. What sort of help could be expected in short span of time?

If the pact is not developed. The patient may feel deceived (be false to) and think that nobody is trustworthy. But gradually the patient accepts the pact.

* Status: is another barrier. The nurse may feel hesitant to approach the patient who is a 'doctor'. She thinks he knows everything so how would she help him. She must know that the patient may know about medicines but he needs psychiatric nursing care because he is a sick human being.

* Anxiety level of the patient and the nurse is also a barrier in this phase. Anxious nurse may handle focus on the patient and his needs. Anxious client may not discuss everything with the nurse, in the beginning.

* When either the patient or the nurse perceives the other participant as a significant individual from the past, i.e. transference and counter transference.

Working Phase/Phase of Emerging Identity

Definition

Working phase starts when the nurse and patient are able to overcome the barriers of orientation or introductory phase. Nurse and patient work together towards achievement of goals which are established during orientation phase.

— *Bimla Kapoor (2007)*

Most of the therapeutic work is carried out during this phase. The nurse and the patient explore stresses and promote the development of insight in the patient by linking perceptions, thoughts, feelings and actions. Change in behavior is expected by developing insight.

The working phase enables the nurse and patient to achieve the maximum goals which are set for this phase. The end result leads the patient to verbalize, socialize and identify and face his problems realistically. This is the phase leads to the termination of the nurse-patient relationship.

Barriers of Working Phase

- Testing of nurse
- Slow progress of the patient
- Difficulty in collecting data
- Difficulty in interpreting the data
- Fear of closeness.

Strategies to Overcome Barriers

The nurse can overcome all these barriers by learning the subject in depth, and by talking to supervisor and experts. Discussion with peer group is also helpful.

Termination Phase

Definition

Termination is also called a resolution phase or end phase. The termination phase begins during the orientation phase. The main objective is to bring a therapeutic end to the nurse-Patient relationship.

— *Bimla Kapoor, (2007)*

When to terminate nurse-client relationship?

(Reason for termination)

- The patient may be discharged without the knowledge of the nurse.
- The patient goes on parole and does not come back to hospital.
- The patient experiences relief from the presenting problem.
- The patient's functioning has improved.
- The patient has redeveloped self-esteem and strong sense of identity.
- The patient uses more adaptive coping responses.
- The patient has achieved the planned treatment outcomes.

Problems and barriers of termination

Termination phase is a phase of separation and may associate with a sense of disappointment and feeling of sadness. There are number of problems which a nurse, specially a student nurse may face such as:

- The patient may ask the nurse to wait for him or come back from duty and see him.
- The patient may ask for the address or telephone number of the nurse.
- The patient should be explained that every relationship terminates.
- Gift giving is another problem faced by student nurse. The patient likes to give a gift to the nurse, who had been caring him.
- The nurse may withdraw earlier from the patient due to her own anxiety.

The nurse needs to explore feelings and thoughts about separation from the patient which will help the nurse to accomplish the tasks of the termination phase.

THERAPEUTIC IMPASSES

Therapeutic impasses are blocks in the progress of nurse-patient relationship. They arise for variety of reasons, but all creates stall in the process of nurse-patient relationship. Impasses provokes variety of emotions in both the patient and nurse ranging from anxiety and apprehension to frustration, love, or intense anger.

Therapeutic impasses are:

- Resistance
- Transference
- Counter transference
- Gift giving
- Boundary violations.

Resistance

Resistance is the patient's reluctance or avoidance of verbalizing or experiencing troubling aspects of oneself. The term resistance was initially introduced by Freud to mean the patient's unconscious opposition to exploring or recognizing unconscious or even preconscious material. Resistance is often caused by the patient's unwillingness to change when the need for change is recognized. Patients usually display resistance behaviors during the working phase of relationship, because the greater part of the problems-solving process occurs during this phase.

Resistance also may be a reaction by the patient to the nurse who has moved too rapidly or deeply into the patient's feelings or who has intentionally or unintentionally communicated a lack of respect.

Secondary gain may be another cause of resistance. Secondary gain is a benefit that a patient experiences as result of his or her illness. For example, the development of the illness may result in the patient experiencing favorable environmental, interpersonal, monetary, or situational changes. Specific type of secondary gain include financial compensation, avoiding unpleasant situations, increased sympathy or attention, escape from work or other responsibilities, attempted control of people, and lessening of social pressures. Secondary gain can become a powerful force in perpetuating an illness because it makes the environment more comfortable and change less desirable.

Resistance may Take Many Forms

Wolberg identified forms of resistance displayed by patients. *They are:*

- Suppression and repression of pertinent information
- Intensification of symptoms
- Self-devaluation and a hopeless outlook on the future
- Forced flight in to health where there is a sudden, but short-lived recovery by the patients
- Intellectual inhibitions: Forgetful, late for sessions, silent or sleepy, breaks appointments.
- Acting out or irrational behavior
- Superficial talk.
- Transference reactions.

Transference

Transference is an unconscious response in which the patients experiences feelings and attitudes toward the nurse that were originally associated with other significant figures in his or her life. They may be triggered by a superficial similarity, such as facial feature or manner of speech, or by a personality style trait. These reactions are the patient's attempt to reduce anxiety.

Transference reduces self-awareness by allowing the patient to maintain an inaccurate view of the world in which all people are seen in similar terms. Thus, the nurse may be viewed as an authority figure from the past, such as a parent figure, or as a lost loved person, such as a former spouse. Transference reactions are harmful to the therapeutic process only if they remain ignored and unexamined.

Two types of transference are particularly problematic in the nurse- patient relationship. They are hostile transference and dependent reaction transference.

Hostile Transference

If the patient internalizes anger and hostility; this resistance may be expressed as depression and discouragement. The patient may ask to terminate the relationship on the grounds that there is no chance of getting well. If the hostility is externalized, the patient may become critical, defiant, and irritable and may express doubts about the nurse's training, experience, or competence. The patient may attempt to compete with the nurse by reading books on psychology and debating intellectual issues rather than working on real life problems.

Hostility also may be expressed by the patient as detachment, forgetfulness. An extreme form of an uncooperativeness and negativism is evident in prolonged silence. The nurse's talk is to understand the meaning of the patient's silence and how to deal with it despite feelings somewhat awkward and uncertain.

Dependent Reaction Transference

This resistance is characterized by patients who are submissive, subordinate, who regard the nurse as a 'godlike' figure. The patient overvalues the nurse's characteristics and qualities' and their relationship become jeopardized because the patient views it as magical. In this reaction, the nurse must live up to the patient's overwhelming expectations, which is impossible because these expectations are completely unrealistic. The patient continues to demand more of the nurse, and when these needs are not met, the patient is filled with hostility and contempt.

Interventions for Resistance and Transference

- The nurse must be prepared for being exposed to powerful negative and positive emotional feelings coming from the patient- feelings that often have an irrational basis. The relationship can become stalled and non-beneficial if the nurse is not prepared to deal with the patient's feelings.
- Make therapeutic contracts, develop a mutually acceptable goals or plans of action, defining the goals, purpose and roles of the nurse and patient in relation.
- Sometimes resistance occurs because the nurse and patient have not arrived at mutually acceptable goals or plans of action. This may occur if the contract was not clearly defined in the orientation stage of the relationship. The appropriate action then is to return to clarifying the goals, purposes and roles of the nurse and patient in the relationship.

Counter Transference

Counter transference is a thera-peutic impasse created by the nurse. It refers to the specific emotional response generated by the qualities of the patient. This response is inappropriate to the content and context of therapeutic relationship and inappropriate in the degree of intensity of emotion. Counter transference is the transference applied to the nurse. **Inappropriateness is the important element of this impasse,** just as it is with transference. For example: The nurse will feel warmth toward or liking for some patients more than others and the nurse will be genuinely angry at times in regard to the actions of certain patients. But in the case of counter transference, the nurse's responses are justified by reality. In this case, the nurse identifies the patient with individuals from his or her past, and the personal needs will interfere with therapeutic effectiveness.

Types of Counter Transference

Counter transference reactions are usually of the following three types:

1. Reactions of intense love or caring.
2. Reactions of intense hostility or hatred.
3. Reactions of intense anxiety often in response to resistance by patient.

Through the use of immediacy, the nurse can identify counter transference in of its various forms.

Forms of Counter Transference Displayed by Nurses

- Difficulty empathizing with the patient in certain problem areas.
- Feelings of depression during or after the session.
- Carelessness about implementing the contract by being late, running overtime, etc.
- Drowsiness during sessions.
- Feeling of anger or impatience because of the patient's unwillingness to change.
- Encouragement of the patient's dependency, praise or affection.
- Arguments with the patient or a tendency to push the patient before he is ready.
- Attempts to help the patient in matters not related to the identified nursing goals.
- Personal or social involvement with the patient.
- Dreams about or preoccupation with the patient.
- Sexual or aggressive fantasies toward the patient.
- Recurrent anxiety, unease or guilt related to the patient.
- Tendency to focus on only one aspect or way of looking at the information presented by the patient.
- Need to defend nursing interventions used with the patient to others.

Interventions to Overcome from Counter Transference

- Constantly lookout for counter transference.
- Utilize counter transference for promoting therapeutic goals.
- Apply self-examination throughout the course of relationship, particularly when the patient attacks or criticizes. Asking oneself the following questions may be helpful:
    - How do I feel about the patient?
    - Do I look forward to seeing the patient?
    - Do I feel sorry for or sympathetic toward the patient?
    - Am I bored with the patient and believe that we are not progressing?
    - Am I afraid of the patient?
    - Do I get extreme pleasure out of seeing the patient?
    - Do I want to protect, reject or punish the patient?
    - Do I dread meeting with the patient and feel nervous during the sessions?
    - Am I impressed by or try to impress the patient?
    - Does the patient make me very angry or frustrated?
- Pursue to find out the source of the problem.
- Exercise control over counter transference.
- Have individual or group supervision.
- Weekly clinical seminars, peer consultation, and professional meetings can also offer emotional support.

Gift Giving

Receiving a gift from the patients make the nurse to inhibit independent decision-making, create a feeling of anxiety or guilt. Gift is that of something of value is voluntarily offered to another person, usually to convey a gratitude.

Gifts can be divided into following five types (Morse, 1991).

1. Gifts to reciprocate for care given.
2. Gifts intended to manipulate or change the quality of care given or the nature of nurse-patient relationship.
3. Gifts given as perceived obligation by the patient.
4. Gifts received by chance.
5. Gifts given to organization to recognize excellence of care received.

Gifts can be in the following form:

Tangible or intangible: Tangible gifts may include box of sweets, a bouquet of flowers or hand painted picture. Intangible gifts can be expression of thanks to a nurse by a patient who is about to be discharged or a family members gratitude at being able to share an emotional burden with another caring person.

Gift giving is a controversial issue in nursing. The taboo against nurse accepting gifts from patients has been long accepted. However, some have questioned the theoretical rationale for this position and suggest that gift giving can sometimes serve discrete therapeutic goals. Whether gift giving is an impasse depends upon the timing of the particular situation, the intent of the giver, and the contextual meaning of the giving of the gift. Occasionally, it may be most appropriate and therapeutic for the nurse to accept a patient's gift; on other occasions it may be quite inappropriate and detrimental to the relationship. In the orientation phase of the relationship, gift giving can be harmful if it meets personal needs rather than therapeutic goals. By giving a gift, the patient may be trying to manipulate the nurse and control the relationship.

In the working phase, gift giving may take on a different significance. For example, the patient offering a cup of coffee can be a sign of respect for the nurse and in their work together. As an isolated incident, the nurse's acceptance of it can enhance the patient's confidence, self-esteem, and a sense of responsibility.

Gift giving most often arises in the termination phase of relationship, and in this phase that the meaning behind it can be the most complex and difficult to determine. At this time, gifts can reflect a patient's need to make the nurse feel guilty, delay the termination process, compensate for feelings of inadequacy or an attempt to transform the therapeutic nurse-patient relationship into social relationship. If feelings are identified and clarified, then a small gift that reflects gratitude and remembrance can be exchanged, accepted and valued.

Boundary Violations

A boundary indicates a border or a limit. It determines the extent of acceptable limits. Many types of boundaries exist. Boundary violations occur when a nurse goes outside the boundaries of the therapeutic relationship and establishes a social, economic or personal relationship with the patient. As a general rule, whenever the nurse is doing or thinking of doing something special, different or unusual for a patient, a boundary violation is involved. A nurse should consider the possibility of a boundary violation if he or she encounters the following:

- Receives feedback that his or her behavior is intrusive with patient or their families.
- Has difficulty in setting limit with a patient.
- Relates to a patient like friend or family member.
- Has a sexual feeling toward a patient.
- Feels that he or she is the only one who understands the patient.
- Receives feedback that he or she is too involved with a patient or family.
- Feels that other staffs are too critical of a particular patient.
- Believes that other staff members are jealous of his or her relationship with a patient.

Possible Boundary Violations Related to Psychiatric Nurses

- The patient takes the nurse out for a lunch or dinner.
- The professional relationship turns to a social relationship.
- The nurse attends a party at a patient's invitation.
- The nurse regularly reveals personal information to the patient.
- The patient introduces the nurse to family members, such as a son or daughter, for the purpose of a social relationship.
- The nurse accepts free gifts from the patient's business.
- The nurse agrees to meet the patient for treatment outside of the usual setting without therapeutic justification.
- The nurse attends social functions that include the patient.
- The patient gives the nurse an expensive gift.
- The nurse routinely hugs or has physical contact with the patient.
- The nurse does business with or purchase services from the patient.

The nurse must carefully consider how to respond to each of these categories based on the possibility of boundary violations. Clinical supervision can be helpful in anticipating and heading off possible boundary violations (Walker and Clark, 1999).

PROCESS RECORDING

Definition

Process recording is a written account or verbatim recording of all that transpired, during and immediately following the nurse-patient interaction.

In other words, it is the recording of the conversation during the interaction or the interview between the nurse and the patient in the psychiatric setup.

Purposes

- Assist the nurse or student to plan, structure and evaluate the interaction in a conscious rather than an intuitive level.

- Assists her to gain competency in interpreting and synthesizing raw data under supervision.
- Helps to consciously apply theory to practice.
- Helps her to develop an increased awareness of her habitual, verbal and nonverbal communication pattern and the effect of those patterns on others.
- Helps the nurse to learn to identify thoughts and feelings in relation to self and others.
- Helps to increase observational skills, as there is a conscious process involved in thinking, sorting and classifying the interaction under the various headings.
- Helps to increase the ability to identify problems and gain skills in solving them.

Pre-requisites for Process Recording

- Physical setting
- Getting consent of the patient for the possibility of cassette recording
- Confidentiality.

Suggested Outlines for Process Recording

Introductory Material

This should include a short description of the patient, his name, age, educational level, health problems and length of stay in the hospital. The date, time, place of interaction and a short description of the milieu of the ward immediately prior to the interaction will be helpful in understanding the thoughts and feelings of the patient. It is also helpful to record the thoughts and feelings of the nurse just before the interaction.

Objectives

They can be different on different days of the interview. For example, in the beginning, setting short-term may be more appropriate. In the second stage (working phase), the objectives can be more long-term in nature, focusing on corrective psychodynamics, including rehabilitation, follow-up and preparing the family for future plans.

Record of Interaction Between Nurse and the Patient

This should include truthful recording of what the nurse said and did and what the patient said and did, including any nonverbal behavior of the patient, such as changing the position, looking at various things, eye contact, biting the nails, pacing, etc.

What the nurse did also means all her non-verbal behavior. The nurse's thoughts and feelings also should be recorded so that a self-evaluation can be made as to how these influence her behavior.

Analysis of the Interaction

An analysis of the interaction should include the interpretation of the verbal and non-verbal behavior and patient's thoughts and feelings as evident from the process. The nurse's thoughts and feelings at the end of the interaction and the plans made for further interactions should be stated.

PROCESS OF RECORDING FORMAT

I. Identification data

1. Name :
2. Diagnosis :
3. Language :
4. Venue :
5. Time :
6. Duration :

II. Brief history of present illness:

III. Objectives:

1. According patient view :
2. According to student nurse :

Person	Verbatim	Nonverbal communication	Inference

Nature of termination: Signature: ....

Evaluation by the student: Date: ....

List of Inferences; Problems identified: ....

5 Treatment Modalities and Therapies in Mental Disorders

The treatment of psychiatric disorders in past had often constituted of merely the admission in an asylum or mental hospital. With the emergence of newer techniques the treatment of psychiatric disorders were made easy now. Some of the treatment modalities are discussed in this chapter.

The treatments of mental disorders can be classified as following:

- **Physical/Somatic therapies:**
  - Electroconvulsive therapy
  - Psychopharmacology
  - Psychosurgery
- **Psychosocial therapies:**
  - Psychotherapy
  - Behavior therapy
  - Other psychosocial therapy
- **Occupational therapy.**

PHYSICAL THERAPIES

Electroconvulsive Therapy (ECT)

Brief History

- 1933—Manfred Sakel developed insulin coma therapy—treated opioid dependent patients first, later schizophrenia.
- Sakel later claimed to have invented convulsive therapy, but this is disputed.
- 1934—Ladislas Meduna induced seizures using *camphor* in oil initially and later, IV Metrazol. Treatment was based upon a theory of opposition between epilepsy and schizophrenia.
- 1938—***Ugo Cerletti*** and ***Lucio Bini*** induce seizures in Rome using electrical stimuli. They called it as EST (Electroshock therapy).
- 1940—Renato Almansi and David Impasto administer ECT at Columbus Hospital in New York City. Lothar Kalinowsky starts giving ECT at Psychiatric Institute.
- 1940—AE Bennett uses curare for muscle relaxation with Metrazol convulsive therapy.
- 1952—Holmberg uses succinylcholine as a muscle relaxant with ECT.

Box 5.1: Misconceptions of electroconvulsive therapy (ECT)

- Dangerous procedure.
- Causes serious brain damages.
- Involves a high voltage (110–220 V) current. Some traditional healers tried 110 V current with some patients assuming that it is the same procedure used by psychiatrist (ECT), leading to serious complications.

Definition

Electroconvulsive therapy is the artificial induction of a grandmal seizure through the application of electrical current to the brain.

Mechanism of ECT

- The exact mechanism of action is not known.
- There are several possible explanations as to how ECT works. The one that seems to be most accepted however is the neurotransmitter theory.
- ECT possibly affects the catecholamine pathways in between diencephalon and limbic system, also involving the hypothalamus.

Types/Methods/Techniques of ECT

There are two methods used to administer ECT, they are:

1. **Direct ECT:** ECT is given in the absence of anesthesia and muscular relaxation. This not commonly using now.
2. **Modified ECT:** Modified ECT—ECT is modified by drug induced muscular relaxation and general anesthesia.

Electrode Placement

- **Bilateral (BL):** Most commonly used, most effective. Each electrode is placed 2.5–4.0 cm (1–1 ½ inch) above the midpoint, on a line joining the tragus of the ear and the lateral canthus of the eye.
- **Right unilateral (RUL):** Electrodes are placed only on one side of head, usually right side. Less cognitive effect and may be less clinically effective.
- **Bifrontal (BF):** Electrodes are placed on the frontal region of head (forehead) may be as effective as BL with less cognitive effect.

Amount of Current

The passage of an electrical stimulus of 70–120 volts for 0.7–1.5 seconds to produce grandmal seizure.

Frequency of ECT

Usually 6–10 treatments are sufficient, although up to 15 treatments can be given if needed. 20–25 ECT's may be required for chronic cases. The treatments should be spaced, so that no more than 3 ECTs are given per week.

ECT does not prevent the relapse of symptoms, so maintenance treatment should be done with drugs and therapies.

Indications

- Major depression with suicidal risk, with stupor
- Melancholia with psychotic features
- Severe catatonia
- Severe psychosis
- Organic psychosis
- Bipolar disorders
- Uncooperative patient with excitement
- Poor drug compliance in major depression.

Contraindications

- **Absolute:**
  - Raised ICP
- **Relative:**
  - Cerebral aneurism
  - Cerebral hemorrhage
  - Brain tumor
  - Acute myocardial infarction
  - Congestive heart failure
  - Pneumonia
  - Retinal detachment.

Side effects

- **Common:** Transient confusion, headache, nausea, myalgia, retrograde and anterograde amnesia.
- **Uncommon***:* Cardiac arrest, unstable arrhythmias, ischemia, severe hypertension or hypotension, stroke, prolonged apnea, aspiration, laryngospasm, prolonged seizures (status), fractures, malignant hyperthermia.
- **Death:** 1:80,000 treatments (1:10,000 patients). ECT does not cause any brain damage.

ECT team

ECT team comprises the following members:

- Psychiatrist
- ECT technician
- Anesthesiologist
- Trained nurses
- Nursing aids.

Treatment Facilities

There should be a suite of three rooms consists of the following:

- Pre ECT room
- ECT room
- Post ECT room

Pre ECT Room

It is a pleasant and comfortable waiting room.

ECT Room

It is the room where ECT is given. It should be equipped with ECT machine, anesthetic machine, suction apparatus, face masks, oxygen cylinders, tongue depressors, mouth gags, resuscitation apparatus, emergency drugs and defibrillator.

Post ECT Room

A wel-equipped recovery room.

Role of Nurse in ECT

Role of nurse before ECT

- Detailed medical and psychiatric history.
- Get an informed consent.
- Give adequate explanations to patient and family members.
- Assess baseline vital signs.
- ECT is usually given in the morning after overnight fast (patient should be in NPO for 4–6 hours prior ECT).
- Withhold night doses of drugs.
- Withhold oral medications.
- Remove jewelers, prosthesis, dentures, contact lens, tight clothing, etc.
- Empty bladder and bowel before the treatment, as incontinence can occur during the induced seizure.
- Administer 0.6 mg atropine IM or SC 30 minutes before ECT or IV just before ECT. This is to decrease the oral secretions and to prevent vagal stimulation which can cause cardiac arrest.

Role of nurse during ECT

- Shift the patient from pre ECT to ECT room.
- Patient is placed supine position on a hard bed which is well insulated.
- Assist in administering the anesthetic agent (thiopentone sodium 2–5 g/kg body weight) and muscle relaxant (1 mg/kg body weight succinylcholine).
- Maintain airway of the patient.
- Mouth gag should be placed between teeth.
- The place of electrode placement should be cleaned with normal saline or 25% bicarbonate solution or a conducting gel is applied.
- Monitor voltage, intensity and duration of electrical stimulus given
- Monitor seizure activity.
- 100% oxygen should be provided.
- Monitor vitals, ECG, oxygen saturation during seizure activity.
- Record the findings.

Role of nurse after ECT

- Monitor vital signs.
- Continue oxygen till spontaneous respiration starts.
- The patient should be observed for a period of 30 min or more in the recovery room till he is wide awake and responds to call.
- Take safety precautions to prevent injury.
- Turn the patient to one side to drain the secretions.
- Reorient and reassure the client.
- Give clear fluid as the client tolerate and give breakfast.
- Encourage normal daily activities.
- Document any findings as relevant in the patient's record.

Monitoring Seizure Activity

The therapeutic adequacy of the treatment is noted by the occurrence of the tonic-clonic seizure lasting for not less than 25–30 seconds. This can be ensured by the following:

- Observing the seizure in direct ECT.
- EEG recording in modified ECT.
- Occluding the circulation of one extremity with a BP cuff, before giving succinylcholine. Thus, the whole body is paralyzed but one extremity convulses and can be directly observed.
- Observing plantar extension and eyelid contractions which may be seen despite the muscular relaxation. It is not a reliable method.

PSYCHOPHARMACOLOGY

Before the advent of modern psychotropic drugs, the mentally ill were treated with psychoanalysis, insulin or electroshock, psychosurgery, etc. All of these had some limitations.

The role of drugs in treating mental illness was minimal until the 1950's. However, when the development of two drugs reserpine and chlorpromazine revolutionized the use of chemotherapy in mental illness. Since, then the development of psychoactive drugs has been rapid; today there are numerous compounds classified as psychoactive agents. As a result of this wide range of drugs to choose from fewer adverse reactions and rapid effect, chemotherapy is often the first treatment of choice for the mentally disturbed client.

Box 5.2: Psychotropic drugs

Medication that affects psychic function, behavior, or experience.

Classification

Psychotropic drugs can be broadly classified as follows:

- Antipsychotics
- Antidepressants
- Mood stabilizers
- Anxiolytics and hypnosedatives

- Anticonvulsants
- Antiparkinsonian agents
- Miscellaneous.

Antipsychotic Drugs

Antipsychotics agents are also known as neuroleptics/major tranquilizers/D-2 receptor antagonists/antischizophrenic/ataractics. This group of drugs has a major clinical use in the treatment of psychosis. Psychosis is a state in which person's ability to recognize reality to communicate and to relate to others in securely impaired.

Types

- **Typical antipsychotics**
  - **Phenothiazines**
    e.g. Chlorpromazine, fluphenazine, triflupromazine, thioridazine
  - **Butyrophenones**
    e.g. Haloperidol, droperidol
  - **Thioxanthenes**
    e.g. Chlorprothixen, thiothixene
- **Atypical antipsychotics**
  - Risperidone
  - Clozapine
  - Olanzapine.

Mechanism of Action

The exact mechanism of action is not known. Antipsychotic agents are thought to block the dopamine receptor, dopamine is a chemical which is released in the brain and cause psychotic thinking.

Increased production of dopamine transmits in the nerve impulses to the brain stem faster and normal. This results strange thoughts, hallucination and bizarre behavior. Antipsychotic drugs help in blocking or reducing the activity of dopamine.

Pharmacokinetics

- Antipsychotics when administered orally are absorbed variably from the intestinal tract. They are highly bound to plasma as well as tissue proteins. Brain concentration is higher than plasma concentration.
- They are metabolized in the liver and excreted mainly through the kidneys.
- Most of the antipsychotics tend to have a therapeutic window. If the blood cell below this window the drug is ineffective. If the blood cell is higher than the upper limit of the window, there is toxicity or the drug is again ineffective.

Indications

Indications of antipsychotics are as follows:

Organic psychiatric disorders:

- Delirium
- Dementia
- Delirium tremens
- Drug induced psychosis
- Other organic mental disorders.

Nonorganic psychiatric disorders:

- Schizophrenia
- Schizoaffective disorder
- Acute psychosis
- Mania
- Major depression

Childhood psychiatric disorders:

- Attention deficit disorder with hyperactivity
- Infantile autism
- Conduct disorders.

Neurotic and other psychiatric disorders:

- Severe intractable and disabling anxiety
- Treatment refractory obsessive compulsive disorder
- Anorexia nervosa.

Medical disorders:

- Huntington's chorea
- Intractable hiccups
- Nausea and vomiting
- Tic disorders
- Impaired hepatic functions.

Contraindications

- Children under 3 years of age
- Comatose patients
- Hypersensitivity
- Angle-closure glaucoma
- Bone marrow depression
- History of epilepsy
- Pregnancy
- Parkinson's disease
- Peptic ulcer
- Circulatory collapse

Side Effects

Side effects of antipsychotics drugs with its nursing managements are summarized in the Box 5.3:

Box 5.3: Side effects of antipsychotics

Side effects	Probable cause	Management
A. Autonomic side effects		
Dry mouth	Muscarinic cholinergic blockade	Usually none; Provide the client with sugarless candy or gum, ice, and frequent sips of water. Ensure that client practices strict oral hygiene. Occasionally, pilocarpine 2%
Constipation	*– do –*	Fiber rich diet; encourage increase in physical activity and fluid intake. Bulk laxatives.
Cycloplegia	*– do –*	Usually none; occasionally pilocarpine 2%.
Mydriasis	*– do –*	Usually none; occasionally pilocarpine 2%.
Urinary retention	*– do –*	Instruct the client to report any difficulty in urinating; monitor intake and output.
Delirium	*– do –*	Physostigmine; diazepam sometimes supportive care.
Orthostatic hypotension	α_1 Adrenergic blockade	Instruct the client to rise slowly from a lying or sitting position. Monitor blood pressure (lying and standing) each shift.
Impotence	*– do –*	
Impaired ejaculation	*– do –*	Decrease dose. If severe, change medication.
B. Extra pyramidal side effects (EPSE)		
Pseudoparkinsonism (tremor, shuffling gait, drooling, rigidity). Seen 1–5 days following initiation of therapy.	Dopaminergic (D2) receptor blockade in striatal areas	Antiparkinsonian medication for treatment; also for prevention if needed.
Akathisia (Motor restlessness) occur 50–60 days following initiation of therapy.	*– do –*	Change of medication or reduction; Beta-blockers such as propranolol; Benzodiazepines.
Acute dystonia (involuntary muscular movements of face, arms, legs, and neck) This occurs most often in men and in people younger than 25 years of age.	*– do –*	Antiparkinsonian medication.
Rabbit syndrome perioral tremor develops after months or years of treatment	*– do –*	Antiparkinsonian medication.

Contd...

Contd...

Side effects	Probable cause	Management
Tardive dyskinesia (Bizarre facial and tongue movements, stiff neck, and difficulty swallowing) long term use and are potentially irreversible	*– do –*	Prevention crucial; treatment unsatisfactory
Neuroleptic Malignant Syndrome: (Include severe parkinsonian muscle rigidity, hyperpyrexia up to 107°F, tachycardia, tachypnea, fluctuations in blood pressure, diaphoresis, and rapid deterioration of mental status to stupor and coma. This is a rare, but potentially fatal	Not known	Stop the medication; Bromocriptine, dantrolene, Baclofen, general supportive care. Occasionally ECT.
C. Other CNS side effects		
Sedation	Histaminergic blockade	This side effect may be beneficial. Otherwise decrease dose. Change drug. Give single dose only at night.
Seizures	Decreased seizure threshold	Decrease dose. Change to a safer antipsychotic.
D. Metabolic side effects		
Weight gain	H_1 Blockade	Change drug. Dietary control. Exercises.
Diabetes	Unknown	Change drug. Dietary control.
Galactorrhea	Increased prolactin secretion	Change drug.
E. Hypersensitivity reactions		
Cholestatic jaundice	Hypersensitivity reaction	Change drug. Supportive care.
Agranulocytosis	Hypersensitivity reaction	Stop drug immediately. Treat infection. General supportive care. Filgrastim may be useful.
F. others		
ECG changes	Anticholinergic effect	Change drug if severe.
Ocular side effects	Not known (probably photosensitivity	Change drug.
Contact dermatitis	Allergic reactions	Avoid handling. Report to physician, Symptomatic treatment.

Treatment Adherence

Many patients with schizophrenia can be uncooperative, with a poor treatment adherence. Therefore, it may be difficult to ensure adequate administration of antipsychotics on an outpatient basis. Since, discontinuation of antipsychotic medication often leads to relapse, long-acting preparations are valuable in the treatment. They may be given in a depot form, either intramuscularly or administered orally.

Box 5.4: Dosage of selected antipsychotics

Class	Examples	Trade name	Oral mg/day	Parenteral (mg)
Phenothiazines	Chlorpromazine	• Megatil • Largactil	300–1500	50–100 IM
	Triflupromazine	• Siquil • Thioril	100–400	30–60 IM
Thioxanthenes	Flupentixol	• Procinate	3–18	–
Butyrophenones	Haloperidol	• Senorm • Serenace	5–30	5–20 IM
Atypical	Clozapine	• Lozapin, • Clozaril	50–900	12.5–5 IM, 4–6 Hourly
	Risperidone	• Sizodon, • Zyprexa	2–8	2–5 IM

Nurse's Responsibility

- Close observation especially when the antipsychotics are just started. Look for the possible side effects.
- Extrapyramidal reaction. These symptoms are reduced or treated with careful observation.
- Observe for drowsiness, medicine should be administered at bed time report if the drowsiness, persists for a very long time.
- Educate the patient not to use hazardous machinery
- Record the medicine and side effect accurately.
- Observe the patient regularly for abnormal movements.
- Take all seizure precautious.
- Advise the patient to use sunscreen measures for photo sensitive reactions.
- Advice the patient to get up from the bed or chair very slowly.
- Advice to take fiber rich diet and fluid management.

Antidepressant Drugs

Antidepressants/mood elevators/thymoleptics are the drugs, which are used for the treatment of depressive illness. It is used to correct neurochemical imbalances that affect mood.

Isoniazid (INH) was found to have mood elevating properties in some patients suffering from tuberculosis in 1951. Iproniazid, a MAO inhibitor and a derivative of INH, was later

(1958) introduced for the treatment of depression. The first tricyclic antidepressant (TCA) *imipramine* was used in 1958 by Thomas Kuhn.

Types, Dosage and Mechanism of Action

Types and mechanism of action of antidepressants are given in the Box 5.5 below.

Pharmacokinetics

Antidepressants are highly lipophilic and protein bound. The half-life is long and usually more than 24 hours. It is predominantly metabolized in liver.

Indications

The indications of antidepressants include:

- Depression:
  - Depressive episode
  - Dysthymia
  - Reactive depression
  - Secondary depression
  - Abnormal grief reaction
- Childhood psychiatric disorders:
  - Enuresis
  - Separation anxiety disorder
  - Somnolence
  - School phobia
  - Night terrors
- Other psychiatric disorders:
  - Agoraphobia and social phobia
  - Panic attack
  - Obsessive compulsive disorder with or without depression
- Medical disorders:
  - Chronic pain (in low dose)
  - Migraine (as an adjuvant).

Box 5.5: Types and mechanism of action of antidepressants

Class	Example	Oral dosage (mg/day)	Mechanism of action
Tricyclic antidepressants (TCA)	• Imipramine	75–300	Blocks the reuptake of Nor epinephrine (NE) and 5-HT (serotonin) at the nerve terminals
	• Amitriptyline	75–300	
	• Clomipramine	75–250	
	• Desipramine	75–300	
Monoamine oxidase inhibitors (MAOI)	• Isocarboxazid	10–60	Increases the amount of NE to release catecholamine and larger amount of NE to react with receptor

Contd...

Contd...

Class	Example	Oral Dosage (mg/day)	Mechanism of action
Selective serotonin reuptake inhibitors (SSRI)	• Fluoxetine	20–60	Block the reuptake of 5-HT into presynaptic nerve from which it originally released
	• Sertraline	50–200	
	• Citalopram	20–40	
Atypical antidepressants	• Amineptine	100–400	Block the transporter site for NE and 5-HT
	• Mianseril	25–50	

Side Effects

Side effect of antidepressant drugs includes the following:

- Autonomic side effects:
  - Dry mouth
  - Constipation
  - Mydriasis
  - Urinary retention
  - Orthostatic hypotension
  - Impotence
  - Impaired ejaculation
  - Delirium
- CNS effects:
  - Sedation
  - Tremor
  - Withdrawal symptoms
  - Seizures
- Cardiovascular system:
  - Tachycardia
  - ECG changes
  - Arrhythmias
  - Direct myocardial depression
  - Decreased conduction time
- Allergic reactions:
  - Agranulocytosis
  - Cholestatic jaundice
  - Skin rashes
  - Systemic vasculitis
- Others:
  - Hypertensive crisis
  - Hepatic necrosis
  - Hyperpyrexia
  - Weight gain.

Nurses Responsibility

- Observation, monitoring and recording of side effects to prevent complications.
- Give plenty of fluid to reduce dryness of mouth. Lemon or chewing gum can be also given to prevent dryness of mouth.
- Give antidepressants drugs after giving something to reduce nausea and vomiting and irritation to the mucosa.
- Maintain I/O chart to check whether there is retention of urine.
- Encourage the patient to get up from bed or chair slowly. Dizziness can be reduced which may result due to orthostatic hypotension while getting up.
- Maintain record of vital signs that is BP and pulse.
- Record and report the side effects.
- Explain to the patient that the effect of drugs will be seen within four to eight weeks. Hence, patient must continue taking drugs.

Ensure that the psychiatrist is informed and drugs are stopped immediately if patient complains of pressure of speech, increased motor activity, elated mood or sexual dysfunction.

ANTIMANIC DRUGS

These drugs are usually effective in treatment of mania and therefore the word *antimanic* is often used to them. But as they are effective in preventing mood swings in bipolar disorder, the better term is *mood-stabilizing agent* or a *prophylactic agent*. Antimanic drug reduces the effect of norepinephrine and serotonin which effects on emotions:

Currently accepted mood stabilizers fall into three families: (1) lithium, (2) a subset of antiepileptic drugs (anticonvulsants), and (3) all of the second-generation or atypical antipsychotics. Common drugs used in the treatment of manic episode include:

- Lithium
- Anticonvulsants
  - Carbamazepine
  - Sodium valproate
- Antipsychotics
  - Risperidone
  - Olanzapine

Lithium

Lithium is an element with atomic number 3 and atomic weight 7. It was discovered by *Arfeudson* in 1817. It has been used for the treatment of gout. It was rediscovered by *F J Cade* in 1949. Lithium is effective in long-term prophylaxis of both mania and depressive episodes in 70% of BAD patients.

Mechanism of Action

Not fully understood, but may enhance reuptake of norepinephrine and serotonin, decreasing the levels in the body, resulting in decreased hyperactivity (may take 1–3 weeks for symptoms to subside). It affects the Na^+–K^+ ATP-ase and accumulates intracellularly as a substitute of Na^+.

Pharmacokinetics

Lithium is readily absorbed orally. Peak plasma levels occurring 2–4 hours after a single dose. Lithium is protein bound and distributed rapidly in liver, kidney and slowly in muscles, bone and tissues. Elimination is through kidney.

Indications

- Treatment of acute mania
- Prophylaxis of bipolar disorder
- Manic depressive psychosis
- Recurrent mania
- Acute hypomania
- Schizoaffective disorder
- Impulsivity and aggression
- Treatment of cyclothymia

Contraindications

- Pregnancy and lactation
- Cardio vascular disorders
- Renal impairment
- Severe dehydration
- Thyroid disorders
- Hepatic disorders
- Obesity
- Diabetes
- Brain trauma

Side effects

- **Digestive system:** Reduced appetite, nausea, vomiting, diarrhea, metallic taste
- Thyroid abnormalities, goiter, weight gain
- Leukocytosis
- Polyuria/polydipsia secondary to ADH antagonism.
- Hair loss, acne
- **Neurological:** Seizure, cognitive slowing, tremor, muscular weakness, motor hyper activity
- **Teratogenicity**
- **Lithium toxicity**

Box 5.6: Blood lithium levels

- Therapeutic levels = 0.6–1.2 mEq/L (for the treatment of acute mania)
- Prophylactic levels = 0.6–1.0 mEq/L (for relapse prevention in bipolar disorder)
- Toxic lithium levels = > 2.0 mEq/L.

If the lithium level increases than the therapeutic level it produces toxicity. Mild levels, 1.5–2.0 see vomiting, diarrhea, ataxia, dizziness, slurred speech, and nystagmus.

In moderate, 2.0–2.5 nausea, vomiting, anorexia, blurred vision, clonic limb movements, convulsions, delirium, and syncope. Severe, > 2.5 generalized convulsions, oliguria, renal failure, coma.

Management of Lithium Toxicity

- Discontinue the medication and report to the doctor immediately
- Induce emesis, gastric lavage or administer activated charcoal
- Check serum Li^+ levels
- Monitor ECG
- Maintain fluid and electrolyte balance
- If serious manifestations, hemodialysis should be initiated.

Dosage

- Lithium carbonate: 300 mg tablets
- Lithium citrate: 300 mg/5 ml
- The usual dosage per day in acute mania is 900–2100 mg in 2–3 divided dosage.

Nurses responsibility

- Medicine should be given after meal to reduce gastric irritability.
- Record and report side effects.
- Check for serum lithium reports and ensure that it is done regularly.
- Check for edema, maintain weight record.
- Intake/output chart should be maintained to check renal functioning.
- Maintain proper intake of diet.
- See that patient does not miss any dose.

Carbamazepine

It is a tricyclic compound synthesized in 1953 by Schindler. It has a structure similar to TCAs. The onset of action can be faster as compared to lithium, but slower compared to valproate. It is structurally similar to imipramine and a first-line agent for acute mania and mania prophylaxis.

Indicated for rapid cyclers and mixed patients. This drug is absorbed slowly from gut. Peak plasma level reached 2–8 hours. Metabolized in liver and excreted through kidneys

Side Effects

- Rashes
- Nausea, vomiting, diarrhea, anorexia
- Sedation, dizziness, ataxia, confusion
- AV conduction delays
- Aplastic anemia and agranulocytosis
- Water retention due to vasopressin-like effect which can result in hyponatremia
- Drug-drug interactions–neurotoxicity develops if it combines with lithium and antipsychotics.

Dosage

The usual dose is 600–1600 mg/day orally, in divided doses. The treatment is best monitored with repeated blood levels. The therapeutic blood levels are 4–12 μg/ml and the toxic blood levels are usually reached at >15 μg/ml.

Valproate

Valproic acid was first synthesized by *Burton* and used as an organic solvent. In 1963, *Meunier* discovered the antiepileptic properties of valproic acid, while *Lambert* reported in 1966 that valpromide (a valproic acid analogue) might be effective as an antimanic.

Valproate and lithium have been widely used as first line drugs for treatment of mania as well as for prophylaxis of bipolar mood disorder.

Sodium valproate is converted to valproic acid in the stomach and completely absorbed from the GI tract.

Indications

- Acute mania
- Schizoaffective disorder
- Seizures
- Useful in psychotic symptoms in schizophrenia and organic disorders.

Side Effects

- Thrombocytopenia and platelet dysfunction
- Nausea, vomiting, weight gain
- Sedation
- Tremor
- Increased risk of neural tube defect 1–2% vs 0.14–0.2% in general population secondary to reduction in folic acid
- Alopecia
- Jaundice, thrombocytopenia

Dosage

The usual dose of valproate is 1000-3000 mg/day orally in divided doses. The therapeutic blood level is 50–125 mg/ml. Oral loading strategies (20–30 mg/kg/day) are rapidly effective in the management of acute mania.

Drug Interactions

Certain drug may increase (such as aspirin, cimetidine, ibuprofen, erythromycin, fluoxetine, fluvoxamine,phenothiazines) or *decrease* (such as carba mazepine,phenytoin, phenobarbital, ethosuxi mide, rifampicin, mefloquine) the serum levels of valproate.

In addition, valproate *increases* serum levels of other drugs (such as lamotrigine, tricyclic antidepressants, zidovudine, tolbutamide).

Anxiolytics, Hypnotics And Sedatives

Anxiety is a state which occurs in all human beings at sometime. Hypnotics are drugs which produce sleep resembling natural sleep. Sedatives are drugs which reduce excitement without producing sleep.

Anxiolytic Drugs

Anxiolytic drugs, also called anti-anxiety drugs and minor tranquilizers. These drugs are used to relieve anxiety. It also relieves moderate or severe tension.

Hypnosis

It is a state of altered consciousness where the subject is highly suggestible.

Hypnotics

These drugs which cause sleep with little analgesia, e.g. barbiturates.

Sedatives

These drugs cause mild depression with calm and quiet excitement without sleep, e.g. Bromides

Classification

- **Barbiturates:** Phenobarbital, pentobarbital, thiopentone
- **Non-barbiturates:** meprobamate, glutethimide, ethanol, diphenhydramine
- **Benzodiazepines:**
  - **Very short acting:** Triazolam, midazolam
  - **Short acting:** Oxazepam, Lorazepam, alprazolam
  - **Long acting:** Diazepam, clonazepam, flurazepam, nitrazepam.

Mode of Action

These drugs act as central nervous system depressants. It is helps to increase the inhibitory neurotransmitter action of GABA. This GABA mediates both presynaptic and post synaptic inhibition all areas of central nervous system.

Indications

- Generalized anxiety disorder
- Panic disorder and school phobia
- Depression
- Insomnia
- Narcoanalysis
- Psycho somatic disorder
- Bipolar I disorder
- Alcohol withdrawal
- Substance induced and psychotic agitation.

Side Effects

- Nausea, vomiting
- Drowsiness, vertigo, weakness
- Ataxia, Confusion
- Dry mouth
- Retrograde amnesia
- Depression
- Blurring of vision.

Dosage

- Alprazolam: 0.5–6, PO
- Oxazepam: 15–120, PO
- Lorazepam: 2–6, PO/IV/IM
- Diazepam: 2–10, PO/IV/slow IV
- Clonazepam: 0.5–20, PO/IM
- Chlordiazepoxide: 15–100.

Nurses Responsibility

- If the sleep pattern is disturbed provide calm and quiet environment, a cup of hot milk, good back care or reading of magazine will induce sleep.
- Daily dose should be given at bed time to induce sleep.
- I/M injection should be given deep intra-muscular to prevent tissue irritation.
- Observe record and report any side effect.
- If patient feels drowsy, do not allow him/her to do any activity.
- Patient should be checked if she is developing drug dependence.
- Record vital signs and symptoms.

Antiparkinsonian Drugs

Antiparkinsonian drugs are the specific drugs to treat the extra pyramidal side effects of antipsychotic agents.

Anticholinergic drugs block the secretion, thereby reducing the symptoms of akathesia and acute dystonia. It is not effective against tardive dyskinesia.

Antihistamines have effects like anticholinergic drugs. Amantadines are doparnine releasing agents from central neurons. Studies show that this drug may affect some clients with tardive dyskinesia.

Side Effects

The side effects are dry mouth, dry skin, blurred vision, drowsiness, dizziness, anorexia, nausea, vomiting, slurred speech, insomnia, inability to concentrate.

Box 5.7: Common drugs and dosage

Class	Example	Dosage Mg/day
Anticholinergic	Benztropine	0.5–6.0
	Trihexyphenidyl	2–12
Antihistamine	Diphenhydramine	75–100

Contd...

Contd...

Class	Example	Dosage Mg/day
Dopamine Drugs	Levodopa	2–3 g
	Amantadine	100–200

Nurses Responsibility

- Observation
- Maintain an intake output chart
- Encourage adequate intake of fluids and roughage in the diet
- Record vital signs
- Advise the patient not to get up quickly from a lying-down position to sitting.

GERIATRIC CONSIDERATIONS

Due to age related changes in brain; old aged people are more sensitive to the psychotropic drugs. Pharmacokinetics of the drugs also varies with the changes in absorption. For elderly people, high potency neuroleptic in small doses are preferred. Antidepressants are safer to start in small doses and maintain on low doses.

Psychosurgery

Psychosurgery is a surgical intervention, to several fibers connecting one part of brain with another, or to remove, destroy or stimulate brain tissue, with the intent of modifying behavior, thought or mood disturbances, for which there is no underlying organic pathology.

Indications

- Chronic incapacitating depression, which has not responded to all available treatments.
- Chronic, severe, incapacitating obsessive compulsive disorder (OCD), which has not responded to all available treatments.
- Chronic, severe, incapacitating anxiety disorder, which has not responded to all available treatments.
- Schizophrenia with severe depressive component, which has not responded to all available treatments.
- Severe, pathological and uncontrolled aggressive behavior associated with a psychiatric or neurological illness.

Techniques

The currently employed procedures include:

- **Stereotactic Subcaudate Tractotomy:** A large subcaudate lesion is produced. It is recommended for severe depression, severe anxiety, severe OCD and schizoaffective disorder.
- **Stereotactic Limbic Leucotomy:** A small subcaudate lesion is made, in addition to a lesion in cingulate bundle. It is used for treatment of intractable OCD and schizophrenia.
- **Amygdalotomy:** This is used for severe, pathological, uncontrolled and intractable aggression associated with neuropsychiatric disorders.

Side Effects

With the use of stereotactic procedures, side effects are very rare. These include a less than 1% risk of seizures, a very uncommon risk of personality change (which used to be frequent with earlier procedures) and a 1:1,000–1:10,000 mortality risks.

It is an extremely uncommon procedure now a day. Most psychiatrists would have never referred any patient for the procedure.

PSYCHOSOCIAL THERAPIES

It therapy is one of the important treatment modalities used for the patients with mental disorders. It is given along with other therapies or separately.

Psychotherapy

Psychotherapy is defined as a form of treatment of an emotional nature in which trained person purposefully develops a professional relationship with objective of removing, modifying or reducing the presenting symptoms.

Psychotherapy is sometimes used to mean all forms of psychological treatments.

Goals

The goals of psychotherapy are to:

- Establish therapeutic relationship with the patient.
- Change specific maladaptive patterns of behavior.
- Reduce or eliminate environment which may be causing such behavior.
- Help patient to develop sense of self-identity.
- Help patient to improve in his/her interpersonal and communication skill.

General Indications of Psychological Treatments

Based on diagnosis:

- Neurotic illness (acute - chronic)
- Personality disorders
- Psychoactive substance abuse
- Childhood disorders
- Chronic psychosis

Based on presenting features:

- Subjective symptoms, e.g. anxiety, phobia.
- Interpersonal difficulties, e.g. over-dependency, marital discord.

Psychotherapies can be conducted either verbal or non verbal means. There are different types of psychotherapies. The important types include the following.

Psychoanalytical Psychotherapy

Psychoanalysis is considered by many to be the foundation for individual psychotherapy. It was originated by Freud in the early 20th century. In psychoanalysis, a major goal is for the client to gain insight and understanding about current relationships and behavior patterns by confronting unconscious conflicts that surface in the transference relationship with the analyst.

Psychoanalysis is a lengthy and costly type of treatment. Some of the techniques used in psychoanalysis are described in the following:

- Free Association
- Dream Analysis
- Hypnosis
- Catharsis

Free Association

In free association, the patient is allowed to communicate unguided i.e. the patient is allowed to say whatever comes to mind in response to a word that is given by the therapist. The therapist remains passive with a non-directive approach but therapist interprets patient's feelings behavior and relationship with the therapist.

For example, the therapist might say 'mother' and the client would give a response, also typically one word. The therapist then looks for a theme or pattern to the client's 11 responses. If the client responds 'evil' to the word 'mother' the therapist might pick up one potential theme, but if the client responds 'kind' to the word 'mother' therapist might hear a completely different theme. The theme may give the therapist an idea of the cause of the client's emotional disturbance.

Dream Analysis

Freudians believe that behavior is rooted in the unconscious and that dreams are the repressed feelings. Psychoanalysts believe that dreams truly are the mirror to the unconscious. Monitoring and interpreting dreams is an important technique of psychoanalysis.

The client is asked to keep a 'dream log' by writing in a notebook as much as he or she can remember of both pleasant and particularly disturbing dreams. The dreams are then interpreted in much the same way as free association. Significant people or situations in the dreams are explored with the client, and possible meanings are offered by the therapist.

Hypnosis

Hypnotherapy is sometimes used in for 'past life regression.' Hypnosis is very deep relaxation during which the trained therapist asks certain questions of the client. Guided imagery also may be used to help the client envision the situation in an effort to find the cause of the problem.

At the end of the session, while the individual is still in the trance state, the therapist may offer some posthypnotic suggestions. These typically include positive, affirming statements regarding the changes in behavior he or she wants to accomplish.

Catharsis

Catharsis is 'the expression of ideas, thoughts, and suppressed material that is accompanied by an emotional response that produces a state of relief in the patient.' Catharsis is used in psychoanalysis to allow the client to purge the repressed mental contents from the psyche. Maladaptive symptoms may be resolved by bringing unconscious thoughts and feelings into consciousness. Sometimes the individual not only may recall the painful experience, but also actually *relives* it, accompanied by the feelings and emotions associated with the event. This process is called *abreaction*.

Individual Psychotherapy

This method helps the patient by encouraging him to discover the reasons for his behavior. To produce limited but worthwhile changes within a short time seldom more than six months and considerably less. Because treatment is focused upon specific problems, the term focal psychotherapy is sometimes used.

Indications

Neurotic disorders, stress-related disorders, alcohol and drug dependency, sexual disorders and marital disharmony.

Role of Nurse

- Promote positive personality growth and development through the intimate relationship with client.
- Facilitate the expression of thoughts and feelings as a way to use more effective behaviors in dealing with stress.

Supportive Psychotherapy

This is a very directive method of psycho therapy, with the focus clearly on existing symptoms and/or current life situations.

Aims

- Correction of the situational problem.
- Symptom rectification.
- Restoring or strengthening defenses.
- Prevention of emotional breakdown.
- Teaching new coping skills.

Techniques

- ***Ventilation:*** It is a free expression of feelings or emotions. This technique allows the release of bottled up emotions of the client.
- ***Persuasion:*** The therapist urges the patient repeatedly changes his behavior or to try new methods of dealing his problems.
- **Abreaction:** It is a process of exploring the repressed emotions in high degree.
- **Reassurance:** It is a supportive approach that anyone can give.
- **Explanation:** Explanations should be given to remove misconceptions and to provide proper understanding of the problems.
- **Recreation:** It helps to break monotony of the work.

- **Work as a therapy:** Work is an important form of therapy for many types of the emotional problems. When a person engages in work, his/her problems get lessened.
- **Guidance:** Involves offering direct advice on handling particularly difficult situation in real life of the patient. He/she may be advised on how and when should seek the help in future.

Unwanted Effects of Psychotherapy

- Patients may become excessively dependent on therapy or therapist.
- Intensive psychotherapy may be distressing to the patients.
- Ineffective psychotherapy wastes time, money and damages patient's morale.

Behavior Therapy

The first use of the term behavior modification was by *Edward Thorndike* in 1911. Through early research in the 1940's and the 1950's, the term was used by *Joseph Wolpe's* research group.

In 1960, behavior therapy emerged as a system and comprehensive approach to psychiatric disorders.

Definition

'Behavior therapy is a type of psychotherapy through the application of principles of learning to the analysis and treatment of disorders of behavior.'

Assumptions of Behavioral Therapy:

- Faulty learning can result in psychiatric disorders.
- Behavior is modified through the application of principles of learning.
- Maladaptive behavior is considered to be excessive or deficient, thus behavior therapy seeks to promote appropriate behavior and eliminates inappropriate behavior.
- One's social environment is a source of stimuli that support symptoms; therefore, it can also support changes in behavior through appropriate treatment measures.

Indications

- Anxiety disorder
- Mood disorder
- Schizophrenia
- Somatoform disorders
- Eating disorders
- Psychosexual disorders
- Substance use disorders
- Childhood disorders–Enuresis, conduct disorder, autism, habit disorder, etc

Contraindications

- Any disorder with acute symptomatology.
- Pervasive disorders with external influence triggering the symptoms.

Techniques of Behavior Therapy

The various techniques of behavior therapy include:

- Systematic desensitization
- Flooding
- Aversion therapy
- Operant conditioning to increase adaptive behavior
- Operant conditioning to decrease maladaptive behavior.

Systematic Desensitization

Systematic desensitization (SD) is developed by *Joseph Wolpe*. The principle states that if a response incompatible with anxiety is made to occur at the same time as an anxiety provoking stimulus, anxiety is reduced by reciprocal inhibition.

This consists of three main steps:

1. **Relaxation training:** It can be done by progressive muscular relaxation, hypnosis, meditation or Yoga, Mental imagery, biofeedback.
2. **Hierarchy construction:** Here the patient is asked to list all the conditions which provoke anxiety. Then, he is asked to list them in a descending order of anxiety provocation.
3. **Desensitization of the stimulus:** This canbe done either in imagery or in reality/*in vivo.* This is a treatment of choice in phobias and OCD.

Flooding

This is usually the method used in the treatment of phobias. Here, the person is directly exposed to the phobic stimulus, but escape is made impossible. By prolonged contact with the phobic stimulus, therapist's guidance and encouragement, anxiety decreases.

Aversion Therapy

It is the pairing of the pleasant stimulus) with an unpleasant response so that even in absence of unpleasant response (after the therapy is over), the pleasant stimulus becomes unpleasant by association.

The unpleasant aversion can be produced by electric stimulus (low voltage), drugs (such as apomorphine and disulfiram) or even by fantasy (when it is called as *covert sensitization*).

Typically, 20-40 sessions are needed, with each session lasting about one hour. After completion of treatment, booster sessions may be given. It may be indicated for alcohol abuse, Paraphilias, homosexuality.

The current use of aversion therapy has declined sharply in the Western world (and also elsewhere) as it is felt by many that it may violate the human rights of the patient.

Operant conditioning to increase adaptive behavior

These methods include:

- **Positive reinforcement:** Here, the desirable behavior is reinforced by a reward, either material or symbolic.

- **Negative reinforcement:** Here, on performance of the desirable behavior, punishment can be avoided.
- **Modeling:** The person is exposed to 'model' behavior and is induced to copy it. This can also be used to avoid certain behaviors.

Operant conditioning to decrease maladaptive behavior

These methods include:

- **Time-out:** Here, the reinforcement is withdrawn for some time, contingent upon the undesired response. Time-out is often used in therapy with children.
- **Punishment:** Aversive stimulus is here presented, contingent upon undesired response.
- **Satiation:** The undesired response is positively reinforced, so that tiring occurs. A similar technique is *negative practice procedure.*

Other Behavioral Techniques

These include:

- Assertiveness training
- Response prevention
- Token economy
- Thought stopping, etc.

Assertiveness Training

Unassertive persons are usually deficient in expressing their feelings and thought directly to others. Assertiveness training helps unassertive persons to practice appropriate social behavior in everyday life, expressing their honest feelings and thoughts in terms of.

- Verbal (tone of voice, volume and content)
- Non-verbal (posture, eye contact, facial expression).

Token Economy

- Repeated rewards of a desired behavior encourage persons to repeat the behavior.
- It is used with chronic schizophrenic patients to improve their social skills e.g. self-hygiene.
- Also used with children and mentally subnormal people.

Response Prevention

It helps patients with compulsions. Patient is asked to exert efforts to suppress compulsions for enough time (about an hour) until the associated anxiety wanes. Repeated efforts are helpful in diminishing the frequency and intensity of compulsions and associated obsessional thoughts. Patient should be encouraged to overcome the initial rising in anxiety.

Thought Stopping

It is used to treat obsessional thoughts. Obsessional thoughts are interrupted by a noxious stimulus, e.g. an elastic band worn around the wrist (mildly painful). Gradual reduction in the intensity of the thoughts is achieved by repeated interruptions.

Cognitive Behavior Therapy (CBT)

Concept

- Persons' behavior is associated with their own particular cognitive processes (ways of thinking, expectations, attitudes and beliefs).
- Maladaptive cognitive processes are associated with behavioral and emotional problems.
- Correcting maladaptive cognitive processes reduces patient's problems.

Process

Maladaptive thinking is **identified;** the common cognitive errors include:

- Magnification and minimization of events out of proportion to their actual significance, e.g. depressed patient magnifies his faults and minimizes his achievements.
- **Overgeneralization:** Forming a general rule from few instances and applying this rule to all situations no matter how inappropriate.
- **Arbitrary inferences:** Making an inference without backing it up with evidence, or alternatively ignoring conflicting evidences.
- **Arbitrary inferences:** Making an inference without backing it up with evidence, or alternatively ignoring conflicting evidences.
- **Selective abstraction:** Taking a fact out of context while ignoring other significant features and then proceeding to base entire experience on that isolated fact.
- **Dichotomous thinking:** Thinking about events or persons in terms of opposite extremes (all or none).
- **Personalization:** Relating events and incidents to self where such incidents have no personal bearing or significance.

The maladaptive thinking is then **challenged** by correcting misunderstandings with accurate information and pointing out illogical ways of reasoning. Then alternative ways of thinking are sought out and tested.

Cognitive behavioral therapy is mainly indicated in:

- Depressive disorders (mild – moderate)
- Panic disorders.
- Phobic disorders.

Group Therapy

Group therapy (or group psychotherapy) is a less time-consuming procedure, in which usually 8 –10 people can be treated at one time. This was first used by Joseph Pratt (an internist) in 1905, for patients suffering from tuberculosis.

Now, it is known that group therapy is not only time-saving but also especially beneficial for certain group of patients. Group therapy offers patients (and their relatives) an opportunity to realize that many others have and share problems which are very similar to their own problems, and that they are not alone in their suffering.

Selection

- Homogenous group
- Adolescents and patients with personality disorder
- Families and couples where the system needs change.

Contraindications

- Antisocial behavior
- Actively suicidal or severely depressed patients
- Patients who are delusional.

Typically, sessions are held once or twice a week, with each session lasting 1–2 hours (often 1½ hours). The patients usually sit in a circle, with equal opportunities for interaction. Group therapy may utilize psychoanalytic, supportive, transactional or behavioral approaches.

Over the years, many types of group therapies have emerged such as self-help groups (Alcoholics Anonymous for alcoholics, Weight Watchers for obese, Phoenix-House for opiate dependent individuals), Transactional Analysis groups (Eric Berne), Training groups (Kurt Lewin), Psychodrama (Jacob Moreno) and the like.

Marital Therapy

Indications

- Marital discord
- When marital problems act as a maintaining factor of a psychiatric disorder in one or both partners.

The couple and the therapist identify marital problems, such as: Failure to listen to the other partner, failure to express wishes, emotions and thought directly. The couples are then helped to understand each other. The therapist should remain neutral.

Techniques used include:

- Behavioral (reinforcement of positive behavior)
- Dynamic (eliciting and correcting unconscious aspects of interaction)
- Problem solving.

Family Therapy

'A psychotherapeutic approach that focuses on altering interactions between a couple within nuclear family or its members in extended family or between the family and other inter personal systems, with the goal of alleviating problems initially presented by individual family members, family subsystems, the family as a whole or other referral sources'.

Indications

- Relational problems within the family units
- Psychoses
- Schizophrenia.

Components

- Assessment
- Teaching

- Writing behavioral marital contract
- Assignments.

Application of Nursing Process

- **Assessment:** Assessment of family systems, subsystems and individual within the family required.
- **Nursing Diagnosis:** The problems related to relational problems, abuse or neglect or bereavement has to be identified.
- **Nursing Intervention:** Case management, psycho education, appropriate referrals
- **Evaluation:** Nurse Clinician will observe whether the family is able to cooperate in provision of care to meet the client's needs within the family and in society where they are living.

Therapeutic Community

In psychiatry, therapy involving the milieu or the environment may be called milieu therapy, therapeutic community or therapeutic environment. The goal of milieu therapy is to manipulate the environment so that all aspects of the client's hospital experience are considered therapeutic.

The word Milieu is French for 'middle'. The English translation of the word is surroundings or environment.

Definition

A scientific structuring of the environment in order to effect behavioral changes and to improve the psychological health and functioning of the individual (Skinner, 1979)

Goals

- Manipulate the environment so that all aspects of client's hospital experience are considered therapeutic.
- Client is expected to learn adaptive coping, interaction and relationship skills that can be generalized to other aspects of his or her life.
- Achieving client autonomy

Principles of Milieu Therapy

- To promote a fundamental respect for individuals.
- To use opportunities for communication between client and staff for maximum therapeutic benefit.
- To promote socialization.
- To provide opportunities for clients to be part of unit management.
- Individuals are held responsible for own actions.
- Peer pressure is utilized to reinforce rules and regulations.
- Team approach is used.
- Group discussions and temporary seclusions are favoured approaches for acting out behavior.

Strategies

- Distribution of power
- Open communication
- Structured interactions
- Work-related activities
- Community and family involvement in the treatment process
- Adaptation of the environment to meet developmental needs.

Programs within the Milieu:

- **Client government**:
  - Structured meeting
  - Clients have inputs into all unit activities
  - May make decisions related to privileges for other clients
  - Discussion of the problems of everyday living
  - Usually meets once per week
- **Work-related activities:**
  - Work therapy
  - Monetary reward
  - Client should choose the type of work
  - Offer a variety of activities.

Role of Nurse

- Providing and maintaining a safe and conflict free environment
- Sharing responsibilities with patients
- Encourage patient to participate in decision making
- Giving feedback
- Carrying out supervisory functions
- Democratic as opposed to hierarchical
- Rehabilitative rather than custodial.

Relaxation Therapies

Stress is a part of our everyday lives. It can be positive or negative, but it cannot be eliminated. Keeping stress at a manageable level is a lifelong process. Relaxation therapy is an effective means of reducing the stress response in some individuals. Various methods of relaxation are described in the following.

Deep-Breathing Exercises

Deep-breathing exercises involve inhaling slowly and deeply through the nose, holding the breath for a few seconds, then exhaling slowly through the mouth, pursing the lips as if trying to whistle.

Progressive Relaxation

This method of deep-muscle relaxation is based on the premise that the body responds to anxiety-provoking thoughts and events with muscle tension. Each muscle group is tensed for 5–7 seconds and then relaxed for 20–30 seconds, during which time the individual concentrates on the difference in sensations between the two conditions.

Soft, slow background music may facilitate relaxation. A modified version of this technique (called passive progressive relaxation) involves relaxation of the muscles by concentrating on the feeling of relaxation within the muscle, rather than the actual tensing and relaxing of the muscle. (e.g: Jacobson's Progressive Muscular Relaxation Technique).

Meditation

It brings on a special state of consciousness as attention is concentrated solely on one thought or object. During meditation, as the individual becomes totally preoccupied with the selected focus, the respiration rate, heart rate, and blood pressure decrease.

Mental Imagery

Mental imagery uses the imagination in an effort to reduce the body's response to stress. The frame of reference is very personal, based on what each individual considers being a relaxing environment. The relaxing scenario is most useful when taped and played back at a time when the individual wishes to achieve relaxation.

Biofeedback

Biofeedback is the use of instrumentation to become aware of processes in the body that usually go unnoticed and to help bring them under voluntary control. Biological conditions, such as muscle tension, skin surface temperature, blood pressure, and heart rate, are monitored by the biofeedback equipment.

Biofeedback is often used together with other relaxation techniques such as deep breathing, progressive relaxation, and mental imagery.

Play Therapy

Play Therapy is a specific form of therapy in which games, toys and mediums such as clay, drawings and paint are used to help a child or adolescent to express their emotions, thoughts, wishes and needs. It helps them to understand muddled feelings and upsetting events that they have not had the chance or the skills to sort out properly.

Types of Play

- Individual versus group play
- Free versus controlled play
- Directive versus nondirective.

Achievements through Play Therapy

- Play Therapy can be useful for any child of four years and older.
- It can help to become aware of what feelings and how these feelings manifest in behavior or one's body.
- They can learn how to become better at regulating emotions and expressing them in constructive ways.

- They can discover who they are and what their strong and weak points, needs, wishes, thoughts and dreams
- Social interaction is stimulated.

Length of Play Therapy

- This depends on the child's personality. Some children are very shy while others are quick to talk.
- In general, a child or adolescent attends therapy for at least six therapy sessions as this usually gives sufficient time to build a relationship of trust and to have time to discover more about feelings and thoughts.

Role of Nurse

- Carefully select the play materials according to the age group.
- Maintain a trusting relation with the child.
- Promote a positive transference as an educational and therapeutic maneuver.

Occupational Therapy (OT)

Occupation as 'any activity, which engages a person's resource of time and energy and is composed of skills and values'

It is the assessment and treatment of physical and psychiatric conditions using specific, purposeful activity to prevent disability and promote independent function in all aspects of daily life.

Indications

- Depression
- Atypical depression
- Dissociative Disorder
- Conversion reaction
- Adjustment disorder
- Atypical psychosis
- Schizophrenia
- Early onset dementia
- Borderline personality disorder (BPD)
- Obsessive compulsive disorder (OCD)
- Panic disorder/anxiety.

Focus for Occupational Therapy

Occupational therapy works towards people achieving a balance of activities within three key areas:

1. Self-care
2. Productivity (work/education)
3. Leisure.

Common Interventions

Following are some common interventions:

- Life skills training
- Cognitive rehabilitation
- Supported employment
- Supported education
- Social and interpersonal skills training
- Life balance intervention
- Modalities such as biofeedback and mindfulness-enhanced therapy

Benefits of Occupational Therapy

- Improves patients' independence in activities of daily living.
- Improves patients' self-esteem, self-worth and confidence by achievement of activities and goals and engaging in valued occupations.
- Enables patients to develop leisure skills and interests.
- Improves patients' physical fitness through sports/exercise and increasing activity levels.

Recreation Therapy

It is a form of activity therapy used in most of the psychiatry settings. Therapeutic recreation can occur as an informal ping pong and card games, structured soft ball, basket ball, or volley ball, as trips outside the hospital, attending sports, etc.

Recreation therapy provides them useful leisure activities and helps them develop skills in engaging in healthy, competitive interactions.

Types of Recreational Activities

The various forms of play or activity used in recreation therapy are:

- **Motor forms:** These can be further divided into fundamental and accessory, based on whether the motor element is the main purpose of the activity or merely incidental to it. Among the fundamental forms are such games are hockey and foot ball, while the accessory forms are exemplified by play activity and dancing.
- The sensory forms may be visual, e.g. looking at motion pictures, play, etc. or auditory, such as listening to a concert.
- The intellectual forms include such activities as reading, debating, etc.

Aims of recreation therapy

- To train memory and concentration
- To give a sense of responsibility
- To stimulate interest
- To stimulate or recreate self-confidence
- To arouse and develop attention
- To give one opportunity for self-expression
- To replace unhealthy trends by healthy ones
- To substitute encouragement for discouragement

- To improve the appetite
- To improve the circulation
- To improve respiration
- To strengthen the tone of the muscles
- To develop a sense of rhythm
- To develop a good posture.

Recreation therapy may also use community resources to help patients identify socialization activities.

Psychodrama

It is the use of guided dramatic action to examine problems (or) issues raised by an individual. It is a structured, directed dramatization of a patient's emotional problems and experiences. These 'dramas' provide the patient with the opportunity to develop greater awareness of his thoughts, feelings and action of how they affect others. It was devised by Dr Jacob, L Morene in 1914.

Uses

- Facilitates insight, personal growth and integration on cognitive, affective and behavioral levels.
- It clarifies issues increased physical and emotional well-being.
- Enhances learning and developing new skills.

Indications

- Alcoholism and substance abuse
- Marital discord.

Phases

There are three phases of Psychodrama:

1. Warm-up
2. Sharing and presentation of the drama
3. Post action group sharing.

Warm up: This is the first phase. During the warm up the psycho-dramatist involves the group in a discussion of issues deemed important to explore for that seeing.

Once a group concern emerges, a protagonist is supported and encouraged to come forth.

Sharing and presentation: The second phase is composed of the sharing and presentation of the drama. If this stage is conducted properly, the entire group may benefit from the action.

Post action group sharing: The final phase is the post action and group sharing. In this phase, the group members express what events in their own lives were touched on by the action.

Music Therapy

Music therapy is the functional application of music towards the attainment of specific psychiatric therapeutic goals.

Goal

- To reduce psychosocial stress, pain and anxiety.
- It slower heart rate, respiratory rate and blood pressure.

Types of Music Therapy

It is of two modes of presentation. One is passive mode or passive form of music therapy which give importance to listening; the other one is active mode or active form of music therapy, which give importance to participating.

Effects of Music Therapy

- Soothing music initiates relaxation
- Soothing music induces sleep
- Facilitates emotional homeostasis
- Reduces pain, anxiety
- Lowers heart rate, blood pressure, etc.
- Music can encourage socialization, communication and motor development
- Helps to reduce the dosage of tranquilizers

Dance Therapy

It is the effective use of movement and dance for emotional, cognitive, social, behavioral and physical condition.

Indication

- Emotionally disturbed persons
- Suicidal ideations
- Mental retardation
- Substance abuse
- Visually and hearing impaired
- Psychotics.

Advantages

- Helps to develop body awareness
- Facilitates expression of feelings
- Improve socialization
- Increases self-confidence.

Light Therapy

It is the exposure of the patient to artificial therapeutic lighting.

The timing and intensity of the light varies from person to person. Most patients feel relief after 3–5 days, and they relapse equally rapidly after stoppage of light therapy.

Indications

- Seasonal mood disorders
- Premenstrual syndrome
- Non seasonal depression.

Bibliotherapy

Bibliotherapy is the use of literature to help the persons to identify and express feelings.

This can be done mainly by arranging a library in the psychiatric set up. While selecting the books, the nurse has to consider the age group of the persons. For example, while selecting books for small children consider the book containing more pictures that holds the child's attention.

Nurse should also think about client's situation and try to select a book that describes real life situation. Observe for the client's response also.

After reading the book nurse can evaluate the usefulness of the intervention.

Art Therapy

This is a form of expressive therapy that uses materials such as paints, chalks and markers.

Purpose

- Improve emotional wellbeing
- Enhance verbal exchange between the person and therapist
- Enhance perception
- Achieves insight and problem solving.

Importance

- Used as a therapeutic and diagnostic measure
- Provides a chance to express fantasies
- Helps patient to relief from anxiety by representing conflict and traumatic experiences through pictures.

Comlementary and Alternative System of Medicine (CAM)

Many individuals today are choosing to move away from traditional medicine by trying a variety of alternative approaches to health care. Some individuals do not completely abandon traditional medicine for alternative therapies. Instead, they may choose to complement the conventional methods with the addition of alternative strategies.

Box 5.8: Alternative system of medicine

Interventions that differ from the traditional or conventional biomedical treatment of disease. 'Alternative' refers to an intervention that is used *instead* of conventional treatment.

Box 5.9: NCCAM categories of complementary and alternative therapies

Category	Description	Examples
Alternative medical systems	Complete systems of health care, apart from the conventional biomedical system used.	• Traditional chinese medicine (TCM) • Ayurveda • Homeopathy • Naturopathy • Siddha • Unani

Contd...

Contd...

Category	Description	Examples
Mind- Body interventions	Therapies that use the mind's ability to affect the physical body. Science of psychoneuroimmunology demonstrates the strength of mind-body connection.	• Relaxation breathing • Prayer • Meditation • Biofeedback • Imagery • Hypnosis • Music therapy • Art therapy • Journaling • Animal-assisted therapy (AAT)
Biologic-Based therapies	Therapies that use substances found in nature for their impact on health and wellness.	• Herbal therapy • Nutraceuticals • Nutritional therapy • Aromatherapy
Manipulative and Body-Based methods	Therapies that manipulate or move one or more parts of the body.	• Chiropractic medicine • Acupressure • Massage therapy • Yoga
Energy therapies	Therapies that use or manipulate energy fields.	• Therapeutic touch • Healing touch • Reiki • Magnet therapy.

Source: NCCAM, National center for complementary and alternative medicine.

Box 5.10: Complementary therapy

A complementary therapy is an intervention that is different from, but used in conjunction with, traditional or conventional medical treatment.

Some commonly used CAM are discussed in this session.

Ayurveda

Ayurveda come from the Sanskrit word *Ayur* means 'life' and *Veda* which means 'knowledge'. It considers the disease results from the accumulation of toxin in the body and an imbalance of emotions. It prescribes individualized diets, detoxification, cleansing from orifices, meditation and yoga.

Origin

Ayurveda Originated in the vedic civilization of India about 4000 years ago. It is a traditional Hindu system of medicine practiced in India since the first century AD.

Approaches

At an early period, Ayurveda adopted the physics of the five elements. They are:
1. Prithvi (earth)
2. Jala (water)
3. Agni (fire)
4. Vayu (air)
5. Akasa (sky).

That composes the universe, including the human body. Ayurveda stresses a balanced of three elemental energies or humors. The three elements are called as *Doshas*. The three domains of dosha in Ayurvedic medicine are.
1. Vata (air and space – 'wind')
2. Pitta (fire and water – 'bile)
3. Kapha (water and earth – phlegm).

Diagnosis

Diagnosis is made by information obtained in a detailed holistic history, review of symptoms and selected physical observations.

The *charaka samhita* recommends a tenfold examination of patient, they are:

- Constitution
- Abnormality
- Essence
- Stability
- Body measurements
- Diet suitability
- Psychic strength
- Digestive capacity
- Physical fitness
- Age
- Observing the effect of therapeutic procedures
- The pathological process.

Hygiene

Hygiene is an Indian cultural value and a central practice of Ayurvedic medicine. Hygienic living involves regular bathing, cleaning of teeth, skin care and eye washing, etc.

Treatment Modalities

- Ayurveda stress the use of plant based medicines and treatment.
- Several animal products may also be used, e.g. milk, bone and gallstones.
- Minerals include sulfur, lead, copper sulfate and gold are also prescribed. This practice of adding minerals to herbal medicine is known as *Rasa Sashtra*.
- Many treatment modalities are specific for each dosha and may include nutrition, exercise, herbs, breathing, meditation, massage, and aromatherapy.

Yoga

Yoga is thought to have developed in India some 5000 years ago and is attributed to an Indian physician and Sanskrit scholar named Patanjali. The objective of yoga is to integrate the physical, mental, and spiritual energies that enhance health and well being Yoga has been found to be especially helpful in relieving stress and in improving overall physical and psychological wellness. Proper breathing is a major component of yoga.

It is believed that yoga breathing—a deep, diaphramatic breathing—increases oxygen to brain and body tissues, thereby easing stress and fatigue, and boosting energy. Another component of yoga is meditation. Individuals who practice the meditation and deep breathing associated with yoga find that they are able to achieve a profound feeling of relaxation.

Unani

The history of Unani system of medicine is traced back to ancient Greece. Centuries of experience and practice, has established that Unani medicine is not only gentle and safe, but also extremely effective in healing numerous acute and chronic diseases.

Unani Principles

Doctrine of naturals: Unani system strongly believes in nature and its healing properties.

Indications

- Stress
- Anxiety
- OCD.

Unani Therapies

The common therapies include:
- Balneology
- Cupping
- Dietetics
- Pharmacotherapy.

Balneology

The application of bath for healing purposes in the traditional Unani medicine system is known as balneology. The bathing therapy is conducted in a bathing room which is referring to as hammam in arabic and ancient.

Cupping

Cupping is a unique therapy in Unani medicine. The therapy is based on the principle of acupuncture and employs glass cups for the same.

Dietetics

The traditional system of medicine, Unani lays stress on the importance of diet on health. According to Avicenna, most of the illnesses arise as a result of prolonged disorder related to diet and regimen.

Pharmacotherapy

Pharmacotherapy in Unani involves the ways of drugs which have natural in nature. This means they can be derived from natural sources like plants, animals, and minerals. With help of these components single as well as compound remedies are prepared.

Siddha

Siddha System of Medicine also known as Siddha Vaidya originated in Tamil Nadu in India is the oldest medical system in the world. It is believed that *Saint Agasthiyar* is the founder of this system and he had given to his 18 disciples known as *Siddhars* (the practitioners in this system are known as Siddhars).

Siddha—Basic Principles

Siddha science considers nature and man as essentially one. According to Siddha medical science, the Universe originally consisted of atoms which contributed to the five basic elements, viz., earth, water, fire, air and sky which correspond to the five senses of the human body and they were the fundamentals of all the corporeal things in the world.

Fundamental Subjects of Siddha Methodology

- Vadham (Alchemy)
- Aithiyam (Medicine)
- Yogam (Yoga)
- Gyanam or Thathuvam (Philosophy)

Siddhars classified the diseases in different topics and accounted the total diseases for human body as 4448 diseases. They mentioned about the curable and incurable diseases along with the symptoms of the body and predicted the concerned, proper medicines also.

Homeopathy

Derived from Greek word homios—similar and pathos—suffering and is developed in 1700s by a German physician, *Samuel Hahnemann.*

Principles

Two main principles:

1. Likes cures like
2. Healing occurs from the inside out.

Homeopathic practices are based on two fundamental laws.

1. **Law of similar:** states that a natural substance that produces a given symptoms in a healthy person will cure it in a sick person.
2. **Law of infinite smalls:** states that the smallest dose possible will have the desired effect.

Treatment

- Homeopathic remedies consist of plant, animal or mineral substances that are diluted in water or alcohol and vigorously shaken.

- The dilution and shaking process can be repeated several times until no chemical trace of the original substance can be detected.
- Paradoxically, the greater the dilution, the more powerful the medication.

TRADITIONAL CHINESE MEDICINE (TCM)

Traditional chinese medicine refers to a broad range of medicine practices sharing common theoretical concepts which have been developed in china and look back on a tradition of more than 2000 years.

It includes various forms of herbal medicine, acupuncture, massage therapy and dietary therapy. TCM is similar to Ayurveda in at least two ways. First, TCM as a healing system is thousands of years old. Second a principle of TCM is that the interaction of people with their environment is most significant in creating health.

TCM partly based on the idea that energy, called *qi* ('chee'), flows along pathways in the body called meridians (Channel). In this belief, if the flow of qi along these meridians is blocked or unbalanced, illness can occur. Causes of qi imbalance are thought to involve:

- External forces, such as wind, cold, or heat.
- Internal forces, such as emotions of joy, anger, or fear.
- Lifestyle factors, such as poor diet, too little sleep, or too much alcohol.

Among the components of TCM are herbal and nutritional therapy, restorative physical exercises, meditation, acupuncture, and remedial massage.

- **Acupuncture:** This uses thin metal needles placed along the body's meridians.
- **Acupressure:** This uses the hands or fingers to apply direct pressure to points along the body's meridians.
- **Chinese herbs:** combinations of herbs, roots, powders, or animal substances to help restore balance in the body.
- **Cupping:** This uses warm air in glass jars to create suction placed on areas of the body to help stimulate *qi.*
- **Diet:** Yin and yang foods can help restore the yin-yang balance in the body.
- **Massage (tui na):** on specific areas of the body or along the body's meridians.
- **Moxibustion:** This uses small amounts of heated plant fiber (moxa, or Chinese mugwort) on specific areas of the body.
- **Qi gong** ('chee-GUNG'): This combines movement, meditation, and regulation of breathing to enhance the flow of qi (vital energy) in the body, improve blood circulation, and enhance immune function..

OTHER CAM'S

Aromatherapy

Aroma therapy is the use of essential oils (e.g. Lavender oil) for therapeutic purposes that encompasses mind, body and spirit

Types

- Holistic aroma therapy
- Medical aroma therapy
- Clinical aroma therapy
- Home aroma therapy
- Armachology.

Modes of Application

- Aerial diffusion
- Direct inhalation
- Topical application.

Materials

- Essential oils (Found in flowers, leaves, bark, wood, roots, seeds and peels)
- Absolutes
- Herbal distillates or hydrosols
- Infusions
- Carrier oils
- Vaporizer (volatized raw herbs).

Therapeutic Effects

- CNS effects
- Metabolic/Endocrine effects
- Psychologic effects
- Increase in μ brain waves
- Lavender—treating wounds, to enhance memory and to aid in sleep.

Chiropractice

It focuses on the relationship between bodily structure (primarily that of the spine) and function, and how that relationship affects the preservation and restoration of health. Chiropractors use manipulative therapy as an integral treatment tool.

Naturopathy

Naturopathic medicine proposes that there is a healing power in the body that establishes, maintains, and restores health. Practitioners work with the patient with a goal of supporting this power, through treatments such as nutrition and lifestyle counseling, dietary supplements, medicinal plants, exercise, homeopathy, and treatments from TCM.

Reiki ('Ray-Kee')

It is a Japanese word representing Universal Life Energy. Reiki is based on the belief that when spiritual energy is channeled through a Reiki practitioner, the patient's spirit is healed, which in turn heals the physical body.

Therapeutic Touch

Therapeutic touch was developed in the 1970s by Dolores Krieger, a nurse associated with the New York University School of Nursing. It is derived from an ancient technique called laying-on of hands. It is based on the premise that it is the healing force of the therapist that affects the patient's recovery; healing is promoted when the body's energies are in balance; and, by passing their hands over the patient, healers can identify energy imbalances.

Massage

Massage is the manipulation of muscle and connective tissue to enhance function of those tissues and promote relaxation and well being. Massage has been shown to be beneficial in the following conditions: Anxiety, chronic back and neck pain, arthritis, sciatica, migraine headaches, muscle spasms, insomnia, pain of labor and delivery, stress-related disorders, and whiplash. Massage is contraindicated in certain conditions, such as high blood pressure, acute infection, osteoporosis, phlebitis, skin conditions, and varicose veins. It also should not be performed over the site of a recent injury, bruise, or burn.

Pet Therapy

The therapeutic value of pets is no longer just theory. Research shows that animals can directly influence a person's mental and physical well being. Petting animals (e.g. dog or cat) enhance a client's mood and social interaction, lower blood pressure,

Psychiatric Rehabilitation

Psychiatric rehabilitation is defined as restoration of the fullest physical, mental, social, vocational, and economic usefulness of which the person suffering from psychiatric disorder is capable.

Most of the psychiatric clients have a poor quality of life, residual symptoms, and long-term disability. Although, early recognition and treatment is the cornerstone of preventing long-term disability, a substantial number of patients may need rehabilitation.

There are several components and methods available for rehabilitation, depending on the type and/or stage of disorder and the type of support available to the patient. Necessarily, a comprehensive assessment is needed before deciding on the individualized rehabilitation for a particular patient.

Methods of Rehabilitation

- Housing Placement:
  - Such as half way homes
  - Supervised housing.
- Vocational Training and Rehabilitation:
  - Activity Therapy
  - Sheltered workshop
  - Transitional/supported employment
  - Vocational-guidance
  - Occupational therapy.

- Treatment
  - Such as ensuring compliance with medication
  - Social skills therapy
  - Family therapy
  - Cognitive remediation.

There is an acute shortage of psychiatric rehabilitation facilities in most parts of India.

6 Nursing Management of Patient with Schizophrenia and other Psychotic Disorders

The term *Schizophrenia* is recent, and it is termed by a Swiss psychiatrist Eugen Bleuler in the year 1908. It is derived from two Greek words '**skhizo**' (split) and '**phren**' (mind).

HISTORY

The physicians of ancient times were aware of conditions with identical symptoms of schizophrenia. Indian writings of 3,500 years ago describe the illness similar to this in which the afflicted wander about naked, body smeared with mud and excreta and who ate food greedy when food was given to them.

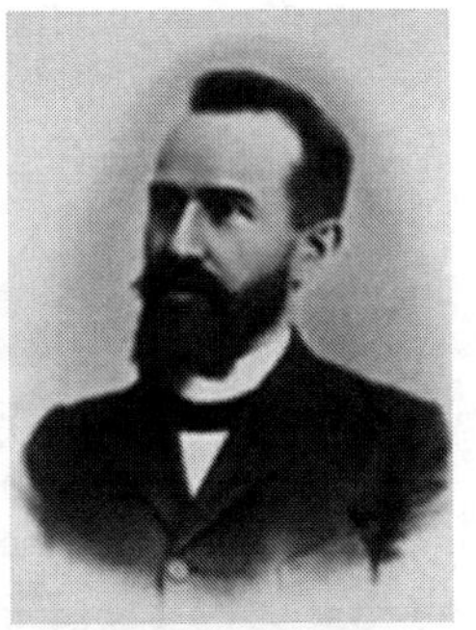

Fig. 6.1: Eugen Bleuler

Emil Kraepelin termed this as ***Dementia praecox*** (Dementia of Puberty). This illness develops relatively early in life, and its course is likely deteriorating and chronic; deterioration reminded dementia, but was not followed by any organic changes of the brain.

Eugen Bleuler renamed dementia praecox as ***schizophrenia*** (1908); he recognized the cognitive impairment in this illness, which he named as a **'splitting'** of mind.

Kurt Schneider, a German psychiatrist (1959) made the diagnosis of schizophrenia more reliable. He listed a series of symptoms which are characteristics of schizophrenia.

Langfeldt, a Norwegian psychiatrist (1993) tried to distinguish the process of schizophrenia from psychoses depending on their prognosis.

DEFINITION

Schizophrenia is a psychotic and a serious mental illness that interferes with a person's ability to think clearly, manage emotions, make decisions and relate to others. This usually leads to social withdrawal.

CLASSIFICATION [INTERNATIONAL CLASSIFICATION OF DISEASES (ICD 10)]

F 20–29: Schizophrenia, schizotypal and delusional disorders

F 20: Schizophrenia

- **F 20.0:** Paranoid schizophrenia
- **F 20.1:** Hebephrenic schizophrenia

F 20.2: Catatonic schizophrenia
F 20.3: Undifferentiated schizophrenia
F 20.4: Post-schizophrenic depression
F 20.5: Residual schizophrenia
F 20.6: Simple schizophrenia
F 20.8: Other schizophrenia
F 20.9: Schizophrenia, unspecified.

EPIDEMIOLOGY

- It is the most common of all psychiatric disorders and is prevalent in all cultures across the world.
- About 15% of new admissions are schizophrenic patients.
- One percent of world population develops schizophrenia.
- 3–4 per 1000 in every community suffer from schizophrenia and the prevalence is equal in both genders.
- Onset 15–25 years for men, 25–35 years for women.
- Two-third cases in age group of 15–30 years.
- The disease is common in low socioeconomic status.

Box 6.1: Myths about schizophrenia

- Schizophrenia refers to multiple personality.
- Schizophrenia is a rare disease.
- People with schizophrenia are dangerous.
- The cause is abnormal parenting.

ETIOLOGY

The cause of schizophrenia is still uncertain. There is no single factor can cause the disease, probably results from a combination of factors including biological, psychological, and environmental.

Box 6.2: Overview of etiology

- Biological influences
- Physiological influences
- Psychological influences
- Environmental influences.

Biological Influences

Genetic Factors

Studies show that relatives of individuals with schizophrenia have a much higher probability of developing the disease than the general population. The siblings or offspring of an identified client have 5–10% risk of developing schizophrenia. How schizophrenia is inherited is uncertain.

Twin Studies

The rate of schizophrenia among monozygotic twins is four times that of dizygotic twins and approximately 50 times that of the general population.

Biochemical Theories

Biochemical hypothesis of schizophrenia orientated towards the role of neurotransmitters and their receptors; dopamine, serotonin, glutamate, gamma-aminobutyric acid (GABA), norepinephrine. Dopamine plays a key role in biochemical hypothesis of schizophrenia.

Box 6.3: Classical dopamine hypothesis

Psychotic symptoms in schizophrenia are a result of increased dopaminergic activity in the brain. It occurs due to increased sensitivity and density of dopamine D2 receptors.

Physiological influences

Viral Infections

- Prenatal exposure to influenza.
- Viral infections of the central nervous system (CNS) during childhood.
- Viral infections during pregnancy and delivery.

Anatomical Abnormalities

Neuroimaging studies shows structural brain abnormalities in individuals with schizophrenia.

- Brains of patients with schizophrenia are lighter and smaller.
- Cortical atrophy in the frontal and temporal lobes of left side is seen in 10–35% cases.
- Larger lateral and third ventricles.

Physical Factors

Researchers reported a link between schizophrenia and epilepsy, head injury in adulthood, alcohol abuse, cerebral tumor and Parkinsonism.

Psychological Influences

Family Theories

Family relationships act as a major influences in the development of illness.

Broken homes, unstable parents and eccentric child rearing practices were seen in many cases. Two family situations leading to the onset of schizophrenia are:

1. **Deviant role relationship:** Marital skew and schism, i.e. the discordant family relation with father and mother.
2. **Discarded communication:** 'Double bind' communication i.e. the parents convey two or more conflicting messages at the same time.

Developmental Theories

The individuals with poor ego boundaries, inadequate ego development, superego dominance, regressed to behavior, love-hate relationships and arrested psychosocial development are prone to schizophrenia.

Environmental Influences

Sociocultural Factors

Statistics have shown that many schizophrenic cases are from the lower socioeconomic classes. This may be due to the conditions associated with living in poverty, such as congested housing accommodations, inadequate nutrition, absence of prenatal care, few resources for dealing with stressful situations, and feelings of hopelessness for changing one's lifestyle of poverty. The incidence is high among migrants due to the effect of new environment and challenges.

Stressful Life Events

There is no scientific evidence to explain that stress causes schizophrenia. Stress may contribute to the severity and course of the illness. The stress can be biological, environmental, or both. Stressful life events may increase schizophrenic symptoms and increased rates of relapse.

PSYCHOPATHOLOGY

The conceptualization of schizophrenia has been subject to considerable debate. Like disorders in medicine there is no known pathophysiological mechanism can be linked to the symptoms of schizophrenia.

Emil Kraepelin and Eugen Bleuler established some modern concept for schizophrenia. Kraepelin's concept was that a variety of psychotic entities could be combining to a single entity consisting of hebephrenic, paranoid deterioration, and catatonia. He used dementia praecox to describe what he perceived as a deterioration process.

Bleuler viewed schizophrenia as a splitting of psychic functions. Thus psychic complexes did not combine in a unified form, like a healthy person. Rather the personality seemed to lose its unity. So that different ideas and drives view split off.

CLINICAL FEATURES

Bleuler's Classification

Bleuler classified the symptoms of schizophrenia into 'primary' or core symptoms (i.e. those related to the splitting) and 'secondary' symptoms, which represented psychological reactions to the primary symptoms. The symptoms are as follows in the box 6.4.

Box 6.4: Bleuler's symptoms of schizophrenia

Primary symptoms: 4A's of schizophrenia

1. **Ambivalence** (the co-existence of strongly conflicting feelings, attitudes and ideas)
2. **Autistic thinking** (withdrawal in thinking and behavior)
3. **Association disturbances** (fragmented thinking)
4. **Affective blunting.**

Secondary symptoms

- Hallucinations
- Delusions
- Catatonic symptoms
- Behavioral abnormalities.

Kurt Schneider's Symptoms of Schizophrenia

Kurt Schneider (1957) described the features of schizophrenia into first rank and second rank symptoms.

First Rank Symptoms

- Audible thought or thought echo
- Voices commenting on him in the third person or voices heard arguing
- Passivity feelings (patient thinks that he is in the grip of a superior force which controls his action)
- Thought withdrawal
- Thought broadcasting
- Delusional perception.

  Other perceptual, motor, and affective symptoms were called second rank symptoms.

Positive and Negative Symptoms

Box 6.5: Negative and positive symptoms of schizophrenia

Negative symptoms 6 As

1. Anhedonia (inability to experience pleasure)
2. Apathy (attentional impairment)
3. Avolition (diminution of will or desire)
4. Alogia (poverty of thinking and speech)
5. Asocial (social withdrawal)
6. Affective flattening

Positive symptoms

- Hallucinations
- Delusions
- Bizarre behavior
- Positive formal thought behavior.

It is very difficult in learning about schizophrenia because the clinical presentations and outcome are so varied. The clinical features of schizophrenia can be studied under the following headings.

- Disturbances of speech and thought
- Disturbances of perception
- Disturbances of mood
- Disturbances of volition and motor behavior
- Other features.

Disturbances of Speech and Thought

Thought disorders are hallmark of schizophrenia. Depends on the type of illness disturbances in form, stream, possession and content of thought are seen. They are as follows:

- Autistic thinking
- Loosening of association (thinking is characterized by speech in which ideas shift from one unrelated subject to another)

- Thought blocking (sudden interruption in thought process)
- Magical thinking (the person believes that the thoughts or behaviors have control over specific situations or people)
- Word salad (a group of words that are put together randomly, without any logical connection)
- Neologisms (the psychotic person invents new words that are meaningless to others but have symbolic meaning to them)
- Poverty of ideation
- Mutism (individual's inability or refusal to speak)
- Perseveration (persistent repetition of the same word or idea in response to different questions).
- Verbigeration (senseless repetition of some words)
- Echolalia (imitation of examiner's words or phrases)
- Delusions (false unshakable beliefs about the self or the environment)

The common types of delusions with schizophrenic patients are:

Box 6.6: Types of delusion

Types of delusion	Definition
Persecution	Belief that others are hostile or trying to harm the individual
Reference	False belief that public events or people are directly related to the individual
Grandiosity	The individual has an exaggerated feeling of importance, power, knowledge, or identity
Control	Belief that one's actions or thoughts are controlled by an external person or force
Somatic Delusion	Belief that one's body is altered from normal structure or function.

Disturbances of Perception

A variety of perceptual disturbances occur in schizophrenia, but the common are hallucinations. Hallucinations occur in all sensory modalities. Auditory hallucinations are the most common.

Hallucination: Hallucinations, or false sensory perceptions not associated with real external stimuli, may involve any of the five senses. This is otherwise known as the imaginary perception.

Auditory hallucinations are common. Visual hallucinations sometimes occur with auditory hallucination. Other types of hallucinations are less common.

Disturbances of Mood/Affect

Affect describes the behavior associated with an individual's feeling state or emotional tone. The affect disturbances in schizophrenia include apathy, inappropriate, blunt or flat affect, Anhedonia.

Disorders of Volition and Motor Behavior

Motor disturbances may be in the form of hyperactivity or hypoactivity. Hypoactivity is common with catatonic schizophrenia. Tics, mannerisms and bizarre posture are also seen with the above type. Stereotypy, echopraxia, negativism and automatic obedience are the other symptoms.

Other Features

Other features of schizophrenia include:

- Personality changes
- Lack of insight
- Decreased functioning in work
- Poor judgment
- Lack of sexual interest
- Poor appetite
- Impulsive behavior.

There are usually no disturbances of consciousness, orientation, attention, memory and intelligence.

Box 6.7: Types of schizophrenia (ICD-10)

Class	Type	Description
F 20.0	Paranoid schizophrenia	• Paranoid schizophrenia is dominated by relatively stable, often paranoid delusions, usually accompanied by auditory hallucinations. • Patient is usually potentially aggressive, angry or fearful, uncooperative and difficult to deal with. • No prominent disorganized behavior or mood. • The onset is usually late and the prognosis is better.
F 20.1	Hebephrenic schizophrenia	• Insidious onset. • Disorganized behavior. • Marked incoherence and loosening of association, inappropriate affect, grimacing and bizarre mannerisms are common.
F 20.2	Catatonic schizophrenia	Presence of one or more of the catatonic features: stupor, mutism, rigidity, negativism, posturing, echopraxia, echolalia, waxy flexibility or purposeless excitement. This may be in the form of catatonic stupor, catatonic excitement and catatonia altering between excitement and stupor. Excited catatonia includes restlessness, agitation, excitement, aggressiveness, increase in speech production, loosening of association. Sometimes, this become very severe and is accompanied by rigidity, hyperthermia and dehydration and can result in death.
		Features of catatonic stupor includes mutism, rigidity, negativism, inappropriate and bizarre posture, stupor (does not react to surroundings and appears to be unaware of them), echolalia, echopraxia, waxy flexibility (maintenance of body posture for a long time in a same position even it is uncomfortable), automatic obedience.
F 20.3	Undifferentiated schizophrenia	Psychotic conditions meeting the general diagnostic criteria for schizophrenia but not conforming to any of the subtypes.
F 20.4	Post-schizophrenic depression	A depressive episode, which may be prolonged, arises in the aftermath of a schizophrenic illness. These depressive states are associated with an increased risk of suicide.
F 20.5	Residual schizophrenia	There has been at least one episode of schizophrenia in the past without prominent psychotic symptoms at present.
F 20.6	Simple schizophrenia	This has insidious onset of social withdrawal, loss of drive and ambition, deterioration of functioning. The negative symptoms are very common. It has a worst prognosis of all types.

Contd...

Contd...

Class	Type	Description
F 20.8	Other schizophrenia	Cenesthopathic schizophrenia, schizophreniform: • Disorder not otherwise specified • Psychosis not otherwise specified, etc.
F 20.9	Unspecified schizophrenia	Unspecified schizophrenia is the mental disorder known as schizophrenia that does not fit any of the generally accepted categories or types of schizophrenia. Symptoms of unspecified schizophrenia may include some or all of the symptoms of the named types of schizophrenia.

Diagnosis

In typical cases, proper history and clinical features differentiate schizophrenia from other illnesses without any difficulty.

Schizophrenia is to be diagnosed clinically based on the psychiatric history collection and mental status examination. There is no single laboratory or brain imaging test for schizophrenia, but they help to rule out multiple factors such as brain tumors, possible medical conditions and other psychiatric diagnoses, such as bipolar disorder.

The requirements for the diagnosis of schizophrenia are as follows:

- Presence of psychotic features for a period of one month or more.
- At least one, two or more of the following symptoms:
  - Thought echo, thought insertion or withdrawal or thought broadcasting
  - Delusional perception
  - Hallucinatory voices
- Symptoms from at least two of the following groups:
  - Persistent hallucinations in any modality
  - Thought disturbances
  - Catatonic symptoms
  - Negative symptoms not attributable to medications
  - Personality deterioration.

Management

There is currently no cure for schizophrenia. Treatment is aimed at reducing symptoms and preventing psychotic relapses. Medication needs to be continued. **Multidisciplinary:** Bio, psycho, social approach is used in treatment of schizophrenia. These include:

- Somatic treatment
- Psychosocial therapies

Somatic Treatment

Pharmacological Management

Uses of antipsychotic drugs have revolutionized treatment in schizophrenia. Conventional or typical antipsychotics like haloperidol control the positive symptoms very effectively. Newer or atypical antipsychotics like clozapine, risperidone, olanzapine, ziprasidone, quetiapine, sertindole is better at treating the negative symptoms.

Electroconvulsive Therapy (ECT)

ECT and medicines given together will bring a quick remission. ECT is helpful in catatonic stupor, uncontrolled catatonic excitement, acute exacerbation not controlled by drugs, severe side effects of drugs in presence of untreated schizophrenia. Positive symptoms usually respond well to ECT. Usually 8–10 ECT's are needed, given three times a week, although up to 18 have been given in poor responders.

Psychosocial Therapy

Psychological methods like individual, family and group therapy are useful along with medications. This helps to improve compliance with treatment and relapse.

- Supportive therapy and counseling
- Rehabilitation
- Social skill training (e.g. self-care)
- Vocational rehabilitation (for more stable cases)
- Token economy: Useful for institutionalized chronic schizophrenics
- Positive and negative reinforcement are used to alter patient's unacceptable behavior. It should be part of a behavioral program.

NURSING MANAGEMENT

Schizophrenia is a difficult and chronic illness requiring understanding and competent care in every facet of the client's life. The application of nursing process for schizophrenia is discussed below.

Assessment

The nurse collects a database regarding the client. This step is very important because without an accurate assessment, problem identification, objectives of care and outcome criteria cannot be accurately determined. Data may be obtained from family members, from old records, or from other individuals familiar with patient.

A proper nursing assessment should include the details of previous psychiatric incidence and episodes of present mental illnesses and these include the following:

- Assess the behavior pattern
- Assess the disturbances in eight areas of cognitive functioning and relationship to the external world, and psychomotor behavior
- Observe for any suicidal ideas.

Nursing Diagnosis

Appropriate nursing diagnoses are formulated from the data collected regarding patient. The possible nursing diagnoses are:

- **Disturbed sensory perception:** Auditory/visual related to panic anxiety, extreme loneliness and withdrawal into the self, evidenced by inappropriate responses, disordered thought sequencing, rapid mood swings, poor concentration, disorientation.
- Disturbed thought processes related to inability to trust, panic anxiety, possible hereditary or biochemical factors, evidenced by delusional thinking or suspiciousness of others.

- Social isolation related to inability to trust, panic anxiety, weak ego development, delusional thinking, regression, evidenced by withdrawal, sad and dull affect, preoccupation with own thoughts, expression of feelings of rejection or aloneness imposed by others.
- **Risk for violence:** Self-directed or other-directed related to extreme suspiciousness, panic anxiety, catatonic excitement, command hallucinations, evidenced by overt and aggressive acts, self-destructive behavior, or active aggressive suicidal acts.
- Impaired verbal communication related to panic anxiety, regression, withdrawal, and disordered, unrealistic thinking evidenced by loose association of ideas, neologisms, word salad, clang associations, echolalia, verbalizations that reflect concrete thinking, and poor eye contact.
- Self-care deficit related to withdrawal, regression, panic anxiety, perceptual or cognitive impairment, inability to trust, evidenced by difficulty carrying out tasks associated with hygiene, dressing, grooming, eating, and toileting.
- **Disabled family coping:** Related to difficulty coping with client's illness evidenced by neglectful care of the client in regard to basic human needs or illness treatment, extreme denial or prolonged over concern regarding client's illness.

Planning

The nursing care for schizophrenia is given in **Box 6.8**. The selected nursing diagnoses with outcome identification and intervention are given in the box.

Evaluation

Evaluation or reassessment is conducted to assess the effectiveness of nursing care. In this final step of nursing process, the nurse has to see that the client developed trust with nurse, regarding existence of hallucination and delusional activity, self-care management, socialization, etc.

Box 6.8: Nursing process for schizophrenia

Nursing diagnosis: Disturbed sensory perception: Auditory/visual related to panic anxiety, extreme loneliness and withdrawal into the self, evidenced by inappropriate responses, disordered thought sequencing, rapid mood swings, poor concentration and disorientation.

Outcome identification	Nursing intervention
Client will be able to reduce or eliminate the occurrence of hallucinations.	• Assess the type of hallucination • Avoid touching the client without warning
	• Show acceptance to the client it will encourage him to share the content of the hallucination • Do not reinforce the hallucination. Use 'the voices' instead of words like 'they' that imply validation • Help to understand the connection between anxiety and hallucinations • Interrupt hallucination and try to bring back to reality.

Nursing diagnosis: Disturbed thought processes related to inability to trust, panic anxiety, possible hereditary or biochemical factors, evidenced by delusional thinking or suspiciousness of others.

Contd...

Contd...

Outcome identification	Nursing intervention
Client will remove pattern of delusional thinking and demonstrate trust in others.	• Assess the content of thought • Assess the intensity and duration of delusion • Do not whisper near to the client • Serve food in family style • Mouth checks for medications • Cautious with touch • Use same staff as much as possible • Meet client needs and keep promises to promote trust • Encourage the client to express the feelings • Encourage client's participation in providing care.
Nursing diagnosis: Social isolation related to inability to trust, panic anxiety, weak ego development, delusional thinking, regression, evidenced by withdrawal, sad and dull affect, preoccupation with own thoughts, expression of feelings of rejection or aloneness imposed by others.	
Outcome identification	**Nursing intervention**
Client will voluntarily spend time with other clients and staff members in group activities.	• Convey an accepting attitude to the client. • Offer to be with client during group activities that he or she finds frightening or difficult. • Give positive reinforcement for client's voluntary interactions with others.
Nursing diagnosis: Risk for violence: Self-directed or other-directed related to extreme suspiciousness, panic anxiety, catatonic excitement, command hallucinations, evidenced by overt and aggressive acts, self-destructive behavior, or active aggressive suicidal acts.	
Outcome identification	**Nursing intervention**
Client will not harm self or others.	• Observe client's behavior frequently. • Remove all dangerous objects from client's environment. • Redirect violent behavior with physical outlets for the anxiety. • Staff should maintain a calm attitude toward client. • Have sufficient staff available to indicate a show of strength to client if it becomes necessary. • Administer tranquilizing medications as ordered by physician. If client is not calmed by 'talking down' or by medication, use of mechanical restraints may be necessary.
Nursing diagnosis: Impaired verbal communication related to panic anxiety, regression, withdrawal, and disordered, unrealistic thinking evidenced by loose association of ideas, neologisms, word salad, clang associations, echolalia, verbalizations that reflect concrete thinking, and poor eye contact.	
Outcome identification	**Nursing intervention**
Client will be able to communicate appropriately with others.	• Attempt to decode incomprehensible communication patterns. Seek validation and clarification by stating, 'Is it that you mean…?' or 'I don't understand what you mean by that. Would you please clarify it for me?' • Facilitate trust and understanding by maintaining staff assignments as consistently as possible • Anticipate and fulfill client's needs until functional communication pattern returns • Orient client to reality as required.

Contd...

Contd...

Nursing diagnosis: Self-care deficit related to withdrawal, regression, panic anxiety, perceptual or cognitive impairment, inability to trust, evidenced by difficulty carrying out tasks associated with hygiene, dressing, grooming, eating, and toileting.	
Outcome identification	**Nursing intervention**
Client will demonstrate ability to maintain a normal activities of daily living (ADL).	• Assess the clients ability to do the self-care activities • Provide assistance with self-care needs as required • Encourage client to perform independently as many activities as possible • Encourage the client to wear appropriate dresses as per the setting • Establish a structured schedule for the client for the ADL.
Nursing diagnosis: Disabled family coping: Related to difficulty coping with client's illness evidenced by neglectful care of the client in regard to basic human needs or illness treatment, extreme denial or prolonged over concern regarding client's illness.	
Outcome identification	**Nursing intervention**
Family will identify more adaptive coping strategies for dealing with client's illness and treatment regimen.	• Identify level of family functioning • Assess communication patterns, interpersonal relationships between members, problem-solving skills, and availability of support systems • Provide information for the family about the client's illness, what will be required in the treatment regimen, and long-term prognosis • With family members, practice how to respond to bizarre behavior and communication patterns and in the event that the client becomes violent.

Patient and Family Education

Explain to the patient and family members regarding schizophrenia and its symptoms especially regarding thought disturbances, mood changes, hallucinations, etc.

Teach about medication compliance and effects of antipsychotic medications.

Instruct the family members that if the patient poses any threat or danger to self-harm or aggressive behavior, hospitalize him immediately.

Teach the patient and family members to recognize family stressors which increase the symptoms and methods to prevent them.

Rehabilitation of Schizophrenic Clients

People who have schizophrenia can have repetitive inpatient hospitalizations. Psychiatric rehabilitation strengthens the self-care and improves the quality of life. There are number of services available in community to improve the quality of the life. It may be as follows:

1. Social skill training
2. Vocational rehabilitation
3. Day hospitals
4. Community mental health centers
5. Wellness centers, etc.

Nurses should be familiar with the services available in the community and link the client with these services.

OTHER PSYCHOTIC DISORDERS

The term psychosis is defined as gross impairment in reality, marked disturbance in personality with impaired social and occupational functioning and presence of characteristic symptoms like delusions and hallucinations. In addition to schizophrenia and mood disorders, there are other psychoses, labeled as third psychoses or other psychotic disorders.

These disorders are as follows:

F22 Persistent delusional disorders

F23 Acute and transient psychotic disorders

F24 Induced delusional disorders

F25 Schizoaffective disorders

F28 Other nonorganic psychotic disorders

F29 Unspecified nonorganic psychosis.

Persistent Delusional Disorders

These include a variety of disorders, in which long-standing delusions constitute the only, or the most conspicuous clinical characteristic and which cannot be classified as organic, schizophrenic or affective. Their origin is probably heterogeneous, but it seems, that there is some relation to schizophrenia.

The patient presents with non-bizarre delusional beliefs but most often the mental status examination is otherwise fairly normal. The delusional ideas are restricted to a specific subject and do not contaminate other mental processes.

Clinical Features

- Persistent delusion at least for 3 months
- Absence of significant or persistent hallucinations
- Absence of organic mental disorders
- Associated symptoms are rare but may include mood or anxiety symptoms.

Subtypes/Specifiers

- **Erotomanic type/Clerambault's syndrome:** The patient erroneously believes that another person is in love with him/ her.
- **Grandiose type:** The patient erroneously believes that he/she possesses enormous wealth, power, authority and knowledge.
- **Jealous type/Infidelity/Othello syndrome:** The patient erroneously believes that his/ her partner is unfaithful.
- **Persecutory type:** The patient erroneously believes that he/she is targeted for punishment or retaliation.
- **Somatic type:** The patient erroneously believes that he/she has a medical condition or body deformity that is overlooked or misdiagnosed.

- **Mixed type:** Delusions characteristic of more than one of the above types but without any one dominating theme.

Acute and Transient Psychotic Diorders

This type of disorders neither followed the classical course of schizophrenia nor resembled mood disorders in clinical picture. According to ICD-10, these disorders have an abrupt or acute onset.

- The criteria should be the following features:
  - Acute beginning (to two weeks)
  - Presence of typical symptoms (quickly changing 'polymorphic symptoms')
  - Presence of typical schizophrenic like symptoms.
- Complete recovery, usually occurs within a few months, often within a few weeks or even days.
- The disorder may or may not be associated with acute stress, defined as usually stressful events preceding the onset by one to two weeks.

Induced Delusional Disorders

This is an uncommon psychotic disorder. In this type, the delusional ideas are shared by two or more people with close emotional links. Only one of the people suffers from a genuine psychotic disorder; the delusions are induced in the other(s) and usually disappear when the people are separated.

Sometimes the delusional ideas are shared between two members ***(folie a deux)*** or more persons ***(folie a trios, folie a quatre, folie a famille).***

Schizoaffective Disorder

This is a disorder which lies on the borderline between schizophrenia and mood disorder. In which both affective and schizophrenic symptoms are prominent but do not justify a diagnosis of either schizophrenia or depressive or manic episodes.

Patients suffering from periodic schizoaffective disorders, especially with manic symptoms, have usually good prognosis with full remissions without any remaining defects.

There are three types described:

1. Schizoaffective disorder-manic type
2. Schizoaffective disorder-depressive type
3. Schizoaffective disorder-mixed type.

The course is usually episodic, although chronic courses in some patients are described. The prognosis is better than that in schizophrenia but it worse than that in mood disorders.

Capgras Syndrome (The Delusion of Doubles)

This is a syndrome that is closely related to delusional disorders and is characterized by a delusional conviction that other persons in the environment are not their real selves but are their own doubles.

Four sub types are described:

1. **Typical Capgras syndrome:** This is otherwise known as *illusion des sosies.* Here, the patient sees a familiar person as a complete stranger who is imposing on him as a familiar person.
2. **Illusion de Fregoli:** Patient falsely identifies stranger as familiar person.
3. **Syndrome of subjective doubles:** The patient's own self is perceived as being replaced by a double.
4. **Intermetamorphosis:** The patient misidentifies not only the external appearance but also the complete personality.

Reactive Psychosis

It is characterized by:

- Sudden onset
- Presence of major stress before the onset
- A clear relation between stress and the onset of psychotic symptoms
- No evidence of organic causes

The usual duration of illness is less than one month and recovery is usually complete.

7 Nursing Management of Patient with Mood Disorders

Manic-depressive illness is known since the era of Hippocrates (460–357 BC), Galen (131–201 AD) and Areteus from Cappadocia, and is described in ancient medical texts. Some authors believe that King Saul was also suffering from this disease and David used to relieve his depression by playing music for him. The ancient Greeks and Romans coined the terms 'melancholia' and 'mania.' Hippocrates was the first to describe melancholia which is the Greek word for 'black bile'.

Kraeplin (1921) established the separateness of affective disorders from other major psychoses by developing the concept of manic-depressive illness.

Broadly speaking, the emotions can be described as two main types:

- **Affect** (objective appearance of mood) which is a short-lived emotional response to an idea or an event.
- **Mood** (person's subjective emotional state) which is a sustained and pervasive emotional response which colors the whole psychic life.

Although anxiety is a variant of normal mood, anxiety disorders are not considered as part of mood disorders in the modern classification.

The mood disorders are so called because one of their essential features is abnormality of mood with associated psychotic features.

DEFINITION

Mood disorders, also called affective disorders, are pervasive alterations in emotions that are manifested by depression, mania, or both. They interfere with a person's life, plaguing him or her with drastic and long-term sadness, agitation, or elation.

Mood disorders are characterized by a disturbance of mood, accompanied by a full or partial manic or depressive syndrome, which is not due to any other physical or mental disorder.

Most of these disorders tend to be recurrent, and the onset of individual episodes is often related to stressful events or situations.

The mood disorders may be subdivided into *unipolar* and *bipolar* types: those that are characterized by depression only or those that are characterized by manic episode either alone or in combination with depression.

CLASSIFICATION (ICD 10)

F 30–39: Mood Disorders

- **F 30** Manic Episodes
- **F 32** Depressive Episodes
- **F 31** Bipolar Mood Disorder
- **F 33** Recurrent Depressive Disorders
- **F 34** Persistent Mood Disorder
- **F 38** Other Mood Disorders
- **F 39** Unspecified mood disorder

Epidemiology

The prevalence of mood disorders is 1.5% and it is uniform throughout the world.

MANIC EPISODES (F 30)

Mania is a mood disorder characterized by elevation of mood, increased psychomotor activity and self important ideas.

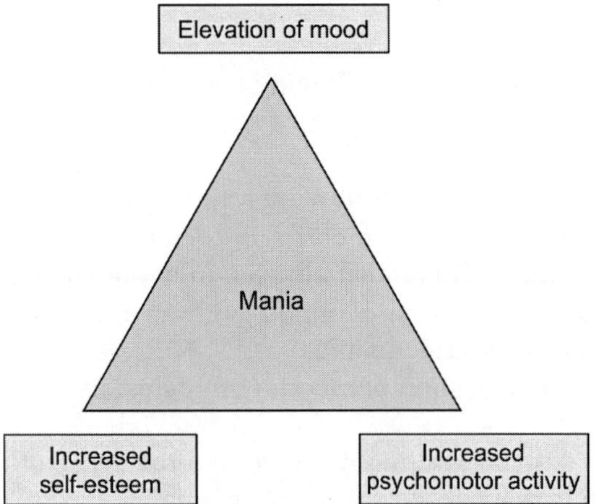

Fig. 7.1: Triad symptoms of mania

Epidemiology

- The life-time risk of manic episode is about 0.8–1%.
- This disorder tends to occur in episodes lasting usually 3–4 months, followed by complete clinical recovery.
- The future episodes can be manic, depressive or mixed.

Etiology

Genetic Factors

Affective disorders are known to have a marked genetic predisposition. Studies of first degree relatives of elderly manic patients have found a quarter to a half are affected.

Monozygotic twins have a higher degree of chance than dizygotic. Siblings and first degree relatives are having a higher degree of incidence. 5–10% chance in first degree relatives. 40–70% chance in identical twins.

Biochemical Factors

Biochemical hypothesis of manic episode is related to the excessive levels of serotonin, norepinephrine and dopamine.

Psychodynamic Theories

This includes faulty family dynamics during the early years of life and as a defense against denial of depression.

Brain Diseases

All studies that have systematically assessed the prevalence of cerebral organic disorders in elderly people with mania have found a significant association between brain disease and mania. Cerebrovascular disease, chronic alcohol misuse, head injury, right-sided lesions may contribute to manic disorders.

Clinical Features of Mania

Manic episode is characterized by the following features.

Elevated, Expansive or Irritable Mood

The elevated mood can pass through following four stages:

Stage I **Euphoria:** Mild elevation of mood), an increased sense of psychological well-being and happiness. This is usually seen in hypomania.

Stage II **Elation:** Moderate elevation of mood with an increased psychomotor activity. Elation is classically seen in mania.

Stage III **Exaltation:** Severe elevation of mood, with delusions of grandeur; seen in severe mania.

Stage IV **Ecstasy:** Very severe elevation of mood, intense sense of rapture or blissfulness; typically seen in delirious or stuporous mania.

Psychomotor Activity

There is an over activity with excessive energy, restlessness, manic excitement where the person is 'on-the-toe-on-the-go', (i.e. involved in ceaseless activity). The activity is usually goal-oriented and is based on external environmental cues. Rarely, a manic patient can go into a stuporous state (*manic stupor*).

Speech and Thought

The person is more talkative than usual; develops pressure of speech; uses playful language with punning, rhyming, joking and teasing; and speaks loudly. Flight of ideas develops. Expansive ideas (inflated self-esteem or grandiosity). Distractibility (reduced concentration).

There can be delusions (or ideas) of grandeur with markedly inflated self-esteem.

Delusions of persecution may sometimes develop. Hallucinations (both auditory and visual), often with religious content, can occur.

Since these psychotic symptoms are in keeping with the elevated mood state, these are called *mood congruent psychotic features.*

Others

- Decreased need for sleep
- Increased libido (may lead to sexual indiscretions)
- Unusually alert
- Increased social communication
- Poor judgment
- Insight is absent
- Decreased food intake
- Suicidal ideas in BMD

Types of Mania

F30.0 Hypomania
F30.1 Mania without psychotic symptoms
F30.2 Mania with psychotic symptoms
F30.8 Other manic episodes
F30.9 Manic episode, unspecified

Hypomania

It is delineated from mania on grounds of severity (Mild form) which includes both symptomatic features and social incapacity. The episode is not severe enough to cause marked impairment in social or occupational functioning or to necessitate hospitalization. There are no psychotic features. Otherwise the features are basically those of mania; elevated mood, grandiosity, over activity, etc.

Mania without Psychotic Features

Symptoms are severe and disturb social and occupational life. Last for at least 1 weak, elation is accompanied by increased energy, resulting in over activity, pressure of speech, and a decreased need for sleep. Normal social inhibition are lost, attention cannot be sustained, and there is often marked distractibility.

Self-esteem is inflated and grandiose or over-optimistic ideas are freely expressed. The individual may embark on extravagant and impractical schemes, spend money recklessly, or become aggressive, amorous, or factious in inappropriate circumstances.

Mania with Psychotic Features

It is the more severe form and psychotic features like hallucination and delusion may develop. This stage disturbs social and occupational life of the patient. Sustained physical activity and excitement may result in aggression or violence, and neglect of eating, drinking, and personal hygiene may result in dangerous states of dehydration and self-neglect.

Diagnosis

- Psychiatric history collection
- Mental status examination
- Psychological tests such as young mania rating scale

Treatment Modalities

- Lithium : 900–2100 mg/day
- Carbamazepine: 600–1800 mg/day
- Sodium valproate: 600–2600 mg/day
- Electroconvulsive therapy

Nursing Management

Assessment

Assessment includes the severity of the manic symptoms. Data should be relevant and should be collected from client and from the relevant sources. Assess the objective and subjective signs of manic episode.

Diagnosis

Possible nursing diagnoses for the client with bipolar disorder (mania) include:

- Risk for injury related to extreme hyperactivity evidenced by increased agitation and lack of control over purposeless and potentially injurious movements
- Risk for violence: Self-directed or other-directed related to manic excitement, delusional thinking, hallucinations
- Imbalanced nutrition: Less than body requirements related to refusal or inability to sit still long enough to eat evidenced by loss of weight, amenorrhea
- Disturbed thought processes related to biochemical alterations in the brain evidenced by delusions of grandeur and persecution
- Disturbed sensory perception related to biochemical alterations in the brain, possible sleep deprivation, evidenced by auditory and visual hallucinations
- Impaired social interaction related to egocentric and narcissistic behavior evidenced by inability to develop satisfying relationships and manipulation of others for own desires. Disturbed sleep pattern related to excessive hyperactivity and agitation, evidenced by difficulty falling asleep and sleeping only short periods.

Box 7.1 Nursing care plan for mania

Nursing diagnosis: Risk for injury related to extreme hyperactivity evidenced by increased agitation and lack of control over purposeless and potentially injurious movements

Outcome identification	Nursing intervention
Client will not experience injury	• Reduce environmental stimuli • Assign single room and keep lighting and noise level low • Remove hazardous objects and substance • Stay with the client who is hyperactive and agitated • Provide physical activities • Administer tranquilizing medication as ordered by physician

Contd...

Contd...

Nursing diagnosis: Risk for violence self-directed or other-directed related to manic excitement, delusional thinking, hallucinations	
Outcome identification	**Nursing intervention**
Client will not harm self or others	• Maintain low level of stimuli • Observe client's behavior at least every 15 minutes. • Ensure that all sharp objects have been removed from client's environment. • Redirect violent behavior. • Encourage client to express his anger verbally • Have sufficient staff to indicate a show of strength to client if necessary. • Administer tranquilizing medication. If client refuses, use of mechanical restraints may be necessary. • Observe the client in restraints every15 minutes. • Remove restraints gradually, one at a time.
Nursing diagnosis: Impaired social interaction related to egocentric and narcissistic behavior evidenced by inability to develop satisfying relationships and manipulation of others for own desires	
Outcome identification	**Nursing intervention**
Client will interact appropriately with others	• Recognize that manipulative behaviors help to reduce feelings of insecurity by increasing feelings of power and control. • Set limits on manipulative behaviors. • Explain what is expected and the consequences if limits are violated. • Discourage the client to argue, bargain, or charm his or her way out of the limit setting. • Give positive reinforcement for non manipulative behaviors. • Discuss consequences of client's behavior and how attempts are made to attribute them to others. • Help client identify positive aspects about self, recognize accomplishments, and feel good about them.
Nursing diagnosis: Imbalanced nutrition less than body requirements related to refusal or inability to sit still long enough to eat evidenced by weight loss, amenorrhea	
Outcome identification	**Nursing intervention**
Client will maintain normal nutritional status	• Assess the nutritional status of the client • Provide high-protein, high-calorie, nutritious diet. • Have juice and snacks on the unit at all times. • Maintain record of intake, output. • Ask clients like, and dislikes about foods. • Supplement diet with vitamins and minerals. • Be with client while he or she eats.

DEPRESSIVE EPISODE (F 32)

The common cold of psychological disorders and a widespread psychiatric problem is affecting many people. It is characterized by depressed mood or loss of interest or pleasure in usual activities.

Epidemiology

- Lifetime risk in males 8–12% and in females 20–26%.
- Lifetime prevalence is in the range of 15–25 %.
- The mean age of onset is about 40 years (25–50 years).
- It may occur in childhood or in the elderly.
- It occurs twice as frequently in women as in men.
- It is commonly associated with a variety of medical conditions.

Types of Depression

F32.0: Mild depressive episode.
F32.1: Moderate depressive episode
F32.2: Severe depressive episode without psychotic symptoms
F32.3: Severe depressive episode with psychotic symptoms
F32.8: Other depressive episodes
F32.9: Depressive episodes, unspecified
F33: Recurrent depression disorder.

Etiology

Etiological factors of depression include Biological factors, Psychological factors.

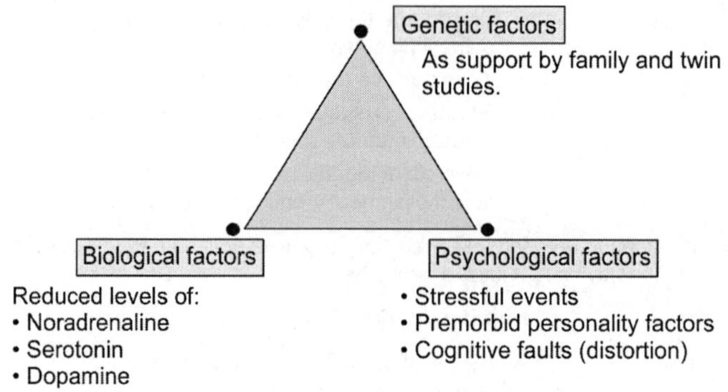

Fig. 7.2: Important causes of depression

Biological Theories

Genetics

A genetic link has been suggested in numerous studies; however no definitive mode of genetic transmission has proved yet. Twin studies suggest that about 50 percent of monozygotic twins and 10–25 % of dizygotic twins are at risk of mood disorders. Major depression is 1.5 to 3 times more common among first degree relatives of people with mood disorder than general population.

Biochemical

Depressive illness may be related to a deficiency of the neurotransmitters norepinephrine, serotonin, and dopamine. Marked disturbance in mood is observed with the endocrine diseases also.

Brain Imaging

Neuroimaging studies (CT, MRI) shows include ventricular dilatation, white matter hyper-intensities, and changes in the blood flow and metabolism in several parts of brain (such as prefrontal cortex, anterior cingulate cortex, and caudate).

Psychosocial Causes

Psychoanalytical theory: Sigmund Freud observed that melancholia occurs after the loss of a loved object, actually by death or emotionally by rejection, or the loss of another abstraction of value to the individual.

Object loss theory: This theory suggests that depressive illness occurs as a result of having been abandoned by or otherwise separated from a significant other during the first 6 months of life. The concept of 'anaclitic depression' was introduced in 1946 by psychiatrist René Spitz to refer to children who became depressed after being separated from their mothers for an extended period of time during the first year of life.

Cognitive theory: This theory suggests that the following reasons leads to depressive features:

- Negative expectations of the environment
- Negative expectations of the self
- Negative expectations of the future

With these the individual feels inadequate, worthless, and rejected by others and become pessimistic and hopeless.

Stress: Increased number of stressful life events before the onset or relapse has a formative rather than a precipitating effect in depression though they can serve a precipitant role in mania. Increased stressors in the early period of development are probably more important in depression.

Other Causes

Medications

Certain medications used alone or in combination can cause side effects much like the symptoms of depression. Examples of these include the anxiolytics, antipsychotics, and sedative hypnotics. Certain antihypertensive medications, such as propranolol and reserpine, have been known to produce depressive symptoms. Use of alcohol or other drugs can lead to or worsen depression.

Neurological Disorders

Neurological disorders like cerebrovascular accident (CVA), brain tumors, particularly in the area of the temporal lobe, often cause symptoms of depression.

Nutritional Deficiencies

Deficiencies in vitamin B_1 (thiamine), vitamin B_6 (pyridoxine), vitamin B_{12}, niacin, vitamin C, iron, folic acid, zinc, calcium, and potassium may produce symptoms of depression. Excessive levels of sodium bicarbonate or calcium can produce symptoms of depression, as can deficits in magnesium and sodium.

Major Illnesses

Major Illnesses such as heart attack, stroke or cancer may trigger depression.

Clinical Features

Depressed Mood

One of the important feature of depression is the sadness of mood or loss of interest and/or pleasure in almost all activities (pervasive sadness), present throughout the day (persistent sadness). Other features related to mood include:

- Lack of enjoyment and inability to experience pleasure (anhedonia)
- Irritability
- Frustration
- Tension

Depressive Ideation/Cognition

Sadness of mood is usually associated with pessimism, which can result in following ideas:

- **Present:** Patient sees the unhappy side of every event.
- **Past:** Unjustifiable guilt feeling and self-blame.
- **Future:** Gloomy preoccupations; hopelessness, helplessness, death wishes (may progress to suicidal ideation and attempt).

The other features are poor attention and concentration, poor memory (subjective), lack of initiative and energy. Thoughts of death and preoccupation with death are not uncommon. Suicidal ideas may be present in severe cases. Delusions of nihilism may occur.

Psychomotor Activity

In younger patients psychomotor retardation is more common and is characterized by slowed thinking and activity, decreased energy and monotonous voice. In a severe form, the patient can become stuporous *(depressive stupor).*

In the older patients (e.g. post-menopausal women), agitation is commoner. It often presents with marked anxiety, restlessness (inability to sit still, hand wriggling, picking at body parts or other objects) and a subjective feeling of unease. Anxiety is a frequent accompaniment of depression. Irritability may present as easy annoyance and frustration in day-to-day activities, e.g. unusual anger at the noise made by children in the house.

Psychotic Features

About 15–20% of depressed patients have psychotic symptoms such as delusions, hallucinations.

Delusions

Delusion of guilt (patient believes he deserves severe punishment), Nihilistic delusion (patient believes that some part of his body ceased to exist or function, e.g. bowel, brain...), delusion of poverty and impoverishment. Persecutory delusion (patient accepts the supposed persecution as something he deserves, in contrast to schizophrenic patient).

Hallucinations

Usually second person auditory hallucinations (addressing derogatory repetitive phrases). Visual hallucinations (scenes of death and destruction) may be experienced by a few patients.

Appearance and Behavior

- Neglected dress and grooming.
- Facial appearance of sadness: Turning downwards of corners of mouth, tearful eyes, and reduced rate of blinking, head is inclined forwards.
- Psychomotor retardation (sometimes agitation).
- Lack of motivation and irritation.
- Social isolation and withdrawal.
- Delay of tasks and decisions.
- Loss of interest in work and pleasure activities.

Biological Features (Neurovegetative Signs)

- Change in appetite (usually reduced but in some patients increased).
- Change in sleep (usually reduced but in some patients increased).
- Early morning (terminal) insomnia; walking 2–3 hours before the usual time, this is usually associated with severe depression.
- Fatigability, low energy level, (simple task is an effort)
- Low libido and/or impotence.
- Change in bowel habit (usually constipation).
- Weight loss
- Change in menstrual cycle (amenorrhea).
- Diurnal variation of mood (usually worse in the morning).

Diagnosis

- Detailed psychiatric history
- Mental status examination
- History of medication uses, neurological disorders, etc.
- Psychological tests like depression scale.

Management

- **Hospitalization** is necessary for the client with depression and is indicated for:
  - Suicidal or homicidal patient.
  - Patient with severe psychomotor retardation who is not eating or drinking.

   - Diagnostic purpose (observation, investigation).
   - Drug resistant cases.
   - Severe depression with psychotic features.
- **Psychopharmacology:** Antidepressants (discussed detail in psychopharmacology), Tricyclics (TCA)/ Monoamino oxidase inhibitors (MAOI), selective serotonin reuptake inhibitors (SSRIs) are useful.
   - After a first episode of a unipolar major depression, treatment should be continued for six months after clinical recovery, to reduce the rate of relapse.
   - If the patient has had two or more episodes, treatment should be prolonged for at least a year after clinical recovery to reduce the risk of relapse.
   - Lithium carbonate can be used as prophylaxis.

Antipsychotics are an important adjunct in the treatment of mood disorder. The commonly used drugs include risperidone, olanzapine, quetiapine, haloperidol, and aripiprazole.

- **Electroconvulsive therapy (ECT):** The indications for ECT in depression include:
   - Severe depression with suicidal risk.
   - Severe depression with stupor, severe psychomotor retardation, or somatic syndrome.
   - Severe treatment refractory depression.
   - Delusional depression (psychotic features).
   - Presence of significant antidepressant side effects or intolerance to drugs.
- **Psychosocial treatment**
   - **Cognitive behavior therapy:** Cognitive behavior therapy (CBT) aims at correcting depressive negative ideations such as hopelessness, worthlessness, helplessness and pessimistic ideas, and replacing them by new cognitive and behavioral responses.
   - **Interpersonal therapy:** Interpersonal therapy (IPT) helps to explore interpersonal stressors, role disputes and transitions, social isolation, or social skills deficits, which act as precipitants for depression. It is useful in the treatment of mild to moderate unipolar depression, with or without antidepressants.
   - **Psychoanalytic psychotherapy:** These techniques are helpful in the treatment of selected patients such as dysthymic disorder, depression co-morbid with personality disorders, or depression with history of childhood loss/child abuse.
   - **Behavior therapy:** This includes the various short-term modalities such as behavioral modification, social skills training; problem-solving techniques, assertiveness training, self control therapy, activity scheduling and decision-making techniques.
   - **Group therapy:** Group psychotherapy can be useful in mild cases of depression. It is a very useful method of psychoeducation in both recurrent depressive disorder and bipolar disorder.
   - **Family and marital therapy**: Educate the family about the nature of illness and the usefulness of somatic treatment. Family therapy can help decrease the intra-familial and interpersonal difficulties and help in a faster and more complete recovery. Their main use is to ensure continuity of treatment.

NURSING MANAGEMENT

Assessment

Assess the symptoms of depressive feature including suicidal ideations. Assess for grief reactions if any. Assess the stage of depression.

Diagnosis

From the data collected from relevant sources following nursing diagnosis are formulated:

- Risk for self-directed violence related to depressed mood, feelings of worthlessness, anger turned inward on the self.
- Dysfunctional grieving related to real or perceived loss, bereavement overload, evidenced by denial of loss, inappropriate expression of anger, inability to carry out activities of daily living.
- Self-esteem disturbance related to learned helplessness, feelings of abandonment by significant other, or impaired cognition fostering negative view of self, evidenced by expressions of worthlessness, hypersensitivity to a slight or criticism, and a negative, pessimistic outlook.
- Powerlessness related to dysfunctional grieving process or lifestyle of helplessness, evidenced by feelings of lack of control over life situation, overdependence on others to fulfill needs.
- Social isolation related to developmental regression, egocentric behaviors, fear of rejection or failure of the interaction, evidenced by being uncommunicative and withdrawn, seeking to be alone, and dysfunctional interaction with peers, family, or others.
- Disturbed thought processes related to underdeveloped ego or impaired cognition fostering negative perception of self or environment, evidenced by delusional thinking, confusion, etc.
- Imbalanced nutrition, less than body requirements related to depressed mood, loss of appetite, or lack of interest in food, evidenced by weight loss, poor muscle tone and weakness.
- Disturbed sleep pattern related to depressed mood, anxiety, and fears, evidenced by difficulty falling asleep, awakening earlier or later than desired, and verbalizations.
- Self-care deficit related to depressed mood, feelings of worthlessness, evidenced by poor personal hygiene.

Planning

Detailed nursing care plan for depression is given below.

Box 7.2: Nursing care plan for mania

Nursing diagnosis: Risk for self-directed violence related to depressed mood, feelings of worthlessness, anger turned inward on the self.

Outcome identification	Nursing intervention
Client will not harm self	• Assess for suicidal ideations • Do not allow the client to be alone in the ward.

Contd...

Contd...

	• Remove all the sharp instruments, ropes from the vicinity of the client. • It may be desirable to place the patient near nursing station for close observation. • Do not allow the client to put bolt on his side door and bathroom. • Encourage the client to express feelings.
Nursing diagnosis: Dysfunctional grieving related to real or perceived loss, bereavement overload, evidenced by denial of loss, inappropriate expression of anger, inability to carry out activities of daily living.	
Outcome identification	**Nursing intervention**
Client will be able to verbalize normal behaviors associated with grieving and begin progression toward resolution	• Assess stage of fixation in grief process • Develop trust. Show empathy, concern, and unconditional positive regard. • Explore feelings of anger and help client direct them toward the intended object. • Promote the use of large motor activities for relieving pent-up tension. • Teach normal behaviors associated with grieving. • Help client with honest review of relationship with lost object.
Nursing diagnosis: Self-esteem disturbance related to learned helplessness, feelings of abandonment by significant other, or impaired cognition fostering negative view of self, evidenced by expressions of worthlessness, hypersensitivity to a slight or criticism, and a negative, pessimistic outlook.	
Outcome identification	**Nursing intervention**
Client will interact appropriately with others.	• Develop a trusting relationship with client • Encourage the client to become involved with staff and other clients through interaction • Explore feelings of anger and help client direct them toward the intended object or person. • Encourage the client for recreational activities • Provide simple activities and shift gradually to complex activity • Give positive feedback for each accomplished activities • Explore with the client his or her personal strengths, making a written list is sometimes helpful.
Nursing diagnosis: Powerlessness related to dysfunctional grieving process or lifestyle of helplessness, evidenced by feelings of lack of control over life situation, overdependence on others to fulfill needs.	
Outcome identification	**Nursing intervention**
Client will be able to solve problems of real life situation	• Allow client to participate in goal setting and decision-making regarding own care. • Ensure that goals are realistic and that client is able to identify areas of life situation that are realistically under his or her control. • Encourage client to verbalize feelings about areas that are not within his or her ability to control.

BIPOLAR DISORDERS

This disorder, earlier known as manic depressive psychosis (MDP), is characterized by recurrent episodes of mania and depression in the same patient at different times. People with MDP changes back and forth between periods of depression and mania.

Epidemiology

The lifetime prevalence is between 0.5 and 1 %. Suicidality is about 19%. Comorbidity increases with alcohol and drug abuse. The first episode may occur at any age from childhood to old age.

The current episode in bipolar mood disorder may be of the following (ICD-10):

F31.0 Bipolar disorder current episode hypomania
F31.1 Bipolar disorder current episode mania without psychotic symptoms
F31.2 Bipolar disorder current episode mania with psychotic symptoms
F31.3 Bipolar disorder current episode mild or moderate depression
F31.4 Bipolar disorder current episode severe depression, without psychotic symptoms
F31.5 Bipolar disorder current episode severe depression, with psychotic symptoms
F31.6 Mixed, or in remission.

Types

Bipolar mood disorder is classified in to

- **Bipolar I:** It is characterized by episode of severe mania and severe depression.
- **Bipolar II:** It is characterized by hypomania and severe depression.

Etiology

- Exact cause is unknown
- Genetic, biochemical and psychosocial causes may have a role
- Stressful life events
- Sleep deprivation and endocrine factors.

Treatment

- Lithium
- Valproic acid
- Carbamazepine
- Antidepressants
- Antipsychotics

Rapid Cycling Bipolar Disorder

This is characterized by alternating episodes (4 or more) of depression, mania or hypomania in the previous 12 months, separated by intervals of 48–72 hours. It is usually more

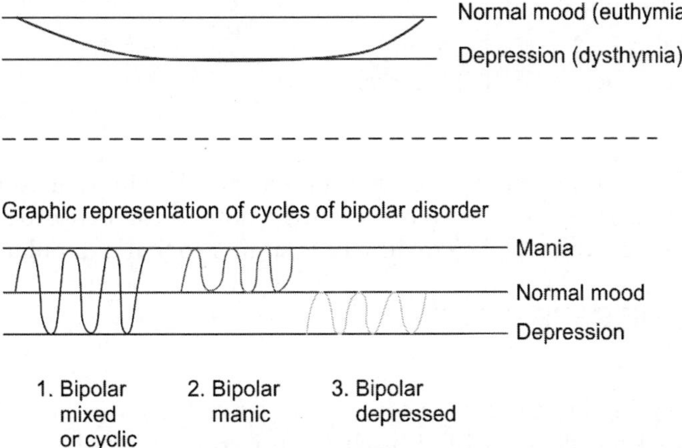

Fig. 7.3: Graphic representation of bipolar disorder

chronic than non-rapid cycling disorders. Around 80% are lithium-treatment failures. Carbamazepine or sodium valproate is usual agents of choice.

RECURRENT DEPRESSIVE DISORDER

This disorder is characterized by recurrent (at least two) depressive episodes (unipolar depression). The current episode may be mild, moderate, severe without psychotic symptoms, or severe with psychotic symptoms.

PERSISTENT MOOD DISORDER

These disorders are characterized by persistent mood symptoms which last for more than 2 years (1 year in children and adolescents) but are not severe enough to be labeled as even hypomanic or mild depressive episode.

If the symptoms consist of persistent mild depression, the disorder is called as *dysthymia*; and if symptoms consist of persistent instability of mood between mild depression and mild elation, the disorder is called as *cyclothymia*.

Dysthymia

Dysthymia was introduced in 1980. It was also called *'depressive neurosis/neurotic depression/ exogenous depression'* compared to major depression (psychotic or endogenous depression).

In this a mild depression that lasts for at least 2 years in adult and 1 year in children. It is twice common in women as in men.

Dysthymia/Neurotic depression is usually characterized by the following:

- Presence of mild to moderate depression.
- Depressive symptoms usually occur in response to a stressful situation.
- Other 'neurotic' symptoms such as anxiety, obsessive symptoms, phobic symptoms, and multiple somatic symptoms, are often present.
- The typical course of neurotic depression is chronic, with fluctuations.
- Delusions, hallucinations and other psychotic features are characteristically absent.

Treatment

- Short-term psychotherapy
- Behavioral therapy
- Group therapy
- Antidepressants such as SSRI, TCA, etc.

Cyclothymia

Less severe bipolar mood disorder with continuous mood swings; alternating periods of hypomania and moderate depression. It is non-psychotic chronic disorder. It starts in late adolescence or early adulthood. The treatment is similar to that of bipolar mood disorder.

OTHER TYPES OF DEPRESSION

Melancholia

Described by Kraeplin, this is a form of severe depression which occurs in the involutional period of life (i.e. 40–65 years of age). It is characterized by marked agitation, presence of psychotic features (such as delusions of persecution, tactile and auditory hallucinations) and multiple somatic symptoms (or hypochondriacal delusions).

Masked Depression

In masked depression, the depressive mood is not easily apparent and is usually hidden by somatic symptoms. This is especially common in the elderly, where the somatic symptoms range from chronic pain, insomnia, atypical facial pain, and paraesthesia. The depressive symptoms can also be masked by drug and/or alcohol misuse.

Double Depression

This is a major depressive episode superimposed on an underlying dysthymia or neurotic depression. The response to treatment is usually poor.

Agitated Depression

This is a type of severe depression with marked motor restlessness or agitation. It is either seen alone or along with involutional melancholia. It is more common after the age of 40 years.

Secondary Depression and Secondary Mania

Both depressive and manic episodes can occur secondary to certain physical diseases and drugs.

Substance-induced Mood Disorder

Characterized by prominent and persistent disturbance in mood that is judged to be a direct physiological consequence of a drug abuse, toxin exposure, or a medication.

Mixed Anxiety Depressive Disorder

This disorder is characterized by the presence of depressive and anxiety symptoms which result in significant distress or disability in the person. The symptoms should not meet the criteria of either an anxiety disorder or a mood disorder.

Seasonal Mood Disorder

This is either a bipolar mood disorder or recurrent depressive episode which tends to occur in the same season on each occasion. It is usually more commonly seen in women. For example the depression begins in the fall or winter, or when there is a decrease in sunlight. Mania would occur in the month of summer.

Seasonal affective disorder is characterized by atypical features of depression, hypersomnia, hyperphagia (carbohydrate craving), weight gain, and increased fatigue. This is related to abnormal melatonin metabolism. It can be treated with exposure to light (artificial light for 2–6 hours a day). It may occur as part of bipolar I or II disorders.

8 Nursing Management of Patient with Neurotic, Stress-Related and Somatization Disorders

Neurotic, stress-related, and somatoform disorders have common historical origin with the concept of neurosis and association of a substantial proportion of these disorders with psychological causation.

With the exception of social phobia their frequency is higher in women than in men.

Anxiety disorder is a blanket term covering several different forms of abnormal, pathological anxiety, fears, and phobias.

Anxiety and fear are ubiquitous emotions. The terms anxiety and fear have specific scientific meanings, but common usage has made them interchangeable.

Anxiety disorders are otherwise called neurotic disorders. They differ from psychotic disorders in some specific characteristics like:

- Distressing to person and unacceptable because of ego dystonia.
- Does not lose touch with reality.
- The symptoms tend to be relatively enduring or recurring unless effective treatment is obtained.
- Does not violate social norms or rules and regulations.
- There is no demonstrable organic etiology and are all functional.
- Differ from personality disorders with discrete onset rather than a continuous development from early life.

PSYCHOPATHOLOGY

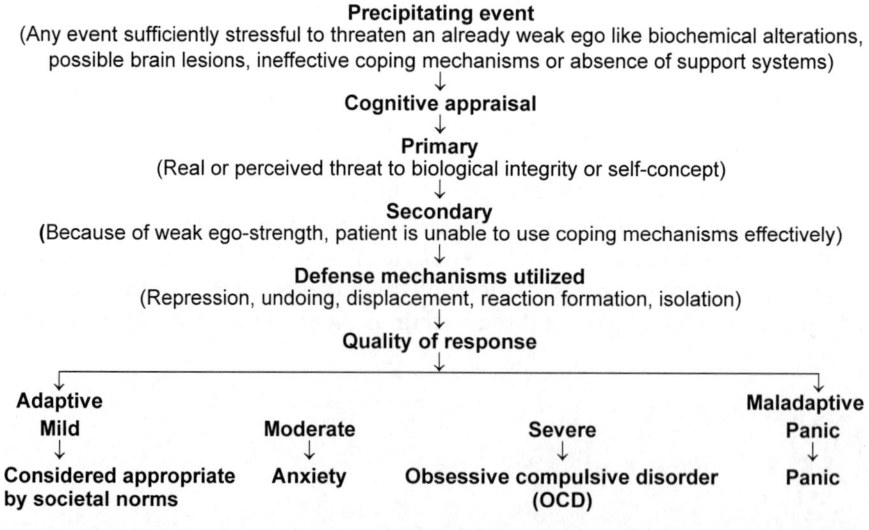

Precipitating event
(Any event sufficiently stressful to threaten an already weak ego like biochemical alterations, possible brain lesions, ineffective coping mechanisms or absence of support systems)
↓
Cognitive appraisal
↓
Primary
(Real or perceived threat to biological integrity or self-concept)
↓
Secondary
(Because of weak ego-strength, patient is unable to use coping mechanisms effectively)
↓
Defense mechanisms utilized
(Repression, undoing, displacement, reaction formation, isolation)
↓
Quality of response
↓

Adaptive			Maladaptive
Mild	**Moderate**	**Severe**	**Panic**
↓	↓	↓	↓
Considered appropriate by societal norms	**Anxiety**	**Obsessive compulsive disorder (OCD)**	**Panic**

Box 8.1: Role of neurotransmitters in mental illness

- Disturbances in serotonin, norepinephrine and gamma aminobutyric acid (GABA) appear to be most significant.
- Serotonin is thought to be decreased and norepinephrine is thought to be increased in anxiety disorders.
- GABA is decreased in anxiety disorders, allowing for increased cellular excitability.

Box 8.2: Core meaning

Neurotic disorder	Stress-related disorder	Somatization disorder
An emotional illness in which the person experiences strong feelings of fear or worry (a relatively mild mental illness that is not caused by organic diseases, involving symptoms of stress but not a loss of touch with reality).	Stress is a psychological process initiated by events that threaten, harm or challenge an organism or that exceed available coping resources and it is characterized by psychological response that are directed towards adaptation.	Somatization disorder is a psychiatric condition marked by multiple medically unexplained physical, or somatic symptoms which are serious enough to interfere significantly with a person's ability to perform important activities and leads the person to seek medical treatment.

Box 8.3: Understanding the concept between psychosis and neurosis

Specifications	Psychosis	Neurosis
Genetic factors	More important	Less important
Stressful life events	More	Less
Behavior	Severely affected	Not affected
Thinking and perception	Disturbed	Not disturbed
Judgment	Impaired	Intact
Insight	Lost	Present
Drugs	Major tranquilizers	Minor tranquilizers
Electroconvulsive therapy (ECT)	Very useful	Not needed
Prognosis	Bad	Good

Box 8.4: Tips to understand difference between normal fear and anxiety

Normal fear of an individual	Anxiety state of an individual
Fear is a state where in a person feels a strong sense of dread, with autonomic nervous system responses that are focused on a specific object or event like fear of a tornado, fear of surgery, fear of failing in a job.	Anxiety is a state where in a person feels a strong sense of dread, frequently accompanied by physical symptoms of increased heart rate, respiratory rate, elevated blood pressure (autonomic nervous system response), without having specific source or reason for the emotions.

Box 8.5: ICD-10 classification of neurotic, stress-related and somatization disorders (F40–F48)

F40. Phobic anxiety disorders
F41. Other anxiety disorders (simple anxiety disorder)
F42. Obsessive-compulsive disorder
F43. Reaction to severe stress, and adjustment disorders
F44. Dissociative (conversion) disorders
F45. Somatoform disorders
F48. Other neurotic disorders.

DESCRIPTION

Now we study above classified disorder one by one according to International classification of diseases (ICD)-10 classification in simple concept.

F40. PHOBIC ANXIETY DISORDER

Almost everyone has an irrational fear; for example, annual dental check-up. For most people, these fears are minor. But when fear becomes so severe and they cause tremendous anxiety and interfere with your normal life, they are called phobias or phobic anxiety disorders. The good news is that phobias can be managed and cured.

What is Phobic Anxiety Disorder or a Phobia?

A phobia is an intense fear of something that, in reality, poses little or no actual danger. Common phobias and fears include closed-in places, heights, highway driving, flying insects, snakes, and needles. Most phobias develop in childhood, but they also develop in adults. It includes 3 types:

1. F40.0: Agoraphobia
2. F40.1: Social phobias
3. F40.2: Specific phobias

Box 8.6: Classification and explanation of F40. phobic anxiety disorder

F40.0	**Agoraphobia**	Agoraphobia means extreme fear of open or public places. ***Definition:*** Agoraphobia is characterized by an irrational fear of being in places away from the familiar setting of home where escape is impossible. ***Signs and symptoms:*** • Fear of being alone in any situation • Fear of being in crowded places • Fear of losing control in public places • Fear of being in places where it may be hard to leave, such as an elevator or train • Inability to leave own home (housebound) • Fears of entering shops, crowds • Fear of traveling alone in trains, buses, underground or planes. ***Important considerations:*** • The avoidance behavior causes sometimes that the sufferer becomes completely housebound • Most sufferers are women. Onset—early adult life. • The lifetime prevalence—between 5–7%. • High comorbidity with panic disorder; depressive and obsessional symptoms and social phobias may be also present.
F40.1	**Social phobia (Now called social anxiety disorder)**	***Definition:*** Social phobia is the fear of interaction with other people that brings on self-consciousness, feelings of being negatively judged and evaluated and as a result leads to avoidance. ***Signs and symptoms:*** • Fear of being introduced to other people • Fear of being teased or criticized
		• Fear of being the center of attention • Fear of being watched while doing something • Fear of meeting well-known or important people • Fear of most social encounters, especially with strangers

Contd...

Contd...

		• Fear to public speaking, or to encounters with the opposite sex • Direct eye-to-eye confrontation may be stressful • Low self-esteem and fear of criticism. ***Physical symptoms accompany social phobia:*** • Intense fear • Racing heart • Excessive sweating and blushing (turning red) • Trembling (shaking of hands) and palpitations • Stammering along with rapid speech. ***Important considerations:*** • Symptoms may progress to panic attacks • Avoidance—almost complete social isolation • Usually start in childhood or adolescence • Lifetime prevalence—between 10–13 % • It is equally common in both sexes • Secondary to alcoholism.

F40.2	**Specific phobias (isolated)**	***Definition:***
		A specific phobia, formerly called as a simple phobia, is a lasting and unreasonable fear caused by presence or thought of a specific object or situation that usually poses little or no actual danger.
		Exposure to the object or situation brings an immediate reaction causing the person to get nervousness or to avoid the object or situation entirely.
		Common types of specific phobias:
		• **Fears to particular animals**
		  - Spiders (arachnophobia)
		  - Insects (entomophobia)
		  - Snakes (ophidiophobia)
		• **Fears of specific situations such as**
		  - Heights (acrophobia)
		  - Thunder (keraunophobia)
		  - Darkness (nyctophobia)
		  - Closed spaces (claustrophobia)
		• **Fears of diseases, injuries or medical examinations visiting a dentist:**
		  - The sight of blood (hemophobia) or injury (pain —odynophobia)
		  - The fear of exposure to venereal diseases
		  - AIDS-phobia or (syphilidophobia).
		Important considerartions:
		• Adults with specific phobia recognize that the fear is excessive or unreasonable, yet are unable to overcome it.
		• Usually arise in childhood or early adult life and can persist for decades if they remain untreated.
		Lifetime prevalence—between 10–20%.

Epidemiology

The lifetime prevalence of agoraphobia ranges from 0.6 to 6%. In community samples, half of the agoraphobic patients have panic disorder. Specific phobia is the most common mental disorder among women and the second most common in men.

The typical age of onset of phobias is usually in childhood and adolescence. The age of onset is earliest in animal phobias, intermediate in social phobias and latest in agoraphobia.

Patients with social phobia have an increased rate of suicidal ideation, financial dependency and having sought medical treatment.

Etiology

They are often linked to frightening event or stressful situation. However, it is not always clear why some phobias occur. There are various assumptions which explain reason behind phobic anxiety disorder. They are:

Neurobiological Causes

Some areas of the brain—the prefrontal cortex, medial prefrontal cortex and amygdale store and recall dangerous or potentially deadly events. In future occasions, if a very similar event is confronted those areas retrieve that same memory and body reacts if there were a recurrence.

Behavioral Factors

Stimulus response model

Anxiety is aroused by a naturally frightening stimulus that occurs when two stimuli are paired on several occasions; the originally neutral stimulus takes on the capacity to arouse anxiety by itself. The neutral stimulus, therefore, becomes a conditioned stimulus for anxiety production.

Operant conditioning theory

In the classic stimulus response theory, the conditioned stimulus gradually loses its potency to arouse a response, if it is not reinforced by a periodic symptoms, the attenuation of the response to the phobic stimulus (i.e. de-conditioning of stimulus) does not occur. The symptom may last for years without any apparent external reinforcement.

Psychoanalytic theories

According to the psychoanalytic theory, the major function of anxiety is a signal to the ego, that a forbidden unconscious drive is pushing for conscious expression, thus altering the ego to strengthen and marshal its defences against the threatening instinctual force.

In social and specific phobia, the conflict is regarding sexual arousal, leading to castration anxiety. When repression fails to be entirely successful, the ego must call on auxiliary defences. These defences in social and specific phobia are of displacement, symbolization and avoidance. In agoraphobia, it is the separation anxiety playing a central role.

Genetic-environmental factors

Genetic and environmental factors can cause phobias. Children who have a close relative with an anxiety disorder are at risk for developing a phobia.

Other Possible Causes of Certain Phobias

Simple phobias can often be linked to an early negative childhood experience. For example, if during childhood trapped in a confined space, he/she may develop a fear of enclosed spaces (claustrophobia) when grow older.

It is also thought that phobias can sometimes be 'learnt' from an early age. For example, if someone in family has a fear of spiders (arachnophobia), same fear also develops in another person of the family.

Treatment

Treatment for phobias can involve therapeutic techniques, medications, or a combination of both.

Psychotherapy

Talking with a trained mental health professional can help to deal with phobias. Several types of psychotherapy, also called talk therapy, may be effective.

- **Desensitization or exposure therapy:** Focuses on changing the response to the object or situation that one fear and may be helpful for phobias. Gradual, repeated exposure to the cause of phobia may help the patient, learn to conquer anxiety. For example, if patient afraid of elevators, therapy may progress from simply thinking about getting into an elevator, to looking at pictures of elevators, to going near an elevator, to stepping into an elevator. Next, to take a one-floor ride, then ride several floors and then ride in a crowded elevator.

Example: Systematic desensitization therapy model for patient having fear of dog.

Box 8.7: Facing a fear of dog: Climbing a fear ladder
• **Step 1:** Look at pictures of dogs.
• **Step 2:** Watch a video with dogs in it.
• **Step 3:** Look at a dog through a window.
• **Step 4:** Stand across the street from a dog on a leash.
• **Step 5:** Stand 10 feet away from a dog on a leash.
• **Step 6:** Stand five feet away from a dog on a leash.
• **Step 7:** Stand beside a dog on a leash.
• **Step 8:** Pet a small dog that someone is holding.
• **Step 9:** Pet a larger dog on a leash.
• **Step 10:** Pet a larger dog off leash.

- **Flooding:** Prolonged exposure to a fearful situation or experience.

Cognitive Behavioral Therapy

Cognitive behavioral therapy (CBT) is the most commonly used therapeutic treatment for phobias. It involves exposure to the source of the fear, but in a controlled setting. This treatment can de-condition people and reduce anxiety.

The therapy focuses on identifying and changing negative thoughts, dysfunctional beliefs, and negative reactions to fear. New CBT techniques use virtual reality technology to safely expose people to the sources of their phobias.

Medical Management

Antidepressants and anti-anxiety medications can help both emotional and physical reactions to fear.

- **Beta blockers:** These medications work by blocking the stimulating effects of adrenaline on body, such as increased heart rate, elevated blood pressure, pounding heart, and shaking voice and limbs that are caused by anxiety. Short-term use of beta blockers can be effective in decreasing symptoms when taken before an anticipated event. For example, before a performance for people who have severe stage fright.
- **Antidepressants:** Antidepressants called selective serotonin reuptake inhibitors (SSRIs) like ***celexa, paxil, prozac, lexapro, and zoloft*** are commonly used in the treatment of phobias. These medications act on the chemical serotonin, a neurotransmitter in brain that believed to influence mood.
- **Sedatives or anti-anxiety drugs:** Medications called benzodiazepines help to relax by reducing the amount of anxiety one feel. Sedatives need to be used with caution because they can be addictive and should be avoided if history of alcohol or drug dependence present.

Box 8.8: Treatment choices: Treatment depends on the type of phobia

- Specific phobias usually are treated with exposure therapy.
- Social phobias may be treated with exposure therapy or with anti- depressants or beta blockers.
- Agoraphobia, especially when it's accompanied by a panic disorder, is usually treated with exposure therapy or with SSRIs.

Nursing Management

(N.B: Nursing management explained below is common for all neurotic, stress related and somatoform disorder and care plan is separately given under each condition**).**

The application of nursing process for neurotic, stress-related and somatoform disorder is discussed below:

Assessment

Patient Should be Assessed for

- Anticipatory anxiety (when thinking about the phobic object)
- Panic anxiety (when confronted with the phobic object)
- Avoidance behaviors that interfere with relationships or social or occupational functioning
- Recognition of the phobia as irrational
- Embarrassment over the phobic fear.

The nurse collects a database regarding the client. This step is very important because without an accurate assessment, problem identification, objectives of care and outcome criteria cannot be accurately determined. Data may be obtained from family members, from old records, or from other individuals familiar with patient.

Nursing Diagnosis

Appropriate nursing diagnoses will be formulated according to the data collected from the patient. The possible nursing diagnoses are;

- Fear related to perceived threat that is consciously recognized as a danger (e.g. fear of being alone in public places, snakes, spiders, dark, heights, stormy weather) evidenced by physiologic symptoms.
- Anxiety [severe to panic] related to unidentified stressor(s) contact with feared object/situation evidenced by physical, mental, and cognitive behaviors indicative of panic.
- Social isolation related to morbid fear to be in public places, open places and fear to interact with other people as evidenced by staying alone and refuse to leave room or home.
- Powerlessness may be related to: Real or perceived threat to physical integrity or self-concept (may or may not be able to identify the threat) evidenced by persistent feelings of apprehension and uneasiness.
- Coping related to: Level of anxiety being experienced by client evidenced by maladaptive coping skills.
- Risk for ineffective role performance related to psychological stress evidenced by repetitive uncontrollable obsession behaviors.
- Disturbed sleep pattern related to psychologic stress (anxiety, depression with recurring disruptive dreams) evidenced by verbal reports of difficulty in falling asleep, reports of sleep disturbances (e.g. nightmares, dreams of personal death, disaster-related dreams, flashbacks, intrusive/trauma images, fear of re-experiencing the event).
- Disturbed thought processes related to Psychological conflict, threat to physical integrity/self-concept evidenced by memory loss/deficit, inability to recall selected events.
- Risk for violence, directed at self/others related to dissociative state/conflicting personalities evidenced by increased motor activity, pacing, excitement, irritability, agitation.
- Disturbed personal identity related to psychological conflicts (dissociative state[s]), memory loss (unable to recall selected events/own identity) as evidenced by presence of more than one personality within the individual.

Planning

Despite the differences among the anxiety disorders, the major goals for nursing care have applicability to each of them. These goals are concerned primarily with the client learning about anxiety and how to cope with it. They are:

- To accept the experience of anxiety as inevitable and normal.
- To increase self-awareness with regard to fluctuations in anxiety level.
- To reduce shame about exhibiting signs of anxiety.
- To learn and apply self-help techniques designed to reduce anxiety.
- To increase problem-solving and coping skills.

Intervention

To help the client reach the planned goals, the nurse needs to establish a supportive relationship with the client. This relationship is establishing trust, respect, and empathy on the client by nurse. Intervention of anxiety disorders depend on the nursing diagnosis of each types of anxiety disorder which is explained under each types of anxiety disorder.

Evaluation

Evaluation or reassessment is conducted to assess the effectiveness of nursing care. The extent to which nursing care for client's anxiety disorder is effective is based on the client's subjective report of his/her feelings state as well as change in the client's behavior. Behavior changes indicating improvement, such as decreased muscular tension and tremors, normal physiological functions, and increased attention span and concentration, may be first signs that the client has begun to improve. Additionally, the reduction of cardinal symptoms associated with anxiety disorders and their replacement with adaptive behavior indicates improvement.

Box 8.9: Nursing process for phobic anxiety disorder

Nursing diagnosis: Fear related to perceived threat that is consciously recognized as a danger (e.g. fear of being alone in public places, snakes, spiders, dark, heights, stormy weather) evidenced by physiologic symptoms.

Outcome identification	Nursing intervention
• Client will be able to: – Verbalize feelings of fear and discomfort – Demonstrate understanding through use of effective coping behaviors.	• Allow the client to express feelings openly. • Provide for client's safety (e.g. secure environments, staying with the client, letting the client know the nurse will provide for safety). • Discuss the process of thinking about the feared object/situation before it occurs. • Encourage to stop, wait, and not rush out of feared situation as soon as experienced. Support use of relaxation exercises (e.g. breath control, muscle relaxation, self-hypnosis). • Explore things that may lower fear level and keep it manageable (e.g. use of singing while dressing, practicing positive self-talk while in a fearful situation). • Expose client to a predetermined list of anxiety-provoking stimuli rated in hierarchy from the least frightening to the most frightening. • Pair each anxiety-producing stimulus (e.g. standing in an elevator) with arousal of another affect of an opposite quality (e.g. relaxation, exercise, biofeedback) strong enough to suppress anxiety. • Administer antianxiety medications as indicated: BZDs, e.g. alprazolam (Xanax), clonazepam (Klonopin), diazepam (Valium), lorazepam.

Nursing diagnosis: Disturbed sleep related to psychological stress as evidenced by reports of difficulty in falling sleep and not feeling rested.

Contd...

Contd...

Outcome identification	Nursing intervention
• Client will be able to: – Verbalize understanding of relationship of anxiety and sleep disturbance. – Report improvement in sleep pattern, increased sense of well-being, and feeling well-rested.	• Determine type of sleep pattern disturbance present, including usual bedtime, rituals/routines, number of hours of sleep, • Provide quiet environment, comfort measures (e.g. back rub, wash hands/face, bath), and sleep aids, such as warm milk. • Discuss use of relaxation techniques/thoughts, visualization. • Involve client in exercise program, avoiding exercise within 2 hour of going to bed. • Avoid use of sedatives, when possible. • Administer medications as indicated, e.g. zolpidem (Ambien).
Nursing diagnosis: Social isolation related to morbid fear to be in public places, open places and fear to interact with other people as evidenced by staying alone and refuse to leave room or home.	
Outcome identification	**Nursing intervention**
• Client will be able to: – Voluntarily attends activities alone. – Verbalizes signs and symptoms of escalating anxiety. – Demonstrates techniques to disrupt escalating anxiety	• Convey acceptance and unconditional positive regard. • Attend activities with client. • Be cautious with touch. • Administer tranquilizers. • Discuss signs and symptoms of increasing anxiety and ways to intervene. • Give recognition for voluntary interactions with others.

F41. OTHER ANXIETY DISORDERS (SIMPLE ANXIETY DISORDER)

Disorders in which manifestation of anxiety is the major symptom and is not restricted to any particular environmental situation. Depressive and obsession symptoms, and even some elements of phobic anxiety, may also be present, proved that they are clearly secondary or less severe.

Box 8.10: Further classification
F41.0: Panic disorder [episodic paroxysmal anxiety] without agoraphobia
F41.1: Generalized anxiety disorder
F41.2: Other mixed anxiety disorders
F41.3: Other specified anxiety disorders
F41.4: Anxiety disorder, unspecified

F41.0: Panic Disorder without Agoraphobia

Definition

Panic disorder is characterized by recurrent attacks of severe anxiety (panic attacks), which are not restricted to any particular situation or set of circumstances and are therefore unpredictable.

Epidemiology

- Lifetime prevalence estimates range from 1.5–5% for panic disorder and 3–5.6% for panic attacks
- Women are more likely to be affected than men by a 2–3 fold factor
- Highest incidence is in late adolescence and second peak in mid 30s.

Etiological Factors

Biological

Major neurotransmitter systems involved are:

Box 8.11: Major neurotransmitter systems involved

System	Panic-inducer
Noradrenergic	Yohimbine
Serotonergic d-	Fenfluramine
GABA	Flumazenil

- **Genetic factors:** The concordance rate in monozygotic twins of patients with panic disorder is 80%.
- **Biochemical factors:** (reduction in GABA activity in brain).
- **Brain abnormality:** Malfunctioning of brain structure such as amyldala and hormonal/ adrenaline glands.
- **Brain imaging:**
  - PET scanning shows abnormal increases in right para-hippocampal area
  - Increased blood flow
  - Increased blood volume
  - Increased O_2 metabolism.

Psychosocial

- **Separation:** There is an increase in frequency of separation of parents and separation from mother before the age of 17 in patients with panic disorder.
- **Cognitive Behavioral:** Theories states that anxiety is a learned response and the genesis and maintenance of panic attacks is explained by a combination of classical conditioning and the negative catastrophic thoughts that patients have during attacks.
- **Psychoanalytical models:** This model view panic attacks as arising from unsuccessful attempts to defend against anxiety provoking impulses.
- **Medical conditions**: Hypoglycemia, hyperthyroidism, mitral valve prolapse, labirinthitis can aggravate panic disorder.
- **Stressful life events**: Life transitions and environment play a role in the onset of panic disorder.

Clinical Features

- Sudden onset of palpitations
- Chest pain, choking sensation
- Sweating

- Trembling or shaking
- Sensation of shortness of breath
- Feeling of choking
- Nausea/butterflies
- Dizziness/light headedness
- Derealization/depersonalization
- Fear of losing control
- Fear of dying
- Paraesthesia
- Chills or hot flushes.

Associated Symptoms

- There is often also a secondary fear of dying, losing control, or going mad.
- Individual attacks usually last for minutes only. The frequency of attacks varies substantially.
- Frequent and predictable panic attacks produce fear of being alone or going into public places.
- The afflicted persons used to think that they got a serious somatic disease.

Box 8.12: Diagnostic criteria

In order to make a diagnosis of panic disorder, the patient should have experienced at least three panic attacks within a three week period. The attacks should occur:
- In circumstances where there is no objective danger
- Without being confined to known or predictable situations
- With comparative freedom from anxiety symptoms between attacks (although anticipatory anxiety is common)

Management

Psychological

Cognitive Behavioral Therapy: Combines both exposure to the feared stimulus with relaxation, and work around the patient's false cognition and giving information about the panic attack.

Pharmacotherapy

Antidepressants of most classes are useful in the treatment of panic disorder.

The most frequently used are:

- Imipramine, Clomipramine
- Fluoxetine, Phenelzine, Venlafaxine
- They should be given at least 8 to 12 weeks to exert their full effects and be continued for 8 to 12 months.

Benzodiazepines may also be useful adjuncts to treatment, especially during the initial phase of antidepressant treatment.

- Alprazolam
- Lorazapam: 0.5 -1 mg IV/ IM, 1-2 mg PO bid.
- Clonazepam (Klonopin) 0.5-2 mg: bid/tid.

Box 8.13: Psychotherapy: subtypes for panic disorder

- CBT
- Psychodynamic psychotherapy
- Relaxation techniques
- Respiratory techniques

F41.1: Generalized Anxiety Disorder

Definition

It is a common chronic disorder characterized by long lasting anxiety that is not focused on any one subject or situation.

The essential feature is anxiety lasting more than 6 months, which is generalized and persistent but not restricted to, or even strongly predominating in, any particular environmental circumstances. (I.e. it is 'free-floating').

Epidemiology

The estimation of lifetime prevalence moves between 4-6%. Onset is usually from childhood to late adulthood.

This disorder is more common in women, and often related to chronic environmental stress.

Etiology

Biological

- **Genetic causes:** Some twin studies report a monozygotic concordance of 50%, and a dizygotic concordance of 15%. About 25% of first degree relatives of sufferers have Generalized anxiety disorder (GAD).
- **Autonomic nervous system:** James Lange theory states that subjective anxiety is a response to peripheral phenomena. Stimulation of autonomic nervous system causes cardiovascular, respiratory and GI symptoms.
- **Norepinephrine (NE):** Studies have found that, in patients with panic disorder, adrenergic agonists (isoproterenol) and adrenergic antagonists (yohimbine) can produce frequent and severe panic attacks.

Psychosocial

- **Cognitive behavioral theories** suggest that GAD arises from selective attention being given to negative details in the environment, by distortions in information processing, and by an overly negative view of one's ability to cope.
- **Psychoanalytical models** hypothesize that anxiety is a symptom of unresolved unconscious conflicts.
- **Environmental factors** (such as loss of a parent, stressful events, changing jobs or schools.) contribute a higher vulnerability for the development of generalized anxiety disorder than other disorders, such as panic disorder.

Use and withdrawal from addictive substances, alcohol, caffeine, nicotine, etc. can worsen anxiety.

Clinical Feature

- Continuous feelings of nervousness
- Trembling
- Muscular tension
- Sweating
- Lightheadedness
- Palpitations
- Dizziness
- Epigastric discomfort.

Its course uses to be fluctuating and chronic connected with symptoms of frustration, sadness and complicated with abuse of alcohol and other illicit drugs.

Management

Pharmacotherapy

- **Benzodiazepines (valium, librium)** are often useful in the short-term or to allow patients to cope with the psychotherapeutic approaches.
- **Antidepressants** including Imipramine and the SSRIs are often useful.
- Buspirone, a 5-HT1A agonist is effective in around 60–80% of patients (More effective on the cognitive than somatic symptoms.)

Psychological

- **Cognitive behavioral therapy:** Addresses both the distorted negative thought processes and some of the somatic symptoms directly, through relaxation and biofeedback.
- **Supportive therapy** has doubtful long term clinical efficacy, although patients report a lessening of their anxiety if they can discuss their worries with a sympathetic individual.

F41.2 Mixed Anxiety and Depressive Disorder

This category should be used when symptoms of anxiety and depression are both present, but neither is clearly predominant, and neither type of symptom is present to the extent that justifies a diagnosis if considered separately.

(N.B: *When both anxiety and depressive symptoms are present and severe enough to justify individual diagnoses, both diagnoses should be recorded and this category should not be used.***)**

F41.3: Other Mixed Anxiety Disorder

This category should be used for disorders that meet the criteria for generalized anxiety disorder (F 41.1) and also have prominent features of other disorders in F40–F49, although the full criteria for these additional disorders are not met.

Nursing Management

Box 8.14: Nursing process for other anxiety disorder (simple anxiety disorder)

Nursing diagnosis: Anxiety [severe to panic] related to unidentified stressor(s) contact with feared object/situation evidenced by physical, mental, and cognitive behaviors indicative of panic.

Contd...

Contd...

Outcome identification	Nursing intervention
• Client will be able to: – Verbalize a reduction in anxiety to a manageable level.	• Establish and maintain a trusting relationship by listening to the client; displaying warmth, answering questions directly, offering unconditional acceptance; being available and respecting the client's use of personal space. • Be aware and in control of own feelings; explore the cause of own anxiety and use this understanding therapeutically. • Provide simple, clear explanations and instructions. • Verbally acknowledge the reality of the pain of the client's present coping mechanism (panic) without focusing on the symptoms that are being expressed. • Provide feedback about behavior, stressors, and coping responses. Validate what you observe with the client. • Observe for increasing anxiety. Assume a calm manner, decrease environmental stimulation, and provide temporary isolation as indicated. • Identify signs/symptoms of escalating anxiety and appropriate responses (e.g. relaxation, stopping negative self-talk). • Administer medication as indicated • Refer client/family to counseling, psychotherapy, or groups as indicated.
Nursing diagnosis: Anxiety [severe]/powerlessness related to real or perceived threat to physical integrity or self-concept (may or may not be able to identify the threat) evidenced by persistent feelings of apprehension and uneasiness.	
Outcome identification	**Nursing intervention**
• Client will be able to: – Verbalize awareness of feelings of anxiety. – Identify effective coping mechanisms to successfully deal with stress.	• Establish and maintain a trusting relationship through the use of warmth, empathy, and respect. • Be aware of any negative or anxious feelings nurse may have because of client's conscious or unconscious resistance of nurse's helpful efforts. • Help to explore conflictual issues by beginning with nonthreatening topics and progressing to more conflict-laden ones. • Monitor the anxiety level of the nurse/client interaction on an ongoing basis. • Explore how client dealt with anxiety in the past and what methods produced relief. Encourage use of adaptive coping responses that have worked in the past. • Encourage and support more realistic thoughts (e.g. 'I do not know for certain that [blank] will happen.' 'Whatever happens, I can manage.' 'I will delay worrying for now and think about something calming.' • Encourage client to use relaxation techniques (e.g. meditation, massage, breathing techniques, exercises, guided imagery, and biofeedback). • Administer medication as indicated, e.g. buspirone (BuSpar), benzodiazepines (BZDs), e.g. alprazolam (Xanax), clonazepam (Klonopin), diazepam .

Contd...

Contd...

Nursing diagnosis: Ineffective coping related to level of anxiety being experienced by client evidenced by maladaptive coping skills.	
Outcome identification	**Nursing intervention**
• Client will be able to: – Identify ineffective coping behaviors and consequences – Use effective problem-solving techniques.	• Assess current functional capacity, developmental level of functioning, and level of coping. • Determine defence mechanisms used (e.g. denial, repression, conversion, dissociation, reaction formation, undoing, displacement or projection). • Identify previous methods of coping with life problems. • Help client identify maladaptive effects of present coping mechanisms. • Provide information about different ways to deal with situations that promote anxious feelings • Emphasize importance of structuring life to provide adequate exercise/sleep, diversional activities, and nutrition. • Refer to outside resources (e.g. support groups, psychotherapy/counselor, spiritual advisor, sexual counseling) as indicated.

F42. OBSESSIVE COMPULSIVE DISORDER

Many of us occasionally have to go back and double-check that an iron is unplugged or the car door is locked. But for sufferers of obsessive-compulsive disorder (OCD), obsessive thoughts and compulsive behaviors become so excessive that they interfere with daily lives. And no matter what they do, just can not seem to shake them.

What is Obsession and Compulsion Disorder (OCD)?

Obsessive compulsive disorder is an anxiety disorder characterized by uncontrollable, unwanted thoughts and repetitive, ritualized behaviors one feels compelled to perform. Person with OCD, probably recognize that obsessive thoughts and compulsive behaviors are irrational but even so, he feel unable to resist them.

Meaning and Definition

The *DSM IV TR* describes obsessive-compulsive disorder (OCD) as recurrent obsessions or compulsions that are severe enough to be time consuming or to cause marked distress or significant impairment (APA, 2000).

The individual recognizes that the behavior is excessive or unreasonable but, because of the feeling of relief from discomfort that it promotes, he or she is compelled to continue the act. The most common compulsions involve washing and cleaning, counting, checking, requesting or demanding assurances, repeating actions, and ordering (APA, 2000).

Understanding Meaning Between Obsessions and Compulsion

OBSESSION
Obsessions are ideas, images or impulses that enter the individual's mind again and again in a stereotyped form. They are recognized as the individual's own thoughts, even though they are involuntary. Common obsessions include fears of contamination, of harming other persons or sinning against God.

Contd...

Contd...

COMPULSION

Compulsions are repetitive, purposeful, and intentional behaviors or mental acts performed in response to obsessions. Compulsions are meant to neutralize or reduce discomfort or to prevent a dreaded event or situation.

Compulsions are performed in an attempt to make obsessions go away. For example if person afraid of contamination, he might develop elaborate cleaning rituals. However, the relief never lasts. In fact, the obsessive thoughts usually come back stronger, and the compulsive behaviors often end up causing anxiety themselves as they become more time-consuming.

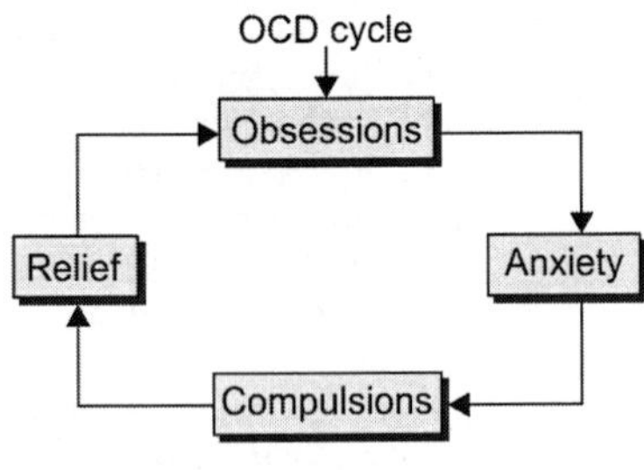

Fig. 8.1: OCD cycle

Abbreviation: OCD = Obsessive–compulsive disorder.

Most People with Obsessive-Compulsive Disorder (OCD) Fall into One of the Following Categories

Box 8.15:

- **Washers** are afraid of contamination. They usually have cleaning or handwashing compulsions.
- **Checkers** repeatedly check things (oven turned off, door locked, etc.) that they associate with harm or danger.
- **Doubters and sinners** are afraid that if everything is not perfect or done just right something terrible will happen or they will be punished.
- **Counters and arrangers** are obsessed with order and symmetry. They may have superstitions about certain numbers, colors, or arrangements.
- **Hoarders** fear that something bad will happen if they throw anything away. They compulsively hoard things that they do not need or use.

Box 8.16: Common examples of obsessive-compulsive disorder (OCD)

Common obsessions	Common compulsions
Contamination fears of germs, dirt, etc.	Washing
Imagining having harmed self or others	Repeating
Imagining losing control of aggressive urges	Checking
Intrusive sexual thoughts or urges	Touching
Excessive religious or moral doubt	Counting
Forbidden thoughts	Ordering/arranging
A need to have things *'just so'*	Hoarding or saving
A need to tell, ask, confess	Praying

Epidemiology

- More common in unmarried males.
- Age of onset in India is late 20s and in the western countries the onset is usually earlier in life.
- Life-time prevalence of OCD is 2–3% high, though the Indian data shows a lower prevalence rate.
- Equally common among men and women.

Etiological Factors

Biological causes

- **Genetics:** Higher in monozygotic twins than for dizygotic twins. 35% of the first degree relatives of OCD patients are affected.
- **Medical illnesses** like encephalitis, basal ganglia lesions, tourette's syndrome causes OCD.
- **Neurotransmitters:** Abnormalities in serotonin level.
- **Brain Imaging:** CT and MRI show increase in ventricular-brain ratio.

Behavior Theory

Compulsions have been described as learned behavior that decreases the anxiety associated with obsessions. This decrease in anxiety positively reinforces the compulsive acts and they become stable learned behavior.

Signs and Symptoms

Most people with obsessive-compulsive disorder (OCD) have both obsessions and compulsions, but some people experience just one or the other.

Obsessive Thoughts

- Fear of being contaminated by germs or dirt or contaminating others.
- Fear of causing harm to oneself or others.
- Intrusive sexually explicit or violent thoughts and images.
- Excessive focus on religious or moral ideas.
- Fear of losing or not having things might need.
- Order and symmetry: The idea that everything must line up 'just right.'
- Superstitions; excessive attention to something considered lucky or unlucky.

Compulsive Behaviors

Common compulsive behaviors in obsessive-compulsive disorder (OCD) include:

- Excessive double-checking of things, such as locks, appliances, and switches.
- Repeatedly checking in on loved ones to make sure they're safe.
- Counting, tapping, repeating certain words, or doing other senseless things to reduce anxiety.
- Spending a lot of time washing or cleaning.
- Ordering or arranging things 'just so.'

- Praying excessively or engaging in rituals triggered by religious fear.
- Accumulating 'junk' such as old newspapers or empty food containers.

Treatment

The most effective treatment for obsessive-compulsive disorder is often cognitive-behavioral therapy.

Antidepressants are sometimes used in conjunction with therapy, although medication alone is rarely effective in relieving the symptoms of OCD.

Psychological

Cognitive behavioral therapy is more effective than pharmacotherapy for OCD:

Involves Two Components

- *Exposure and response prevention:* Involves repeated exposure to the source of obsession. Then patient asked to refrain from the compulsive behavior that he usually perform to reduce anxiety. **For example,** if patient is a compulsive hand washer, he might be asked to touch the door handle in a public restroom and then be prevented from washing. As he sits with the anxiety, the urge to wash hands will gradually begin to go away on its own. In this way, the patient learns that he does not need the ritual to get rid of anxiety and feel that he has some control over obsessive thoughts and compulsive behaviors.
- *Cognitive therapy:* A big part of cognitive therapy for OCD is teaching healthy and effective ways of responding to obsessive thoughts, without resorting to compulsive behavior.

Pharmacotherapy

Antidepressants influencing the central serotoninergic system:

- Selective Serotonin Reuptake Inhibitors (SSRIs): ***Clomipramine, Fluvoxamine and fluoxetine.***
- Tricyclic anti-depressants
- Benzodiazepines
- Atypical-antipsychotics

Higher doses of the drugs are required to treat OCD than depression, and response is often delayed.

(Effective in approx. 50–80% of OCD patients.)

Family Therapy for OCD Treatment

Because OCD often causes problems in family life and social adjustment, family therapy can often be beneficial. Family therapy promotes understanding of the disorder and can help reduce family conflicts.

Group Therapy

Through interaction with fellow OCD sufferers, group therapy provides support and encouragement and decreases feelings of isolation.

Psychosurgery

- Still indicated for severe, intractable OCD
- Most common operation is ***stereotactic cingulotomy:*** Produces symptomatic improvement in about 65%
- **Subcaudate tractotomy** is also used.

Nursing Management

Box 8.17: Nursing process for obsessive compulsive disorder (OCD)

Nursing diagnosis: Anxiety [severe] related to earlier life conflicts (may be reflected in the nature of the repetitive actions and recurring thoughts) evidenced by repetitive action (e.g. handwashing) recurring thoughts (e.g. dirt and germs) and decreased social and role functioning.

Outcome identification	Nursing intervention
• Client will be able to: – Demonstrate ability to cope effectively with stressful situations without resorting to obsessive thoughts or compulsive behaviors	• Establish relationship through use of empathy, warmth, and respect. • Use a relaxed manner with the client; keep the environment calm. • Assist client to teach stress management (e.g. thought-stopping, relaxation exercises, imagery). • Give positive reinforcement for non-compulsive behavior. • Avoid reinforcing compulsive behavior. • Assist client to find ways to set limits on own behaviors. At the same time allow adequate time during the daily routine for the ritual(s). • Limit the amount of time allotted for the performance of rituals. Encourage client to gradually decrease this time. • Administer medications as indicated.

Nursing diagnosis: Risk for ineffective role performance related to psychological stress evidenced by repetitive uncontrollable obsession behaviors.

Outcome identification	Nursing intervention
• Client will be able to: – Identify conflicts within work/family situations.	• Determine client's role within family and extent to which illness-related thoughts and actions affect role relationships. • Discuss client's perceptions of role, how obsessive-compulsive behaviors affect role, and whether perceptions are realistic. • Explore options for changes or adjustments in role and practice behaviors using role-play. • Provide positive reinforcement for movement toward resuming role responsibilities and decreasing ritualistic behaviors.

F43. REACTION TO SEVERE STRESS AND ADJUSTMENT DISORDERS

This category includes disorders, identifiable on the basis of one or other of two causative influences:

1. An exceptionally stressful life event producing an acute stress reaction.
2. A significant life change leading to continued unpleasant circumstances that result in an adjustment disorder.

(Individual vulnerability and coping capacity play an important role in the occurrence and form of this disorder.)

Classification

F 43.0: Acute Stress Reaction
F 43.1: Post Traumatic Stress Disorder
F43.2: Adjustment Disorder

Etiology

Psychodynamic Factor

The client's ego has experienced a severe trauma, often perceived as a threat to physical integrity or self-concept. This results in severe anxiety, which is not controlled adequately by the ego and is manifested in symptomatic behavior.

Biologic

Some studies have revealed abnormalities in the storage, release, and elimination of catecholamines affecting function of the brain in the region of the locus coeruleus, amygdala, and hippocampus. Hypersensitivity in the locus coeruleus may lead to 'learned helplessness.' The amygdala appears to be the storehouse for memories, whereas the hippocampus provides narrative coherence and a location in time and space. Hyperactivation in the amygdala may prevent the brain from making coherent sense of its memories resulting in the memories being stored as nightmares, flashbacks, and physical symptoms.

Box 8.18: More to know

Research is exploring the possibility of a genetic vulnerability including the belief neurologic disturbances in the womb or during childhood may influence the development of Post traumatic stress disorder (PTSD).

Family Dynamics

Types of formal education, family life, and lifestyle are significant forecasters of PTSD. Below average or lack of success in education, negative parenting behaviors, and parental poverty have been identified as predictors for development of PTSD.
Explanation of each disorder

F43.0: ACUTE STRESS REACTION

A transient disorder of significant severity which develops in an individual without any other apparent mental disorder, in response to physical and/or mental stress and which usually subsides within hours or days.

The stressor may be traumatic experience involving serious threat to the security or physical integrity of the individual or of a loved person, (natural catastrophe, accident, criminal assault, etc.) or an unusually sudden and threatening change in social position, or network.

Clinical Features

There must be an immediate and clear connection between the impact of an stressor and the onset of symptoms.

Depression, anxiety, anger, despair, over activity, and withdrawal may all be seen, but no one type of symptom predominates for long.

Duration

Resolve rapidly (within a few hours at the most) in those cases where removal from the stressful environment is possible; in cases where the stress continues the symptoms usually begin to diminish after 24–48 hours and are usually minimal after about 3 days.

Treatment

The condition is self-limiting and therefore supportive treatment is all that is required.

F 43.1: POST-TRAUMATIC STRESS DISORDER

Definition

Post-traumatic stress disorder (PTSD) is an anxiety disorder caused by very stressful, frightening or distressing events which recollects the traumatic event through nightmares and flashbacks, and causes feelings of isolation, irritability and guilt.

Incidence

About 25% exposed to potentially traumatic event develop PTSD.

Conditions which causes PTSD

- Natural or manmade disaster
- Serious accident
- Being a victim of terrorism, rape or other crime
- Military combat
- Being held hostage.

Signs and Symptoms

Fall into three categories:

- **Re-experiencing** of the traumatic event characterized by:
  - Recurrent and intrusive distressing recollections of the event, including images, thoughts, and perceptions.
  - Recurrent distressing dreams of the event.
  - Acting or feeling as if the event was reoccurring.
- **Persistent avoidance of stimuli***:* Associated with the trauma evidenced by:
  - Efforts to avoid thoughts, feelings, or conversations associated with the trauma.
  - Efforts to avoid activities, places, or people that arouse recollections of the trauma.
  - Inability to recall an important aspect of the trauma.

  - Markedly diminished interest or participation in significant activities and a feeling of detachment from others.
  - Restricted range of affect, and a sense of foreshortened future ('doom').
- **Persistent symptoms of increased arousal:** Characterized by:
  - Difficulty falling or staying asleep
  - Irritability or outbursts of anger
  - Hypervigilance
  - Difficulty concentrating
  - Exaggerated startle response.

Box 8.19: Diagnostic guidelines
The disorder should arise within 6 months of a traumatic event of exceptional severity.
There must be a repetitive, intrusive recollection ('flashbacks') or re-enactment of the event in memories, daytime imagery, or dreams.

Etiology

Biological

- Increased autonomic arousal
- Reduced hippocampal volume on MRI scan
- Nor dysfunction may underlie recurrent memories/ flashbacks in PTSD.

Psychological

- The ***cognitive model*** holds that sufferers are unable to process the trauma adequately, and use avoidance techniques to minimize reliving the stressor.
- **The *behavioral model*** holds that PTSD arises through pairing of the stressor with physical or mental reminders of the trauma.
- **The *psychodynamic model*** suggests that the trauma reactivates a previously quiescent, yet unresolved psychological conflict.

Treatment

Pharmacotherapy

Antidepressant medications to treat PTSD and to control the feelings of anxiety and its associated symptoms including:

Selective Serotonin Reuptake Inhibitors (SSRIs)

Paxil, Celexa, Luvox, Prozac, and Zoloft. *Tricyclic antidepressants*: Elavil and Doxepin.

Psychotherapy

Psychotherapy for PTSD involves helping the person learn skills to manage symptoms and develop ways of coping. Therapy also aims to teach the person and his or her family about the disorder, and help the person work through the fears associated with the traumatic event. A variety of psychotherapy approaches are used to treat people with PTSD, including:

- **Cognitive behavioral therapy,** which involves learning to recognize and change thought patterns that lead to troublesome emotions, feelings, and behavior.

- **Exposure therapy,** a type of cognitive behavioral therapy that involves having the person re-live the traumatic experience, or exposing the person to objects or situations that cause anxiety. This is done in a well-controlled and safe environment. Exposure therapy helps the person confront the fear and gradually become more comfortable with situations that are frightening and cause anxiety. This has been very successful at treating PTSD.
- **Family therapy** may be useful because the behavior of the person with PTSD can have an effect on other family members. (It increase support for the sufferer and victims of mass trauma respectively)
- **Group therapy** may be helpful by allowing the person to share thoughts, fears, and feelings with other people who have experienced traumatic events.
- **Eye Movement Desensitization and Reprocessing (EMDR)** is a complex form of psychotherapy that was initially designed to alleviate distress associated with traumatic memories and is now also used to treat phobias.

F43.2: ADJUSTMENT DISORDER

Definition

A maladaptive reaction to a psychosocial stressor. It is maladaptive because it interferes with the affected person's social or occupational functioning.

Clinical Features

- Onset is usually within one month of the stressful event or life change.
- Duration is not longer than six months
  - Brief depressive reaction
- Transient mild depression
- Duration < 1 month
  - Prolonged depressive reaction
- Mild depression in response to chronic stressor
- Duration < 2 years
  - Mixed anxiety and depressive reaction
    - It is the state of subjective distress and emotional disturbance, usually interfering with social functioning and performance, and arising in the period of adaptation to a significant life change or to the consequences of a stressful life event.
    - The manifestations include depressed mood, anxiety, worry, feeling of inability to cope, plan ahead, or continue in the present situation and some degree of disability in the performance of daily routine.
    - Onset is usually within 1 month of the occurrence of stressful event or change, and duration of symptoms usually does not exceed 6 months.

Treatment

Psychological

- *Group therapy:* Reinforce positive coping strategies.
- *Individual therapy.*

Pharmacotherapy

Short courses of medications may be useful for brief symptom relief such as insomnia.

Nursing Management

Box 8.20: Nursing process for reaction to stress, PTSD and adjustment disorder

Nursing diagnosis: Anxiety [severe to panic]/fear related to current memory of past traumatic life event, such as natural disasters, accidental/deliberate manmade disasters, and events such as rape, assault, or combat evidenced by increased tension. Restlessness, helplessness, apprehension, fearfulness, uncertainty/confusion.

Outcome identification	Nursing intervention
• Client will be able to: – Verbalize awareness of feelings of anxiety/sense of control over fearful stimuli. – Identify healthy ways to manage feelings.	• Assess degree of anxiety/fear present, associated behaviors, and reality of threat perceived by client. • Develop trusting relationship with the client. • Observe for and elicit information about physical injury, and assess symptoms such as numbness, headache, and tightness in chest, nausea, and pounding heart. • Identify psychologic responses (e.g. anger, shock, acute anxiety [panic], confusion, denial), expressions of disbelief and/or self-blame. Record emotional changes. • Identify development of phobic reactions to ordinary articles (e.g. knives), situations (e.g. strangers ringing doorbell, walking in crowds of people). • Discuss with client perception of what is causing anxiety. • Give positive feedback when client demonstrates better ways to manage anxiety and is able to calmly and/or realistically appraise own situation. • Administer medications as indicated.

Nursing diagnosis: Powerlessness related to interpersonal interaction (lack of control of traumatic event) being overwhelmed by symptoms of anxiety and poor coping skills evidenced by verbal expression of lack of control over present situation/future outcome; passivity and/or anger.

Outcome identification	Nursing intervention
• Identify areas over which individual has control.	• Identify present/past effective coping behaviors and reinforce use. • Note ethnic background, cultural/religious perceptions and beliefs about the occurrence (e.g. retribution from God). • Encourage client to identify factors under own control as well as those not within own ability to control. • Assist client to identify precipitating factors when feelings of powerlessness and loss of control began. • Explore actions client can use during periods of stress (e.g. deep breathing, counting to 10, reviewing the situation, reframing). • Give positive feedback when client uses constructive methods to regain control. • Promote involvement in group therapy.

Nursing diagnosis: Disturbed sleep pattern related to psychological stress (anxiety, depression with recurring disruptive dreams) evidenced by verbal reports of difficulty in falling asleep, reports of sleep disturbances (e.g. nightmares, dreams of personal death, disaster-related dreams, flashbacks, intrusive/trauma images, fear of re-experiencing the event).

Contd...

Contd...

Outcome identification	Nursing intervention
• Verbalize understanding of sleep disorder problem	• Assess sleep pattern disturbance by observation and reports from client and/or significant others. • Identify causative and contributing factors (e.g. intrusive/ repetitive thoughts, nightmares, severe anxiety level). Note use of caffeine and/or alcohol, other drugs. • Provide a quiet environment; arrange to have uninterrupted sleep as much as possible. • Encourage client to develop behavior routine when insomnia is present (e.g. no napping after noon, having warm bath/milk before bed, relaxing. • Administer sedative, hypnotic, or antianxiety drugs as indicated.

F 44. DISSOCIATIVE [CONVERSION] DISORDERS

Dissociative (conversion) disorder is characterized by a disturbance or alteration in the normally integrative functions of identity, memory, or consciousness.

The individual blocks off part of his or her life from consciousness during periods of intolerable stress. The stressful emotion becomes a separate entity because the individual 'splits' from it and mentally drifts into a fantasy state.

Clinical Feature

For a definite diagnosis, the following clinical features should be present:

- No evidence for a physical disorder that might explain the symptoms.
- Evidence for psychological causation, in the form of a clear association in time with stressful events and problems, or disturbed relationships (even if denied by the patient)
- **Primary gain**: Produces positive internal motivations. ***For example,*** a patient might feel guilty about being unable to perform some task. If he has a medical condition justifying his inability, he might not feel so bad.
- **Secondary gain**: The disorder confers some advantage to the patient. ***For example,*** excused from normal responsibilities.

Box 8.21: Difference between dissociative vs conversion

Dissociative	Conversion
It is characterized by disruption in the normal functioning of memory consciousness, identity, and world around her/him.	Conversion disorder is defined as a mental disorder where central features is the appearance of signs/ symptoms affecting the patients senses or voluntary movements that suggest a neurological or general medical disease or condition.

Box 8.22: More to know: Pseudoneurological

Conversion symptoms affect voluntary motor or sensory functioning suggestive of neurological disease and therefore are sometimes called 'pseudoneurological disorder'.

Etiologic Theories

Psychodynamics

Selective repression of distressing mental contents from conscious awareness is used as a mechanism for protecting the individual from emotional pain or expressing self in dangerous ways. The stressor(s) may arise from external circumstances or internal sources with onset of symptoms sudden or gradual and of transient or chronic nature. Intrapsychic conflict thus uses denial and 'ego splitting' to decrease anxiety.

Physical sensations seen in these disorders may represent forbidden wishes that have been somatized.

Biological causes

Research on the biologic basis of these disorders is increasing as more recognition of the mind-body connection is accepted. Biochemical, physiologic, and endocrine systems have an intimate connection with actual physical changes occurring in all body systems via the autonomic nervous system.

Organic causes of pathologic dissociative experiences that are known or suspected include temporal lobe epilepsy, sensory deprivation, sleep loss, strokes, encephalitis, and Alzheimer's disease.

Drugs may also induce amnesia or depersonalization directly or indirectly in some incidences.

Psychosocial theory

Psychosocial theory states that individuals who develop dissociative disorders have often experienced severe physical, sexual, and/or emotional abuse early in life—stress so severe that the only way to cope with the painful emotions is to detach from them. The child learns to respond to stressful situations in this manner.

Responding to stressful situations with dissociative behaviors then becomes a method of coping for some individuals into adulthood, when there is less control over the dissociative states. The response becomes maladaptive in that the individual escapes from the stressful situation rather than facing it.

Psychopathology

Dissociation is a psycho-physiologic process alters a person's thoughts, feelings, or actions

↓

So that, for a time, certain information is not associated or integrated with other information as it normally is.

↓

Manifests along a continuum of severity, produces a range of clinical and behavioral phenomena involving alterations in memory and identity.

↓

In extreme cases, the process gives rise to a set of psychiatric syndromes known as dissociative disorders.

Box 8.23: Classification
ICD-Classification
F44.0 Dissociative Amnesia
F44.1 Dissociative Fugue
F44.2 Dissociative Stupor
F44.3 Trance and Possession Disorders

Contd...

Contd...

F44.4 Dissociative Motor Disorders
F44.5 Dissociative Convulsions
F44.6 Dissociative Anesthesia and Sensory Loss
F44.7 Mixed Dissociative (Conversion) Disorders
F44.8 Other Dissociative (Conversion) Disorders
• Ganser's Syndrome
• Multiple Personality
F44.9 Dissociative (Conversion) Disorders, Unspecified

CLASSIFICATION AND EXPLANATION OF F44. DISSOCIATIVE (CONVERSION) DISORDER

F44.0	***Dissociative amnesia***	**Definition:** Dissociative amnesia is a sudden inability to recall important personal information that can not be explained by ordinary forgetfulness. ***Types:*** • ***Localized amnesia*** — Failure to recall all events that occurred during a circumscribed time period. • ***Selective amnesia*** — Failure to recall some of the events that occurred during a circumscribed time period. • ***Generalized amnesia*** — Failure to recall all events over the entire life span. • ***Continuous amnesia*** — Failure to recall events subsequent to a specific time up to and including the present. • ***Systematized amnesia*** — Failure to recall certain categories of information. ***Clinical features:*** • Client cannot recall important, usually stressful or traumatic, personal information. • Perplexed and disoriented, wandering aimlessly. • Unable to remember the event that precipitated the episode. • After the episode has ended, the patient is unaware of his illness.
F44.1	***Dissociative fugue***	**Definition:** A dissociative fugue may be present when a person impulsively wanders or a travel away from home and upon arrival in the new location is unable to remember his/her past. **(OR)** Dissociative fugue is a sudden, unexpected, travel away from home or one's customary place of daily activities, with inability to recall some or all of one's past. **Signs and Symptoms:** • Patients suddenly leave their surroundings and begin a journey. Journeys can cover thousands of miles. (Unexpected travel from a person's usual place of living.) • Patients fail to remember some or all of their past. • Confusion about personal identity and may take on a whole new identity. • Patients starting entirely new lives and acting more gregarious and uninhibited than in their previous lives.

Contd...

Contd...

		• Patients who are in a state of dissociative fugue appear normal and healthy to outsiders and do not attract attention. • The flight and amnesia that characterize the fugue not related to physical illness. • The diagnosis can then be made using the patient's history and reconstruction of events that occurred before, during, and after the patient's excursion. • Complete Amnesia. • Unaware that they have forgotten anything. • Mild depression.
F40.2	***Dissociative stupor***	**Definition:** Profound absence of voluntary movements and speech, and of normal responsiveness to light, noise and touch.
F44.3	***Trance and possession disorder***	**Definition:** Possession and trance involves single or episodic alterations in the state of consciousness, characterized by the exchange of the person's customary identity by a new identity usually attributed to a spirit, divine power, deity, or another person. (Conviction that the individual has been taken over by a spirit, power, deity or other person.)
F44.4	***Dissociative motor disorders***	**Definition:** Complete or partial loss of the ability to perform movements those are normally under voluntary control (including speech).
F44.5	***Dissociative convulsions (Pseudo-seizures)***	**Definition:** Sudden and unexpected spasmodic movements, closely resembling any of the varieties of epileptic seizures, but not followed by loss of consciousness, tongue-biting, serious bruising or laceration due to falling, or incontinence of urine.
F44.6	***Dissociative anesthesia and sensory loss***	Partial or complete loss of any or all of the normal cutaneous sensations over part or all of the body (specify: touch, pin prick, vibration, heat, cold). ***Sensory loss:*** Partial or complete loss of vision, hearing or smell (specify).
F44.8	***dissociative (conversion) disorder*** ***a) Ganser syndrome***	**Definition:** Ganser's syndrome is a rare factitious disorder, a mental illness in which a person act as if he or she has a physical or mental illness when in truth, he or she has caused the symptoms is characterized by nonsensical or wrong answers to questions or doing things incorrectly. (In simple meaning the person gives approximate answers for questions being asked) **e.g.: 2+2 = 5** • First described by a neurologist **Mr. Sigbert Ganser** in 1987. • It also called **prisoner psychosis.** • Patients produce symptoms consciously or unconsciously. **Clinical features:** • ***Vorbeireden:*** Approximate answering • ***Clouding of the consciousness:*** Hysterical 'wilight state' cloudiness resolves suddenly leaving only a residual amnesia. • ***Somatic conversion symptoms:*** Headache, abdominal pain. • ***Dreamy appearance*** • ***Confusion*** • ***Stress*** • ***Loss of personality identity*** • ***Echolalia and Echopraxia*** • ***Fugue, amnesia*** • ***Visual hallucinations*** • ***No response to painful stimuli.***

Contd...

Contd...

	b) Multiple personality disorder	**Definition:** The existence of two or more distinct personalities within the individual, only one being evident at a time. • Each personality has its own memories, preferences and behavior patterns, and at some time (and recurrently) takes full control of the individual's behavior. • Inability to recall important personal information, too expensive to be explained by ordinary forgetfulness. ***(Dissociative identity disorder formerly referred to as multiple personality disorder.)*** ***Signs and symptoms:*** • Amnesia and disturbances in time perception. • Family members describe that patient can not recall, alterations in facial presentation, voice, and behavior. • Stress or idiosyncratically meaningful social or environmental cues commonly trigger the transition from one personality to another. • Although usually sudden, the transition can occur over hours or days. • At least two of these identities or personality states recurrently take control of the person's behavior.

Management

Pharmacotherapy

- **Antidepressants**
  - Sertraline
  - Clomipramine
- **Anxiolytics**

Cognitive Therapy

Focuses on changing dysfunctional thinking patterns and the resulting feelings and behaviors.

Behavioral Therapy

Some behavior therapists initially use behavioral treatments such as only responding to a single identity, and using more traditional therapy once a consistent response is established.

Creative Therapies (Art Therapy, Music Therapy)

These therapies allow the patient to explore and express his or her thoughts and feelings in a safe and creative way.

Clinical Hypnosis

It uses intense relaxation, concentration and attention to achieve an altered state of consciousness (awareness), allowing people to explore thoughts, feelings and memories they may have hidden from their conscious minds.

Family Therapy

This helps to teach the family about the disorder and its causes, as well as to help family members recognize symptoms of a recurrence.

Nursing Management

Box 8.24: Nursing process for dissociative (conversion) disorder

Nursing diagnosis: Disturbed thought processes related to psychologic conflict, threat to physical integrity/self-concept evidenced by memory loss/deficit, inability to recall selected events.

Outcome identification	Nursing intervention
• Client will be able to: – Verbalize understanding that loss of memory is related to stress.	• Determine degree/extent of memory deficits. Obtain information about client from family/significant other, • Expose client to stimuli that represent pleasant experiences from the past, such as smells associated with enjoyable activities and music known to be pleasurable. • Engage in further activities that stimulate life experiences as memory returns. • Encourage client to discuss situations that have been especially stressful and to explore the feelings associated with those times. • Explore more adaptive ways to respond to anxiety.

Nursing diagnosis: Risk for violence, directed at self/others related to dissociative state/conflicting personalities evidenced by increased motor activity, pacing, excitement, irritability, agitation.

Outcome identification	Nursing intervention
• Patient will be able to: – Verbalize understanding of why behavior occurs.	• Remain vigilant to behavioral changes that may signal destructive actions. Assess seriousness of suicidal tendency, gestures, threats, or previous attempts. • Structure the environment to reduce stressors, and remove dangerous objects. • Help client identify/recognize precipitants to destructive behaviors. • Active-listen, and encourage the client to seek restraint and/or support, when self-destructive or violent impulses are present. • Assist client to identify alternatives to aggression or self-destructive behaviors (e.g. verbal expression, physical activity, written expression). • Administer antianxiety/antidepressant medication as indicated.

Nursing diagnosis: Disturbed personal identity related to psychologic conflicts (dissociative state[s]) memory loss (unable to recall selected events/own identity) as evidenced by presence of more than one personality within the individual.

Outcome identification	Nursing intervention
Verbalize awareness of all personalities, their thoughts and behaviors (development of co-consciousness).	• Develop trusting relationship with individual (and 'alters' or subpersonalities if present). • Ascertain what client does recall and compare with information obtained from family members/other personalities. • Share information in small amounts over a period of time. • Facilitate identification of stressful situations that precipitate dissociative state/transition from one personality to another. • Provide psychotherapy with feedback relative to behavioral observations. • Engage in activities that reflect life experiences, using occupational/vocational/recreational/physical therapy.

F45. SOMATOFORM DISORDERS

'I am more sick than my doctors think' –Alfred Nobel

Somatoform disorder (also known as ***Briquet's syndrome***) is characterized by physical symptoms that mimic disease or injury for which there is no identifiable physical cause or physical symptoms such as pain, nausea, depression, and dizziness. Somatoform disorders are physical symptoms which present as part of a general medical condition. However, no general medical condition, other mental disorder, or substance is adequately diagnosed. The complaints are serious enough to cause significant emotional distress and impairment of social and/or occupational functioning.

Definition

'Somatoform disorders are those disorders in which physical symptoms suggesting a physical disorder for which there are no demonstrable organic findings or known physiological mechanisms and for which there is strong evidence, or a strong presumption, that the symptoms are linked to psychological or conflicts.'

Box 8.25: It has following subtypes
F45.0 Somatization disorder
F45.1 Undifferentiated somatoform disorder
F45.2 Hypochondriacal disorder includes *body dysmorphic disorder*
F45.3 Somatoform autonomic dysfunction includes *Da Costa's syndrome, irritable bowel syndrome*

Further Classification and Explanation of F45: Somatization Disorder

F45.0	***Somatization disorder***	**Definition:** Somatization disorder is characterized by many somatic symptoms that cannot be explained adequately based on physical and laboratory examinations. ***Specific characteristics of somatization disorder include the following:*** • Onset of unexplained medical symptoms in persons younger than 30 years. • Multiple and chronic complaints of unexplained physical symptoms. • Multiple pain symptoms involving multiple sites, such as the head, neck, back, stomach, and limbs. • At least 2 or more unexplained gastrointestinal symptoms, such as nausea and indigestion. • At least 1 sexual complaint and/or menstrual complaint. • At least 1 pseudo-neurological symptom, such as blindness or inability to walk, speaks, or move. ***Important considerations:*** • lifetime prevalence: 0.1–0.2 % • F:M ratio = 5–20:1 • age of onset: before 30 years old (usually in the teens) **Treatment** **1. Psychological** **a)** ***Psychotherapeutic:*** Some patients may benefit, but only once they have acknowledged some psychological basis for their problems ***b) Consistency:*** Patient should be seen by the same physician each time.

Contd...

Contd...

<table>
<tr><td>F45.2</td><td>Hypochondriacal disorder includes body dysmorphic disorder</td><td>A) Hypochondriacal disorder:
Definition: Hypochondriasis is a somatoform disorder characterized by unexplained physical symptoms related to fear of a specific medical condition, i.e. a complaint of breast pain perceived as being due to breast cancer when no breast cancer is present.
(Includes non-delusional dysmorphophobia - a preoccupation with an imagined bodily defect)
Incidence:
• About 1/5 of patients attempt suicide (in contrast to most patients with hypochondriacal disorder).
• Age of onset usually 20–30 years, but may occur at any age
Signs and Symptoms:
• Preoccupation with the possibility of having one or more serious and progressive physical disorders, and even a disfigurement.
• Preoccupation persists despite medical evaluation and reassurance.
• Fear persists for at least 6 months.
Course and Prognosis:
• Usually episodic, often with long gaps between presentations
• 1/3–½ eventually improve significantly
Treatment: Similar to that for somatization disorder.
B) Body dysmorphic disorder:
Body dysmorphic disorder is a somatoform disorder characterized by a focus on a physical defect that is not evident to others.
Specific characteristics of body dysmorphic disorder include the following:
• Preoccupation with an imagined defect in appearance.
• May be associated with multiple, frantic, and unsuccessful attempts to correct imagined defect by cosmetic surgery.</td></tr>
<tr><td>F45.3</td><td>Somatoform autonomic dysfunction includes: Da Costa's syndrome</td><td>A group of disorders manifested by symptoms of internal organ or organ systems, but not with objectively recorded basis. The complaints can physical disorder of a system or organ that is largely or completely under the influence of the autonomic nervous system, I.e. The cardiovascular, gastrointestinal or respiratory system. Among them is partially and urogenital system. The most frequent and prominent examples relate to the cardiovascular system (the 'heart neurosis'), respiratory system (psychogenic dyspnea and hiccup) and gastrointestinal system ('neurosis of the stomach' and 'nervous diarrhea').
Da Costa's syndrome: Which was colloquially known as soldier's heart, is a syndrome with a set of symptoms that are similar to those of heart disease, though a physical examination does not reveal any physiological abnormalities. In modern times, Da Costa's syndrome is considered the manifestation of an anxiety disorder, and treatment is primarily behavioral, involving modifications to lifestyle and exercise.</td></tr>
<tr><td>F45.4</td><td>Persistent somatoform pain disorder</td><td>Persistent severe and distressing pain, in any part of the body, which cannot be explained adequately by evidence of a physiological process or a physical disorder, and in which pain is the main focus of the patient's attention.
(Symptoms should present for 6 months continuously on most of the days)</td></tr>
</table>

Etiologic Theories

Psychodynamics Theory

This disorder may represent an unconscious transformation of internal conflicts into physical symptoms that can be explained in terms of the ego's ability to control the sensory and motor apparatus, which may have specific meaning for the client. Dependency is common in individuals with somatoform disorders, and fixation in an earlier level of development may be evident.

Biologic

Although biologic and neurophysiologic influences in the etiology of anxiety have been investigated, no relationship has yet been established. However, there does seem to be a genetic influence with a high family incidence.

Family Dynamics

The family contributes to these conditions by initiating, reinforcing, and perpetuating the behavior patterns. The children learn (overtly or covertly) that physical complaints are acceptable ways of coping with stress and obtaining attention, care, and gratification of dependency needs. The client may gain attention and meet these needs by over dramatization of the symptoms, resulting in over involvement of other family members in enmeshed behavior patterns. In the beginning, the client may exaggerate minor symptoms to prove she or he is really ill when others ignore reports of illness.

Box 8.26: Nursing process for somatoform disorder

Nursing diagnosis: Chronic pain related to severe level of anxiety, low-self-esteem; unmet dependency needs evidenced by multiple reports of severe/prolonged pain, facial mask of pain, social withdrawal, history of seeking assistance from numerous healthcare professionals.

Outcome identification	Nursing intervention
• Client will be able to: – Acknowledge relationship between psychological problems and onset of pain. – Verbalize noticeable reduction/relief of pain.	• Note and record duration and intensity of pain. Assess factors that precipitate onset of pain. Observe and report any new or different pattern of pain behavior to physician. • Convey to client a belief that the pain is indeed real, even though no organic pathology can be found. • Provide nursing comfort measures with a matter-of-fact approach that does not provide added attention to the pain behavior (e.g., back rub, warm bath, heating pad). • Assist client with activities that distract from focus on self and pain. • Identify specific situations that cause anxiety to rise, and demonstrate techniques to interrupt the pain response (e.g., visual or auditory distractions, guided imagery, breathing exercises, massage, application of heat or cold, relaxation techniques). • Provide positive reinforcement when client is not focusing on pain.

Nursing diagnosis: Disturbed body image related to low self-esteem; unmet dependency needs evidenced by preoccupation with real or imagined change in bodily functions.

Contd...

Contd...

Outcome identification	Nursing intervention
• Patient will be able to: – Verbalize realistic perception of bodily condition.	• Ascertain client's perception of own body image. Acknowledge that disability is real to the client, even in the absence of evidence of organic pathology. • Help client to see that image is distorted and out of proportion to reality of actual change in structure and/or function. Correct inaccurate perceptions in a matter-of-fact, nonthreatening manner. • Encourage verbalization of fears and anxieties associated with identified stressful life situations. Discuss ways in which client may respond more adaptively in the future. • Encourage and give positive feedback for independent self-care behaviors, while gradually withdrawing attention from dependent behaviors. • Administer medications as indicated, e.g.: antidepressants: like clomipramine (Anafranil), fluoxetine (Prozac).

Nursing diagnosis: Impaired social interaction related to inability to engage in satisfying personal relationships and preoccupation with self and physical symptoms evidenced by preoccupation with own thoughts; repetitive verbalization about self/physical symptoms uncommunicative, sad and dull affect.

Outcome identification	Nursing intervention
• Patient will be able to: – Spend time voluntarily with others in group activities.	• Spend time with client after setting limits on attention-seeking behaviors. Withdraw presence if ruminations about physical symptoms begin. • Increase amount of time/attention given during times when client is not focusing on physical symptoms. • Assist client in learning assertiveness techniques, especially the ability to recognize the difference between passive, assertive, and aggressive behaviors • Encourage attendance in group activities after client is interacting appropriately in the 1:1 relationship. • Provide positive feedback for any attempts at social interaction in which the client's focus is on others rather than self/physical symptoms.

MORE TO KNOW: MUNCHAUSEN SYNDROME

Definition

It is a factitious disorder, a mental disorder in which a person repeatedly and deliberately acts as if he or she has a physical or mental illness when he or she is not really sick.

Most of the symptoms in people with Munchausen syndrome are related to physical illness, symptoms such as chest pain, stomach problems, or fever, rather than those of a mental disorder.

Box 8.27: Origin of the disease

Munchausen syndrome, named for Baron von Munchausen, an 18th century German officer who was known for embellishing the stories of his life and experiences, is the most severe type of factitious disorder.

Causes

The exact cause of Munchausen syndrome is not known, but researchers are looking at the role of biological and psychological factors in its development. Some theories suggest that a history of abuse or neglect as a child, or a history of frequent illnesses that required hospitalization might be factors in the development of the syndrome.

Signs and Symptoms

People with Munchausen syndrome deliberately produces or exaggerate symptoms in several ways. They may lie about or fake symptoms, hurt themselves to bring on symptoms, or alter tests (such as contaminating a urine sample). Possible warning signs of Munchausen syndrome include:

- Dramatic but inconsistent medical history
- Unclear symptoms that are not controllable and that become more severe or change once treatment has begun
- Extensive knowledge of hospitals and/or medical terminology, as well as the textbook descriptions of illnesses
- Presence of multiple surgical scars
- Presence of symptoms only when the patient is with others or being observed.
- Willingness or eagerness to have medical tests, operations, or other procedures
- History of seeking treatment at numerous hospitals, clinics, and doctors offices, possibly even in different cities
- Problems with identity and self-esteem.

Treatment

Although a person with Munchausen syndrome actively seeks treatment for the various disorders he or she invents, the person often is unwilling to admit to and seek treatment for the syndrome itself. This makes treating people with Munchausen syndrome very challenging, and the outlook for recovery poor.

Goal

- When treatment is sought, the first goal is to modify the person's behavior and reduce his or her misuse or overuse of medical resources.
- Another key goal is to help patients avoid dangerous and unnecessary medical diagnostic or treatment procedures (such as surgeries), often sought from different doctors who may be unaware that physical symptoms are either being faked or self-inflicted.
  - Primary treatment for Munchausen syndrome is psychotherapy or talk therapy (a type of counseling). Treatment usually focuses on changing the thinking and behavior of the individual (cognitive-behavioral therapy).
  - Family therapy may also be helpful in teaching family members not to reward or reinforce the behavior of the person with the disorder.
  - There are no medications to treat factitious disorders themselves. Medication may be used, however, to treat any related illness, such as ***depression or anxiety***.

F48. OTHER NEUROTIC DISORDERS

Neurasthenia

Persistent, distressing complaints of feelings of exhaustion after minor mental effort (such as attempting to perform every-day tasks that do not require unusual mental effort).

Persistent, distressing complaints of feelings of fatigue and bodily weakness after minor physical effort.

Clinical Features

- Feelings of muscular aches and pains
- Dizziness
- Tension headaches
- Sleep disturbance
- Inability to relax
- Inability to recover from symptoms after normal periods of rest, relaxation or entertainment.
  (The duration of the disorder is at least 6 months.)

Depersonalization-Derealization Syndrome

- **Depersonalization:** The patient complains of a feeling of being distant, 'not really here' (for example he may complain that his emotions, or feelings, or experience of his inner self are detached, strange, not his own, or unpleasantly lost, or that his emotions or movements feel as if they belong to someone else, or that he feels as if acting in a play).
- **Derealization:** The patient complains of a feeling of unreality (for example he may complain that the surroundings or specific objects look strange, distorted, flat, colorless, lifeless, dreary, uninteresting, or like a stage upon which everyone is acting).

9 Nursing Management of Patient with Substance use Disorder

Substance abuse occurs in almost all countries and in all segments of all societies. Men are more at risk than women and adolescents are most vulnerable. This is commonly associated with low level of education, broken family, personality disorders, criminal records and financial difficulties.

Substance use disorder, also known as drug use disorder, is a condition in which the use of one or more substances leads to a clinically significant impairment or distress. Even though the name substance might refer to any matter, 'substance' in this scenario refers to only psychoactive drugs.

TERMINOLOGIES

- **Abuse:** Self-administration of any substance in a culturally disapproved manner that causes adverse consequences.
- **Intoxication:** The transient effects (physical and psychological) due to recent substance ingestion, which disappear when the substance is eliminated.
- **Withdrawal:** A group of symptoms and signs occurring when a drug is withdrawn or reduced in amount.
- **Tolerance:** The state in which the same amount of a drug produces a decreased effect, so that increasingly larger doses must be administered to obtain the effects observed with the original use.
- **Dependence:** The physiological state of neuro adaptation produced by repeated administration of a drug, necessitating continued administration to prevent the appearance of the withdrawal state.
- **Addiction:** A nonscientific term that implies dependence and associated deterioration of physical and mental health as well as a high tendency to relapse after discontinuation.
- **Abstinent:** Not using substances of abuse at any time
- **Blackout:** A blackout is a period of amnesia or memory loss, typically caused by chronic, high-dose substance abuse.
- **Crack:** Cocaine (cocaine hydrochloride) that has been chemically modified so that it will become a gas vapors when heated at relatively low temperatures.
- **Detoxification:** It is the clearing of toxins from the body. The medical and bio-psychosocial procedure that assists a person who is dependent on one or more substances to withdraw from dependence on all substances of abuse.

- **Relapse:** A breakdown or setback in a person's attempt to change or modify any particular behavior.
- **Remission:** A state in which a mental or physical disorder has been overcome or a disease process halted.
- **Substance use disorders:** A class of substance-related disorders that includes both substance abuse and substance dependence.
- **Toxicity:** Poisonous nature, poisonous quality.

Classification

F10–19 Mental and Behavior Disorders Associated with Psychoactive Substance Use

F10 Mental and behavioral disorders due to use of alcohol
F11 Mental and behavioral disorders due to use of opioids
F12 Mental and behavioral disorders due to use of cannabinoids
F13 Mental and behavioral disorders due to use of sedatives or hypnotics
F14 Mental and behavioral disorders due to use of cocaine
F15 Mental and behavioral disorders due to use of other stimulants, including caffeine
F16 Mental and behavioral disorders due to use of hallucinogens
F17 Mental and behavioral disorders due to use of tobacco
F18 Mental and behavioral disorders due to use to volatile solvents
F19 Mental and behavioral disorders due to multiple drug use and use of other psychoactive substances

Types of Substance-related Disorders

- Substance use disorders (dependence and abuse)
- Substance-induced disorders (intoxication, withdrawal)

Box 9.1: Difference between substance abuse and dependence

Substance use	Substance dependence
'Substance abuse is a maladaptive pattern of substance use manifested by recurrent and significant adverse consequences related to repeated use of the substance. Substance abuse has also been referred to as any use of substances that poses significant hazards to health'. **—DSM-IV TR (APA-2000)**	'A compulsive or chronic requirement. The need is so strong as to generate distress (either physical or psychological) if left unfulfilled'. It is two types: **a. Physical dependence** Physical dependence on a substance is evidenced by cluster of cognitive, behavioral and physiological symptoms indicating that the individual continues use of the substance despite significant substance-related problems. **b. Psychological dependence** An individual is considered to be psychologically dependent on a substance when there is an overwhelming desire to repeat the use of a particular drug in order to produce pleasure or avoid discomfort.

Box 9.2: Substance induced disorders

Substance intoxication	Substance withdrawal
It is defined as the development of a reversible substance-specific syndrome caused by the recent ingestion of (or exposure to) a substance. The behavior change can attributed to the physiological effects of the substance on the CNS and develop during or shortly after use of the substance.	It is the development of a substance-specific maladaptive behavioral change, with physiological and cognitive concomitants, that is due to the cessation of, or reduction in, heavy and prolonged substance use.

COMMONLY USED PSYCHOACTIVE SUBSTANCES

- CNS depressants
  - Alcohol
  - Sedatives, hypnotics or anxiolytics
  - Inhalants (volatile solvents)
- CNS stimulants
  - Amphetamines
  - Cocaine
  - Caffeine
  - Nicotine (tobacco)
- Cannabis
- Opioids
- Hallucinogens
- Phencyclidine
- Others (e.g. anabolic steroids, anticholinergics).

ETIOLOGICAL FACTORS OF PSYCHOACTIVE SUBSTANCE USE

It is difficult to point out the exact causes of drug dependence because of the fact that the cause and the effects of drug dependence are inter-related and closely associated. Some of the predisposing factors are given below.

Genetics

Genetic studies shows the vulnerability especially evident with alcoholism, and less so with other substances. Children of alcoholics are three times more likely than other children to become alcoholics. Twin studies suggest that monozygotic twins have a higher concordance with alcoholism than dizygotic.

Biochemical Factors

Neurotransmitters like dopamine and norepinephrine have a role in cocaine, ethanol and opioid dependence. Alcohol may produce morphine-like substances in the brain that are responsible for alcohol addiction.

Psychodynamic Theory

Many psychodynamic theories have been evolved in the past years to describe the exact causes of substance abuse among individuals. Some of these theories suggest that substance abuse may be an expression of people's sexual energy. It is also described as an ego defense mechanism against anxious impulses or an outward expression of oral regression.

Some psychodynamic theorists suggest that it is caused by a disturbed ego functions and an inability to deal effectively with the reality.

Behavioral Theory

Behavioral theory suggests that drug abuse is a result of conditioning or reinforcement from drug use by avoiding some negative or aversive state such as anxiety, pain or depression.

In social situations, substance use may bring about peer approval and thus acting as a positive reinforcement.

Psychological Factors

Psychological factors include the following:

- Poor impulse control
- Sense of inferiority
- Poor impulse control
- Inability to cope with the real life stresses
- Desire to escape from reality
- Pleasure seeking behavior
- Sexual immaturity

Social Factors

- Peer pressure
- Urbanization
- Poverty
- Unemployment
- Loss of job
- Over crowding
- Poor social support
- Effects of mass medias

Easy Availability of Drugs

- Use of drugs prescribed by doctors (like hypnotics, sedatives)
- Use of drugs that can be bought legally without prescription (nicotine)
- Use of drugs from illicit sources (street drugs).

ALCOHOL USE DISORDERS

Profile of the Alcohol

Alcohol/ethanol/ethyl alcohol is a chemical intoxicating ingredient found in beer, wine, and liquor. Alcohol is produced by the fermentation of yeast, sugars, and starches. It exerts a depressant effect on the CNS, resulting in behavioral and mood changes that are rapidly absorbed from the stomach and small intestine into the bloodstream.

A standard drink equals 0.6 ounces of pure ethanol, or 12 ounces of beer; 8 ounces of malt liquor; 5 ounces of wine; or 1.5 ounces of spirits or liquor (e.g. gin, rum, vodka, or whiskey).

Alcohol use disorder was previously called as *alcoholism*. The hallmarks of this disorder are *addiction* to alcohol, inability to stop drinking, and repeated interpersonal, school or work-related problems that can be due to use of alcohol. Alcoholism can have serious consequences, affecting an individual's health and personal life, as well as impacting society at large.

History of Alcohol use

- Around the world, Fermented grain, fruit juice and honey have been used to make alcohol (ethyl alcohol or ethanol) for thousands of years.
- In early Egyptian civilization fermented beverages existed and there is evidence of an early alcoholic drink in China around 7000 BC.
- In India, an alcoholic beverage called sura, distilled from rice, was in use between 3000 and 2000 BC.
- The Babylonians worshiped a wine goddess as early as 2700 BC.
- Greek literature is full of warnings against excessive drinking.
- Several Native Americans developed alcoholic beverages in pre-Columbian times.
- A variety of fermented beverages were used in the Andes region of South America were created from corn, grapes or apples, called 'chicha.'

Evolution of Alcohol use in India

The evolution of alcohol use can be traced back to historical periods and divided into 3 broad historical periods.

1. In beginning during Vedic era (1500–1700 BC) used alcohol as a mind enhancer. And during this period the writings of the renowned medical practitioners, Charaka and Sushrutha, added new lines of thought, and arguments for 'moderate alcohol use'.
2. The period of Islamic influence (1100–1800 CE), including the Mughal era from the 1520s to 1800, exhibited widespread alcohol use.
3. During 1800 AD to present deep influence of alcohol use by British colonial rule and the recent half century of Indian independence, beginning in 1947 and in modern era there is wide spread of alcoholism everywhere which is considered as major social evil in society.

Different alcoholic beverages and their sources of sugar for the fermentation process are as follows:

- Beer: Malted barley
- Wine: Grapes or berries
- Whisky: Malted grains
- Rum: Molasses.

Patterns of use

According to *Jellinek*, there are five species of alcohol dependence (Alcoholism) on the basis of the pattern of use.

- **Alpha (α) alcoholism**
  - Excessive and inappropriate way of drinking to relieve physical and emotional pain
  - No loss of control over alcohol
  - Ability to abstain present.

- **Beta (β) alcoholism**
  - Excessive and inappropriate drinking
  - Physical complications may occur
  - No dependence.
- **Gamma (γ) alcoholism**
  - Progressive course
  - Physical dependence with tolerance and withdrawal symptoms starts
  - Psychological dependence with inability to control over drinking.
- **Delta (δ) alcoholism**
  - Inability to abstain
  - Tolerance
  - Withdrawal symptoms
  - Amount of alcohol consumed can be controlled
  - Social disruption is minimal
- **Epsilon (ε) alcoholism**
  - Client will reach the stage of compulsive drinking called *dipsomania.*

Stages of Alcohol use

There are basically 3 stages in which all alcoholics may go through, they are:

- **Early stage (stage 1)**
  - To relax, relieve stress
  - Begins to become intoxicated regularly
  - Makes excuses and tries to rationalize drinking behavior frequently.
- **Middle stage (stage 2)**
  - Drinker denies or tries to hide problem.
  - Gradually body develops tolerance.
  - Frequently absent from school or work.
  - Drinking becomes central event in a person's life and drinks daily.
  - Drinks lot when alone
  - Drinks first thing in the morning.
- **Final stage (stage 3)**
  - Person becomes aggressive and isolated in this stage.
  - Person become malnourished because drinker consumes alcohol and does not worry about food.
  - Body is addicted to alcohol.
  - Try to quit leads to *withdrawal*
  - Delirium Tremens: hot/cold flashes, tremors, nightmares, hallucinations, fear of people and animals.

  (No cure-only recovery at this stage)

Blood Alcohol Concentration and its Symptoms

- 25–100 mg% excitement
- 100–200 mg% leads to serious intoxication, slurred speech, in coordination, nystagmus
- 300–350 mg%: Hypothermia, dysarthria, cold sweats

- 350–400 mg%: Coma, respiratory depression
- 400 mg%: Death may occur.

EPIDEMIOLOGY

The studies on alcohol use epidemiology have reported that alcohol use is predominantly seen in males than in females and the rates for female users of alcohol are very low and less than 5% of all the female.

The epidemiological studies of alcohol use in India shows the use of alcohol in general population is 25.6–74.2% and in students it is 21.8 to 58.4% and among medical professionals it is 8.5 to 66.7%

The life time prevalence of alcohol disorders with schizophrenia and affective disorders is 33.7% and 21.8% respectively.

ETIOLOGICAL THEORIES

As of today, no single causative factor is scientifically acceptable to explain reason for alcoholism. The multi-factorial approach of the bio-psycho-social model is acknowledged as being more comprehensive and clinician and patient friendly.

Physiological Theories

Genetic Theory (Goodwin, 1979)

Some workers in the field of theories that alcoholism may be inherited. Alcoholism appears to run in families.

Endocrine Theory

Another major physiological theory of the cause of alcoholism is any dysfunction in the endocrine function. Similarities between the symptoms seen in alcoholic patients and in patients with endocrine disorders suggest that some failure of the endocrine might be causally related to the onset of alcoholism.

Neurological Theory (Gardener EL, 1997)

The substances which are commonly abused act on brain circuits that evoked to sub serve the normal reinforcement functions of the central nervous system, like biologically essential behavior of feeding.

Psychological Theories

Some researcher believes that individuals with alcohol problems possess a number of distinctive traits which together make up the alcoholic personality.

Psychoanalytic Theory

Psychoanalytic explanations of the causes of alcoholism rest on two major theoretical position.

- **The Freudian view:** He expressed by, a number of people related alcoholism to such factors as repressed urges, oral dependency, need for security, self punishment and parental hatred.

- **The Adlerian view:** His view is that alcoholism represents a striving for power, which compensates for a pervasive feeling of inferiority.

Learning Theory

The learning and reinforcement theory explain that alcoholism occurs by considering alcohol ingestion as a reflex response to some stimulus and as a way to reduce an inner drive such as fear or anxiety and tension. In the latter case alcohol ingestion is said to reduce the tension or feelings of unpleasantness and to replace them with a feeling of well-being or euphoria.

Personality Trait Theory

Though it is concerned that all alcoholics need not have the same characteristics. It is postulated that, person need to be evaluated about his pre-alcoholic personality pattern which will correlates with the predisposition towards alcoholism.

Sociological Theories (Johnson BD, 1997)

Alcohol serves vastly different functions within and among societies, cultural, subculture and ethnic and religious groups. So these factors have great influence on individual's behavioral pattern in using alcohol.

Cultural Theory

The cultural theory of alcoholism suggests that within a given society, the attitudes towards drinking the culture produces is the main cause for alcoholism.

Some societies have strict control over alcohol use; therefore have a lower alcoholism rate. Other permits emotional outlets through ceremonies and rituals and thereby provides a culturally accepted means of anxiety reduction.

Process of Alcohol on Human Body

Alcohol is absorbed into the bloodstream via small blood vessels in the walls of the stomach and small intestine

Approximately 20% of alcohol is absorbed through the stomach. Most of the remaining 80% is absorbed through the small intestine

Within minutes of drinking alcohol, it travels from the stomach to the brain, where it quickly produces its effects, slowing the action of nerve cells

Alcohol is also carried by the bloodstream to the liver, which eliminates the alcohol from the blood through a process called 'metabolizing,' where it is converted to a nontoxic substance

The liver can only metabolize a certain amount at a time, leaving the excess circulating throughout the body

Thus the intensity of the effect on the body is directly related to the amount consumed

When the amount of alcohol in the blood exceeds a certain level, the respiratory (breathing) system slows down markedly, and can cause a coma or death, because oxygen no longer reaches the brain

EEFECTS OF ALCOHOL ON THE BODY

Short-term Effects

Depending on how much is taken and the physical condition of the individual, alcohol can cause:

- Upset in stomach
- Headaches
- Breathing difficulties
- Distorted vision and hearing
- Impaired judgment
- Slurred speech
- Drowsiness
- Vomiting
- Diarrhea
- Decreased perception and coordination
- Unconsciousness
- Anemia (loss of red blood cells)
- Coma
- Blackouts (memory lapses, where the drinker cannot remember events that occurred while under the influence).

Long-term Effects

Binge drinking and continued alcohol use in large amounts are associated with many health problems, including:

- Intentional injuries such as sexual assault, domestic violence
- Unintentional injuries such as car crash, falls, burns, drowning
- Increased family problems, broken relationships
- Alcohol poisoning
- High blood pressure, stroke, and other heart-related diseases
- Liver disease
- Nerve damage

- Sexual problems
- Permanent damage to the brain
- Vitamin B_1 deficiency, which can lead to a disorder characterized by amnesia, apathy and disorientation (see next page for its treatment).
- Gastritis and ulcers
- Malnutrition
- Cancer of the mouth and throat.

COMPLICATIONS

Chronic abuse of alcohol results in multi organ impairments. These complications include:

Liver Damage

- **Fatty liver:** Alcohol interferes with body's ability to break down fats. Excess fat blocks blood flow in liver which result in reduced oxygen and cell death. It can be reversed when drinking stops.
- **Cirrhosis of liver:** It is excessive scarring of the liver tissues which result in blockage of blood flow in scarred area *and prevent* liver cells from function and it is irreversible.

The symptoms of alcoholic liver cirrhosis are similar to other alcohol-related liver disorders.

Symptoms include:

- Jaundice
- Portal hypertension, which increases blood pressure in the vein that travels through the liver.
- Skin itching (pruritus).

Delirium Tremens

It is most severe form of alcohol withdrawal syndrome. It occurs usually within 2 to 4 days of complete or significant abstinence from heavy alcohol drinking. It includes:

- Visual and auditory hallucination
- Clouding of consciousness
- Poor attention span
- Tachycardia, fever, sweating
- Hypertension
- Pupillary dilation
- Insomnia and dehydration.

Alcohol Seizure (Rum Fits)

Generalized tonic-clonic seizures occur in about 10% of alcohol dependence patients, usually 12–48 hours after heavy bout of drinking. (Administer anticonvulsants).

Alcoholic Hallucinosis

Alcoholic hallucinosis is a type of hallucination characterized by the presence of hallucinations (usually auditory) during partial or complete abstinence or followed by regular alcohol intake. It occurs in about 2% of patients.

Neuropsychiatry Complications of Chronic Alcohol Use

Wernicke's Encephalopathy

This is an acute reaction which occurs due severe deficiency of thiamine, in chronic alcohol users, because alcohol reduces the absorption ability of thiamine in the stomach which commonly occurs during presence of alcohol content in stomach for long duration of time. The clinical signs are:

- **Ocular signs:** Nystagmus ophthalmoplegia with bilateral external rectus paralysis.
- **Higher mental function disturbance:** Recent memory disturbances, disorientation, confusion, poor attention span and distractibility.

Korsakoff's Psychosis

Most of the time it occurs followed by wernicke's encephalopathy.

Clinically it characterized by gross memory disturbance with confabulation. Insight is often impaired.

Note: Preparation of vitamin B containing 100 mg of thiamine should be administered through parenterally, twice daily for 3–5 days. This should be followed by oral administration of vitamin B_1 for at least 6 months. Thiamine commonly is deficient in alcoholics. Replacement therapy is required to prevent neuropathy, confusion, and encephalopathy.

Marchiafava–Bignami Disease

This is a rare disorders characterized by disorientation, epilepsy, ataxia, dysarthria, hallucination, spastic limb paralysis and deterioration of personality and intellectual functioning.

Other Complications

- Alcohol dementia
- Cerebellar degeneration
- Peripheral neuropathy

Complication of Alcohol Use During Pregnancy: (Fetal Alcohol Syndrome)

Fetal alcohol syndrome (FAS) is a range of disabilities which seen in a child born to mother who used alcohol during her pregnancy.

A child or person with FAS has differences in their face and head. They are smaller or shorter than average, and have learning and behavioral difficulties.

Symptoms

Usually, FAS is diagnosed only when a child has the following major clinical manifestations, or signs:

- Growth retardation
- *Characteristic facial features, such as:*
  - Small eyes with drooping upper lids
  - Short, upturned nose
  - Flattened cheeks

- Small jaw
- Thin upper lip
- Flattened philtrum (the groove in the middle of the upper lip)

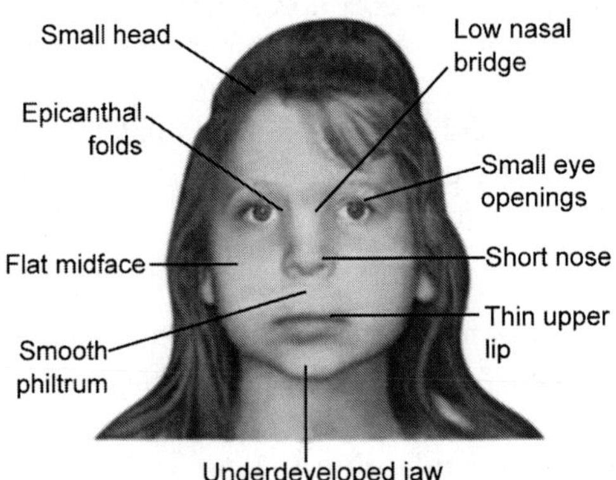

Fig. 9.1: FAS child showing facial features
Abbreviation: FAS = Fetal alcohol syndrome

- *Central nervous system problems:*
  - Mental retardation
  - Hyperactivity
  - Delayed development of gross motor skills such as rolling over, sitting up, crawling and walking
  - Delayed development of fine motor skills such as grasping objects with the thumb and index finger, and transferring objects from one hand to the other
  - Impaired language development
  - Memory problems, poor judgment, distractibility, impulsiveness
  - Problems with learning
  - Seizures.

Treatment

Although there is no cure for FAS, children who are identified and diagnosed early preferably by preschool age have a better chance of overcoming the condition. Because from early on their education can be designed to maximize of their potential.

How much Alcohol is too much during pregnancy? (0 ml)

Ideally no any amount of alcohol is considered as normal during pregnancy, so it is clear that abusing alcohol during pregnancy is dangerous.

CLASSIFICATION OF ALCOHOL–RELATED DISORDER (ICD-10)

Basically alcohol-related disorder classified into two groups such as alcohol use disorder *(includes alcohol abuse and alcohol dependency)* and Alcohol induced disorder *(includes alcohol intoxication and withdrawal)* which is explained in detail below:

Alcohol Use Disorder

Alcohol Abuse and Alcohol Dependency

Alcohol use disorder is a pattern of alcohol use that involves problems in control over drinking, being preoccupied with alcohol, continuing to use alcohol even when it causes problems, having to drink more to get the same effect, or having withdrawal symptoms when person rapidly decrease or stop drinking.

Difference Between Alcohol Abuse and Alcohol Dependence

There are a number of key elements that defines a person who abuses alcohol or who use it in a harmful way and those who are dependent on alcohol. A dependence on alcohol differs from this as the behaviors are linked to physical or mental need for alcohol.

Alcohol Abuse (Harmful Use)

Box 9.3: Core concept

Use of alcohol in an abnormal way which causes harmful to the body and leads to severe physiological and psychological distress.

Alcohol abusers have some ability to control or limit their drinking which is what defines them from an alcohol dependent person.

Health implications for alcohol abusers: When an individual abuses alcohol, they often engage in high-risk behaviors which put themselves and others at risk.

Health issues that can be a direct result of abusing alcohol include the following:

- Alcohol poisoning
- Sexually transmitted diseases
- Unwanted pregnancy
- Liver damage
- Neurological damage
- Sexual dysfunction

Alcohol Dependence

Box 9.4: Core concept

Alcohol dependency can be defined as a physical and/or mental dependency on alcohol which produces specified symptoms including a high level of tolerance to the effects of alcohol.

Alcohol dependence is considered a chronic disease as its symptoms are progressive and can be fatal. Alcohol dependency is characterized by cravings and an increased tolerance to alcohol despite severe medical implications and an inability, physically and mentally, to stop drinking.

Alcoholism is another term for alcohol dependency and according to the *National Institute on Alcohol and Alcoholics (NIAA)*, there are four key symptoms that define this disease:

1. **Craving:** A need or strong desire to drink alcohol.
2. **Loss of control:** An inability to cease drinking, a feeling of no control of the situation.
3. **Physical dependence:** When not drinking, a person will have signs of withdrawals such as nausea, sweating and vomiting.
4. **Tolerance:** A person will need more alcohol to meet cravings and to get drunk.

Box 9.5: Do you know?

An increasingly heavy drinker often says

When I went to quit drinking, I realized that alcohol had taken to my body in such a way that I could not stop. I would shake like I was going to break, I would start to sweat, I could not think until I had another drink. I could not function without it.

Clinical Features

Box 9.6: Explained with the help of ICD-10 diagnostic criteria

Alcohol abuse or harmful use

- Clear evidence that the substance use was responsible for physical or psychological harm, including impaired judgement or dysfunctional behavior.
- The nature of the harm should be clearly identifiable (and specified).
- The pattern of use has persisted for at least one month or has occurred repeatedly within a twelve-month period.
- The disorder does not meet the criteria for any other mental or behavioral disorder related to the same drug in the same time period.

Alcohol dependence

Three or more of the following manifestations should have occurred together for at least one month or if persisting for periods of less than one month then they have occurred together repeatedly within a twelve month period.

- A strong desire or sense of compulsion to take the substance.
- Impaired capacity to control substance-taking behavior as evidenced by: the substance being often taken in larger amounts or over a longer period than intended, or any unsuccessful effort in control of substance use.
- A physiological withdrawal state when substance use is reduced or ceased.
- Evidence of tolerance to the effects of the substance, such that there is a need for markedly increased amounts of the substance to achieve intoxication or desired effect, or that there is a markedly diminished effect with continued use of the same amount of the substance.
- Preoccupation with substance use, as manifested by:
  - Important alternative pleasures or interests being given up or reduced because of substance use.
- Persisting with substance use despite clear evidence of harmful consequences.

—Adopted from WHO, ICD-10 text book

Alcohol-induced Disorder

Alcohol-induced disorder is characterized by appearance of bodily physical and psychological symptoms which occurs due to excessive use of alcohol during short period of time (intoxication) or total cessation of alcohol intake, or reduction in the amount of alcohol intake (withdrawal syndrome), after repeated, and usually prolonged and high-dose use of that substance.

So alcohol induced disorder commonly named as alcohol intoxication and alcohol withdrawal symptom.

Diagnostic Studies

- **Blood alcohol/drug levels:** Blood alcohol level (BAL) may yields following results.
  - In the absence of elevated alcohol tolerance, blood levels in excess of 100 mg/dL are associated with ataxia.
  - At 200 mg/dL the client is drowsy and confused.
  - Respiratory depression occurs with blood levels of 400 mg/dL and death is possible.

- **Complete Blood Count (CBC):** Decreased hemoglobin (Hb)/hematocrit (Hct) may reflect problems such as iron deficiency anemia or acute/chronic GI bleeding.
- **Liver function tests:** LDH and amylase may be elevated, reflecting liver or pancreatic damage.
- **Nutritional tests:** Albumin is low and total protein may be decreased. Vitamin deficiencies are usually present, reflecting malnutrition/malabsorption.
- **Chest radiography:** May reveal right lower lobe pneumonia (common manifestation may be related to malnutrition depressed immune system.
- **Electrocardiogram:** Dysrhythmias, cardiomyopathies, and ischemia may be present because of direct effect of alcohol on cardiac muscles.
- **Urine analysis:** Infection may be present, ketones may present due to breakdown of fatty acids in malnutrition.
- **Other screening studies:** Check for HIV, Hepatitis, TB depend on individual risk factors.

Box 9.7: Difference between alcohol intoxication and withdrawal

Alcohol intoxication	Alcohol withdrawal syndrome
It occurs as a result the amount of alcohol in blood stream increases. The higher the blood alcohol concentration is, the more impaired. **Symptoms include:** • Inappropriate behavior • Unstable moods • Impaired judgment • Impaired attention • Slurred speech • Impaired attention or memory • Poor coordination • Aggression • Lability of mood • Unsteady gait • Difficulty standing • Nystagmus • 'Blackouts,' where person do not remember any events during intoxicated period • Decreased level of consciousness (e.g. stupor, coma). • Very high blood alcohol levels can lead to coma or even death. • Acute alcohol intoxication when severe may be accompanied by hypotension, hypothermia and depression of the gag reflex.	It can occur when alcohol use has been heavy and prolonged and is then stopped or greatly reduced. It can occur within several hours to four or five days later. **Symptoms include:** • Sweating, rapid heartbeat, hand tremors • Problems sleeping (insomnia) • High blood pressure • Nausea and vomiting • Hallucinations • Restlessness and agitation • Anxiety, and occasionally seizures • Symptoms can be severe enough to impair ability to function at work or in social situations (Above symptoms are more noticeable when person wake up with less alcohol in blood) • The most severe type of withdrawal syndrome is known as delirium tremens (DT). Its signs and symptoms include: – Extreme confusion – Extreme agitation – High fever – Seizures (Grand mal convulsions) – Tactile hallucinations, such as having a sense of itching or burning that is not actually occurring. – Auditory hallucinations or hearing sounds that do not exist. – Visual hallucinations, or seeing images that do not exist.

MANAGEMENT

Alcohol Deterrent Therapy

Deterrent agents are those which are given to desensitize the individual to the effects of alcohol and maintain abstinence. The most commonly used drug is disulfiram or *Antabuse.*

What is antabuse?

Antabuse (disulfiram) blocks an enzyme that is involved in metabolizing alcohol intake. Disulfiram produces very unpleasant side effects when combined with alcohol in the body.

Disulfiram: Disulfiram (tetra ethylthiuram disulfide [TETD]) has been used for more than 50 years as a deterrent to ethanol abuse in the management of alcoholism. It is used as a conditioning treatment for alcohol dependence. When taken with alcohol, disulfiram causes many unwanted and unpleasant effects, and the fear of these is meant to condition the patient to avoid alcohol.

Mechanism of action: Disulfiram is an oral drug used for treating alcoholism. Alcohol is converted in the body into acetaldehyde by an enzyme called alcohol dehydrogenase. Another enzyme called acetaldehyde dehydrogenase then converts acetaldehyde into acetic acid.

Flow chart 9.1: Disulfiram mechanism

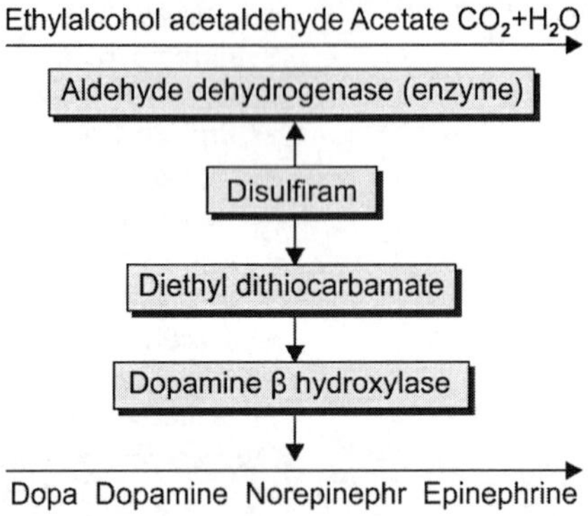

Ethylalcohol acetaldehyde Acetate CO_2+H_2O

Aldehyde dehydrogenase (enzyme)

Disulfiram

Diethyl dithiocarbamate

Dopamine β hydroxylase

Dopa Dopamine Norepinephr Epinephrine

Disulfiram prevents acetaldehyde dehydrogenase from converting acetaldehyde into acetic acid, leading to a build up of acetaldehyde levels in the blood and in presence of alcohol it produces acetaldehyde-alcohol reaction in the body which is an unpleasant feeling to a person.

Warning: Alcohol must not be consumed during treatment and for up to 14 days after discontinuation, as disulfiram prevents the metabolism of ethanol, causing acetaldehyde to accumulate in the body. This can result in a 'disulfiram-alcohol reaction' causing adverse effects.

Disulfiram ethanol reaction (DER): Disulfiram irreversibly inhibits acetaldehyde dehydrogenase. Intake of ethanol during disulfiram therapy will lead to accumulation of acetaldehyde, which is considered the main contributing factor to the disulfiram-alcohol reaction.

- Disulfiram-ethanol reactions often develop within 15 minutes after exposure to ethanol; symptoms usually peak within 30 minutes to 1 hour, and then gradually subside over the next few hours. Symptoms may be severe and life-threatening.

- The disulfiram-alcohol reaction is characterized by:
  - Intense vasodilation of the face and neck causing flushing
  - Increased body temperature
  - Sweating, nausea, vomiting
  - Pruritis, urticaria
  - Anxiety, dizziness, headache
  - Blurred vision
  - Dyspnea, palpitations and hyperventilation.

In severe cases tachycardia, hypotension, respiratory depression, chest pain, arrhythmias, coma and convulsions may occur. *Rare complications* include hypertension, bronchospasm and methemoglobinemia.

Box 9.8: Side-effects

- Psychotic reactions; depression.
- Reduction in libido

Nervous system disorders

- Drowsiness (during initial treatment)
- Peripheral neuritis, optic neuritis
- Encephalopathy

Gastrointestinal disorders

- Nausea, vomiting

Hepatobiliary disorders

- Hepatic cell damage

Skin and subcutaneous tissue disorders

- Allergic dermatitis

General disorders

- Fatigue (during initial treatment)
- Halitosis

Contraindications: Caution should be exercised in the presence of renal failure, hepatic or respiratory disease, diabetes mellitus, hypothyroidism, cerebral damage and epilepsy.

Dosage: In the first phase of treatment, a maximum of 500 mg daily in the form of tablet is given in a single dose for one to two weeks. Usually it is taken in the morning.

Maintenance Regimen: The average maintenance dose is 250 mg daily (range, 125 to 500 mg), it should not exceed 500 mg daily.

Warning: Disulfiram should not be administered until it has been ascertained that the client has abstained from alcohol for at least 12 hours. And effect of disulfiram even after discontinuing remains for about 2 weeks.

Nurse responsibility in disulfiram therapy:

- Educate the patient about disulfiram and obtain informed consent.
- Wait until the patient has abstained from alcohol at least 12 hours and/or breath or blood alcohol level is zero.
- Advice patient to wear ID card which mentioning about Disulfiram treatment, Doctors name and Contact number.

- Advice him not to take alcohol.
- Start Disulfiram after 12 hours of alcohol.
- Advice him to avoid the substances contain alcohol.
- Inform about DER.
- Avoid CNS depressants.
- Avoid driving.
- Advice the patient not to use any alcohol content products like aftershave, spray, etc. while patient is in therapy.

Acamprosate (Preventing Relapse)

It is used to prevent relapse in recovering alcohol-dependent patients. It appears to restore the normal activity of glutaminergic neurons, which become hyper, excited as a result of chronic alcohol exposure. Patients treated with acamprosate report a significantly greater rate of complete abstinence. It is contraindicated in cases of renal insufficiency or severe hepatic failure.

Naltrexone

Naltrexone tablet is indicated for use in alcohol dependence to reduce the risk of relapse, support abstinence and reduce alcohol craving. These drugs only deal with physical symptoms and do not treat the psychological causes of addiction. Naltrexone is contraindicated in case of acute hepatitis or liver failure.

Treatment Alcohol-induced Disorder (Alcohol Intoxication and Withdrawal)

Detoxification Therapy

It is the process by which an alcohol dependent person recovers from the intoxification and withdrawal effects in a supervised manner.

- **Benzodiazepines:** Chlordizepoxide 80–200 mg/day.
- **Diazepam:** 40–80 mg/day to control anxiety, agitation and tremors.
- **Thiamine:** 100 mg intramuscular for 3–5 days followed by vitamin B administration 100 mg OD for at least 6 months.

THERAPIES TO TREAT ALCOHOL DISORDER

- Motivational interviewing
- Individual psychotherapy
- Group therapy
- Counseling
- Aversive conditioning
- Behavior modification techniques
- Family therapy
- Self-help groups

Agencies Concerned with Alcohol-related Problems

- **Alcoholic anonymous (AA):** This is a self-help organization founded in the USA by two alcoholic men, Dr Bob smith and Bill Wilson on 10th June 1935. AA considers alcoholism as a physical, mental and spiritual disease, a progressive one, which can be arrested but not cured.

  Members attend group meetings usually twice a week on a long-term basis. Each member is assigned a support person. From whom he may seek help when the temptations to drink occur. In crisis he can obtain immediate help by telephone.
- **AL-ANDN:** It is a group started by wife of Dr Bob (Mrs. Anne), to support the spouses of alcoholics.
- **AL-ATEEN:** Provides support to their teenage children.
- **HOSTELS:** These are for those rendered homeless due to alcohol-related problems. They provide rehabilitation and counseling.
- **Adult children of alcoholics (ACOA):** Adult who grew up with an alcoholic in the home.
- **Children are people:** School age children with an alcoholic family members.
- **Women for sobriety:** Meant for female alcoholics.

NURSING MANAGEMENT

Assessment

CAGE Question

A good way to assess history and pattern of drinking is to use a short test known as the CAGE test, which consists of four questions:

- Have you ever thought you should *cut down* on your drinking?
- Have people *annoyed* you by criticising your drinking?
- Have you ever felt *guilty* about your drinking?
- Have you ever drunk an *'eye-opener'*, which means: have you ever drunk alcohol first thing in the morning to get over a hangover and steady your nerves?

If answer is 'yes' to one or more of the questions above, it indicate that the person having problem with drinking.

Nursing Assessment

- **History:** Collect brief history of the client, developmental aspects and details about stressors in working environment, work load.
- **Marital history:** Any history of conflicts between partners.
- **Sexual history:** Satisfaction pattern, dissatisfactory life, difficulties in sexual life, transitional periods in life-any life events influencing alcoholism.
- **Social history:** Social environment, peer group influence.
- **Forensic history:** Previous court cases, any imprisonment or pending court cases.
- **Physical examination.**
- **Mental status examination.**

- General appearance and behavior
- Psycho motor activity
- Thought, content, mood, perception
- Orientation, memory, judgment, insight, abstractibility, intelligence.

Box 9.9: Nursing care plan for alcohol-related disorder

Nursing diagnosis: Risk for ineffective breathing pattern related to direct effect of alcohol toxicity on respiratory center and sedative drugs given to decrease alcohol withdrawal symptoms

Outcome identification	Nursing intervention
Client will be able to: • Maintain effective breathing pattern with respiratory rate within normal range.	• Monitor respiratory rate/depth and pattern. Note for periods of apnea, Cheyne-Stokes respirations. • Auscultate for breath sounds. Note presence of adventitious sounds (e.g. rhonchi, wheezes). • Elevate head end of the bed. • Encourage deep-breathing coughing exercises. • Change positions frequently. • Keep suction equipment, airways ready. • Administer supplemental oxygen if needed. • Review serial chest X-rays, arterial blood gases (ABGs)/pulse oximetry as indicated.

Nursing diagnosis: Risk for Injury related to cessation of alcohol and appearance of withdrawal symptoms, Involuntary clonic/tonic muscle activity (seizures), reduced muscle and hand/eye coordination.

Outcome identification	Nursing intervention
Client will be able to: • Demonstrate absence of untoward effects of withdrawal. • Experience no physical injury.	• Monitor for withdrawal symptoms. • Monitor/document seizure activity. • Maintain patent airway. • Provide safety to the patient (e.g. padded side rails, bed in low position). • Assess for gait. • Palpate upper arm to conform actual withdrawal versus medication-seeking behavior. • Assist patient in ambulation and self-care activities as needed. • Administer medications as indicated e.g.: Benzodiazepines (BZDs)

Nursing diagnosis: Anxiety or fear related to physiologic withdrawal, situational crisis (hospitalization) and perceived threat of death as evidenced by feelings of inadequacy, shame, increased helplessness/ hopelessness and increased tension.

Outcome identification	Nursing intervention
Client will be able to: • Verbalize reduction of fear and anxiety. • Demonstrate problem-solving skills and use resources effectively.	• Identify cause of anxiety. • Explain that alcohol withdrawal usually increases anxiety and uneasiness. • Reassess level of anxiety on an ongoing basis. • Develop a trusting relationship with patient through frequent contact being honest and nonjudgmental. • Show an accepting attitude about alcoholism. • Reorient frequently. • Administer medications as indicated, e.g.: BDZs (e.g. chlordiazepoxide [Librium], diazepam [Valium]). • Referral patient for Detoxification and crisis center.

OPIOID USE DISORDERS

The use of opioids has increased markedly for the last few decades. Dried exudates obtained from unripe seed capsules of *Papaver somniferum* has been used and abused for centuries. The natural alkaloids of opium and their synthetic preparations are highly dependence.

This group includes several narcotic substances like opium, heroin, morphine, codeine, pethidine, methadone, and pentazocine. Synthetic preparations are highly dependence producing. These drugs are mainly used as an analgesic, but long term use can produce dependency.

Intoxication of Opioid

Intoxication of opioids includes:

- Psychological effects
  - Euphoria
  - Relaxation
  - Hyperactivity
  - Drowsiness
  - Analgesia
  - Reduced sexual desire
- Physical effects
  - Small pupil
  - Bradycardia
  - Reduced appetite
  - Constipation
  - Respiratory depression

  With increase in dosage tolerance develops rapidly.

Withdrawal of Opioid

Withdrawal of opioid drugs rarely threatens life and does not produce serious effects.

The features are flu-like symptom include:

- Lacrimation
- Running nose
- Muscle and joint pain
- Cold and hot flushes
- Nausea, vomiting and diarrhea
- Piloerection

Intense craving for the drug is a notable feature. This symptom starts 6 hours after the last dosage and peaks within 36–48 hours.

Complications

- With IV users it may develop AIDS, hepatitis, endocarditis, septicemia, acute local infections (cellulitis, thrombophlebitis).
- Involvement in criminal activities.

Treatment

Opioid Intoxication

Opioid overdose can be life-threatening and needs immediate management.

- Naloxone is the antidote used for the detoxification of the opioid overdose.
- Maintain patent airway
- Administer oxygen
- Administer IV fluids for the excretion of the drug
- Monitor vital signs.

Opioid Withdrawal

- Symptomatic treatment is given
- Methadone, clonidine can be used for maintenance.

Other Measures

- Dietary management
- Treat complications
- Antidepressants can be used if the client develops with depressive features
- Supportive psychotherapy, counseling
- Group therapy and family therapy
- Supportive groups.

CANNABINOIDS ABUSE

Cannabis is obtained from *Cannabis sativa*. The dried leaves and flowers are used for abuse. These products often referred as *Ganja or Marijuana.*

Acute Intoxication

The features are as follows:

Psychological

- Person experience a feeling of well-being
- Mild elevation of mood (euphoria)
- Impaired memory
- Impaired psychomotor activity
- Dream like state
- Flash back phenomena

Physical

- Tachycardia
- Reddening of the conjunctiva
- Dry mouth
- Respiratory tract irritation
- Increased appetite

Tolerance can be developed with high doses for a long-term use. Long-term use can give rise to dependence.

Withdrawal Symptoms

Withdrawal from cannabis use gives rise to a syndrome of nausea, anorexia, irritability and insomnia.

Treatment

- Total abstinence form cannabis
- Symptomatic treatment
- Psychological measures like support, counseling
- Follow-up and monitoring.

HYPNOTICS, SEDATIVES AND ANXIOLYTICS

This includes the over use of the following:

- Benzodiazepines (e.g. diazepam, lorazepam)
- Benzodiazepine, like drugs (e.g. zolpidem, zopiclone)
- Barbiturates (e.g. secobarbital)
- Carbamates (e.g. meprobamate)

These substances are brain depressants.

Intoxication

Intoxication features include similar to alcohol like slurred speech, unsteady gait, nystagmus, ataxia impaired attention or memory, stupor or coma.

Withdrawal

These include: Autonomic hyperactivity (e.g. sweating, tachycardia), nausea, vomiting, anorexia, insomnia, anxiety/agitation, perceptual disturbances (e.g. illusion), seizures, delirium.

Treatment

- Induce vomiting if the patient is conscious.
- Administer activated charcoal to reduce absorption.
- Provide symptomatic treatment.

STIMULANTS

These are the drugs that enhance the action of dopamine and noradrenaline.

Some of these drugs include:

- Amphetamine
- Cocaine
- Caffeine
- Nicotine (tobacco)

AMPHETAMINE USE DISORDER

Amphetamines are a group of CNS stimulant. They result in a sense of increased alertness, energy, increased attention span, concentration, social skills, more self-confidence, improved mood, and less appetite.

They are commonly prescribed for Attention deficit hyperactivity disorder (ADHD).

Acute Intoxication

Intoxication symptoms include:
- Aggression, violent behavior or hostility
- Paranoia
- Anxiety
- Emotional numbing with sadness, fatigue and social withdrawal
- Entitlement regarding obtaining positions of power or influence
- Convulsions hallucinations especially hearing voices or conversations that are not real
- Delusions
- Amphetamine induced psychosis
- Confusion.

Withdrawal Symptoms

Amphetamine withdrawal symptoms are classified as follows:
- Fatigue, exhaustion, difficulty staying awake
- Vivid, unpleasant dreams
- Insomnia or hypersomnia at night
- Increased appetite
- Psychomotor retardation or agitation
- Anxiety
- Short-term memory loss
- Inability to concentrate

Treatment

- Absorption of the drug can be reduced by administering activated charcoal, within one hour of ingestion (acute intoxication)
- No effective pharmacological or psychosocial treatment options available to treat Amphetamine dependence
- Complete abstinence from the drug and its sources
- Not using alcohol or other substances
- Being socially active
- Engaging with support groups and self-help groups.

COCAINE USE DISORDER

Cocaine is an alkaloid derived from the coca bush, *Erythroxylum coca*. Commonly cocaine is called as '*crack*'. It is taken orally, intranasal, smoking or by parenterally.

Intoxication features include dilation of the pupil, sweating, nausea and hypomanic features. While withdrawal features include agitation, anorexia, depression, etc.

Treatment

- Antidote amyl nitrite can be administered
- Benzodiazepines-diazepam
- Individual and group psychotherapy.

CAFFEINE

Caffeine is one of the most commonly used drugs worldwide. It is a psycho stimulant readily crosses BBB. Caffeine enhances dopamine and noradrenaline activity and is contained in coffee, soft drinks and some medications.

Uses of 100 mg produce mild euphoria more than 250 mg produces intoxication and the symptoms are as follows:

- Restlessness
- Excitement
- Agitation
- Insomnia
- Diuresis
- GI upset
- Tachycardia
- Muscle twitching
- Flushed face

TOBACCO (NICOTINE)

Nicotine is also having a CNS stimulatory activity by exciting acetylcholine receptors and activating dopamine and noradrenaline.

The effects of nicotine produce improved attention, learning, reaction time, and problem-solving ability. Tobacco is the most common form of nicotine and is smoked in cigarettes, cigars, and pipes. Nicotine dependence develops rapidly.

Withdrawal symptoms occur after abrupt cessation of nicotine. These symptoms include the following:

- Irritability
- Frustration
- Poor concentration
- Insomnia
- Dysphoric mood
- Increase appetite

HALLUCINOGENS

This group of substances alters perception, thinking, or emotional states of individuals. It acts by changing serotonin level in brain.

These drugs may be natural (e.g. magic mushroom) or synthetic (e.g. Lysergic acid diethylamide, LSD).

This group has no medical use and a high abuse is common.

Intoxication

Intoxication of LSD includes marked perceptual distortions like hallucinations, depersonalization, derealization, euphoria, anxiety, panic, tachycardia, hypertension wide pupils, blurred vision, etc.

Treatment

- Symptomatic treatment
- Aggression management
- Supportive therapy

PHENCYCLIDINE (PCP)

This is a synthetic anesthetic substance with hallucinogenic properties. It is no longer used in humans because of delirium, agitation and aggressive behavior. It is often added to other drugs boost their effects.

Intoxication produces hypertensive crisis, status epilepticus, malignant hyperthermia, euphoria and peaceful floating sensations.

Treatment

- Anxiolytics may be given.
- Haloperidol can be used to treat aggressive behavior.

INHALANTS (VOLATILE SOLVENTS)

Inhalants are the organic substances and abused for producing psychotropic effects. These substances include glues, paint, thinner, nail polish remover, varnish etc. These agents generally depress brain and are commonly seen among adolescence and low socio-economic peoples.

Intoxication

Intoxication symptoms include euphoria, excitement, pleasant floating sensations, and disturbance in consciousness, perceptual disturbances, impulsiveness, impaired judgment, sedation and slurred speech.

Complications

Long-term use can cause irreversible multi organ damages. Psychological dependence occurs but physical dependence is unusual. (Withdrawal syndrome does not occur frequently).

Treatment

- Supportive therapy
- Anxiolytics.

10 Nursing Management of Patient with Personality Behavioral, Sexual and Eating Disorders

PERSONALITY DISORDERS

What is Personality?

The personality includes a combination of talents, attitudes, values, hopes, interests, mannerism, philosophies, loves, hates and habits. Personality is the sum total of an individual's traits and characteristic, i.e. the typical way of acting, thanking and feeling that makes each person unique.

Box 10.1: Do you know?

The word personality is derived from the Greek term Persona. It was used originally to describe the theatrical mask worn by some dramatic actors at the time. Over the years, it lost its connotations of pre-tense and illusion and came to represent the person behind the mask–the 'real' person.

Definition of Personality

Box 10.2: Definition of personality

The DSM IV TR (APA, 2000) defines personality traits as enduring patterns of perceiving, relating to, and thinking about the environment and oneself that are exhibited in a wide range of social and personal contexts.

Box 10.3: Definition of personality disorder

'A personality disorder is an enduring pattern of inner experience and behavior that deviates markedly from the expectations of the individual's culture, is pervasive and inflexible, has an onset in adolescence or early adulthood, is stable over time and leads to distress and impairment' (DSM-IV-TR).

Classification of Personality Disorder According to DSM (IV TR) and ICD-10

Box 10.4: Classification of personality disorder

The DSM-IV-TR groups the personality disorders into 3 clusters. These clusters have got individual personality disorders as follows:	International classification of disease [ICD-10]
Cluster A: Odd or eccentric disorder • Paranoid personality disorder • Schizoid personality disorder • Schizotypal personality disorder **Cluster B: Dramatic, emotional, or erratic disorder** • Antisocial personality disorder • Borderline personality disorder • Histrionic personality disorder • Narcissistic personality disorder	**F60 Specific personality disorder** F60.0 Paranoid personality disorder F60.1 Schizoid personality disorder F60.2 Dissocial personality disorder F60.3 Emotionally unstable personality disorder F60.4 Histrionic personality disorder F60.5 Anankastic personality disorder F60.6 Avoidant personality disorder F60.7 Dependent personality disorder F60.8 Other specific personality disorder

Contd...

Contd...

Cluster C: Anxious or fearful disorder	F60.9	Unspecified personality disorder
• Avoidant personality disorder	F61	Mixed and other personality disorders
• Dependent personality disorder	F61.0	Mixed personality disorder
• Obsessive compulsive personality disorder	F61.1	Troublesome personality disorder

Incidence

5–15 percent of adults have one or more personality disorders (PD).

Etiology

Genetics

Genetic factor play an important role in development of personality disorders.

- **Antisocial PD:** Common among first degree biological relatives with the disorder, greater risk if relative is female. Increased risk for children of parents with antisocial personality disorder, whether adopted or biological, suggesting both genetic and environmental factors.
- **Borderline PD:** Five times more common among first-degree biological relatives.
- Among monozygotic twins the concordance for personality disorders are several times higher than dizygotic twins.
- Cluster A personality disorder are more common in the biological relatives of schizophrenia patients.
- Cluster B personality disorders have a genetic base.
- **Antisocial PD:** More common in alcoholics.
- **Borderline PD:** Tends to occur in depression people, Histrionic PD seen more in somatization.

Biological Factors

- Person with personality disorder having the alteration in brain structure and function
- **Hormone:** Increased testosterone, estradiol and estrone
- **Low platelet monoamine oxidase:** Schizotypal disorders
- **Neurotransmitters:** Increased endogenous endorphin levels
- **Reduced serotonin:** Borderline PD. Increased norepinephrine associated with irritability and hostility-Borderline PD.

Psychodynamics

- Parental rejection or indifference
- Unmet need for satisfaction and security
- A lack of ego strength, Id directed behavior.

Family Dynamics

- Absence of parental discipline
- Extreme poverty
- Removal from home

- Lack of parental figures of both sexes
- Inadequate nurturing
- Over protection.

Other Factors

- **Antisocial personality disorder:** Maternal deprivation
- **Borderline personality disorder:** Physical and sexual abuse
- **Histrionic personality disorder:** Failure to resolve oedipal complex and excessive use of repression as a mechanism of defence
- **Dependent personality disorder:** Fixation in oral stage of development
- **Paranoid personality disorder:** Absence of trust-lack of parental affection in childhood and persistent rejection by parents leading to low self-esteem.

Classification of Personality Disorder Based on Clusters and Clinical Pictures, Nursing Management of Each Personality Disorders According to DSM-IV TR

Box 10.5: Cluster wise classification of personality disorder

Cluster		Subtype	Discriminating feature
A	Odd/eccentric	Paranoid	Suspicious
		Schizoid	Socially indifferent
		Schizotypal	Eccentric
B	Erratic/impulsive	Antisocial	Disagreeable
		Borderline	Unstable
		Histrionic	Attention seeking
		Narcissistic	Self-centred
C	Anxious/fearful	Avoidant	Inhibited
		Dependant	Submissive
		Obsessive	Perfectionist

Cluster A: Behavior Regarded as Odd or Eccentric

It includes, 1. Paranoid, 2. Schizoid, 3. Schizotypal

Paranoid personality disorder	**Definition** The *DSM-IV-TR* defines paranoid personality disorder as 'a pervasive pattern of distrust and suspiciousness of others such that their motives are interpreted as malevolent, beginning by early adulthood and present in a variety of contexts' (APA, 2000). **Clinical features** Paranoid personality disorder people are: • Suspects, without sufficient basis, that others are exploiting, harming, or deceiving him or her • Constantly on guard • Hypervigilant • Persistent refusal to forgive insults and slights • Suspiciousness

Contd...

Contd...

	• Suspiciousness concerning fidelity of sexual partner • Has tendencies to experience excessive self-importance • They avoid interactions with other people. • They always feel that others are there to take advantage of them. **Treatment** • Psychotherapy • Role playing • Pharmacotherapy • Antianxiety agent such as diazepam • Antipsychotic to control severe agitation.

Schizoid personality disorder	**Definition**
	DSM-IV defines schizoid personality disorder as a pervasive pattern of detachment from social relationships and a restricted range of expression of emotions in interpersonal settings, beginning by early adulthood and present in a variety of contexts.
	Clinical features
	• Neither desires nor enjoys close relationships
	• Has little, if any, interest in having sexual experiences with another person
	• Takes pleasure in few, if any, activities
	• Lacks close friends or confidants other than first-degree relatives
	• Shows emotional coldness, detachment
	• Preoccupied with fantasy.
	N.B: Does not occur exclusively during the course of schizophrenia, a mood disorder with psychotic features.
	Treatment
	• Gradually increasing social involvement
	• Group therapy
	• Pharmacotherapy
	  – Antipsychotic
	  – Antidepressant
	  – Psycho stimulants
	  – Serentonergic agents
	• Group therapy
	• Family-based interventions.

Schizotypal personality disorder	**Definition** DSM-IV defines schizotypal personality disorder as 'A pervasive pattern of social and interpersonal deficits marked by acute discomfort with, and reduced capacity for, close relationships as well as by cognitive or perceptual distortions and eccentricities of behavior, beginning by early adulthood and present in a variety of contexts' **Clinical features** • Odd beliefs or magical thinking that influences behavior (inconsistent with subcultural norms) e.g: superstitiousness, belief in clairvoyance, telepathy, or 'sixth sense • Unusual perceptual experiences (including bodily illusions) • Odd thinking and speech (e.g. vague, circumstantial, metaphorical, over elaborate, or stereotyped) • Suspiciousness or paranoid ideation • Behavior or appearance that is odd, eccentric • Lack of close friends.

Contd...

Contd...

	N.B: Does not occur exclusively during the course of schizophrenia, a mood disorder with psychotic features. **Treatment** • Low dose of neuroleptics to treat cognitive distortion, depression and anxiety. • Group therapy • Supportive psychotherapy • Social skill training.

Box 10.6: Nursing process for personality disorders

Nursing diagnosis: Anxiety related to inability to trust.

Outcome identification	Nursing intervention
Client will be able to: • Over come from anxiety	• Develop primary nurse patient relationship. • Assist client to identify sources of anxiety and concerns. • Explore present patterns of coping with anxiety and how effective they have been. • Discuss alternatives to current ineffective behaviors. • Encourage implementation of new strategies, giving feedback on effectiveness.

Nursing diagnosis: Social isolation related to disturbed thought process that result in delusional thinking.

Outcome identification	Nursing intervention
Client will be able to: • Verbalize willingness to be involved with others.	• Assess degree of isolation by listening to client's comments about loneliness. • Spend time with client • Plan appropriate time for activities • Assist client to participate in diversion activities • Identify support system available to the client • Assess family relationships, communication patterns, knowledge of client condition • Note client's sense of self-worth and belief about individual identity within milieu and family setting.

Nursing diagnosis: Disturbed thought process related to psychological conflicts.

Outcome identification	Nursing intervention
Client will be able to: • To recognize changes in thinking and behavior	• State reality matter of fatly • Communicate in clear, concise terms with clearly stated rules about what client can do. • Note impulsive behaviors and request to stop. • Gradually involve in learning activities, occupational therapies.

Cluster B: PD (Behavior Regarded as Dramatic, Emotional, or Erratic)

(1. Antisocial personality disorder, 2. Borderline personality disorder, 3. Histrionic personality disorder, 4. Narcissistic personality disorder)

Antisocial personality disorder	**Definition** DSM-IV defines antisocial personality as 'A pervasive pattern of socially irresponsible, exploitative and guiltless behavior, as evidenced by the tendency to fail to conform the law and fail to develop stable relationship'

Contd...

Contd...

	ICD-10 defines antisocial personality as enduring pattern of inability to conform to social norms that result in impaired life functioning. **Clinical features** • Failure to conform to social norms with respect to lawful behavior • Deceitfulness as indicated by repeated lying • Failure to plan ahead • Irritability and aggressiveness • Consistent irresponsibility as indicated by repeated to failure to sustain consistent work • Long standing pattern of socially irresponsible behaviors • Disregard the rights of others • Lying, truancy, running away from home, thefts, fights, substance abuse and illegal activities. **Treatment** • Hospitalization • Self-help group • Therapeutic community • Environmental manipulation • Assertiveness • Pharmacotherapy: Psycho stimulants, e.g. methyl phenidate for attention deficit/ hyperactivity.
Borderline personality disorder	**Definition** DSM-IV defines borderline personality disorder as 'A pervasive pattern of instability of inters personal relationship, self image and affects and marked impulsivity that begins by early adulthood' ICD-10 define borderline personality disorder as 'A pattern of intense and chaotic relationship with affective instability, fluctuating and extreme attitude regarding others people, impulsivity directly self-destructive behavior and a lack of a clear or certain sense of identity or values. **Clinical features** • A pattern of unstable and intense interpersonal relationship • Unstable emotions • Impulsive, directly and indirectly self-destructive, and lack a clear sense of identity • Lack of control on anger • Recurrent suicidal threats or behavior • Chronic feelings of emptiness • Uncertainty about personal identity • Acting out feelings instead of expressing them appropriately or verbally • Affective instability and fluctuating attitudes toward other people • Chronic depression. **Treatment** • Psychotherapy • Behavior therapy • Antipsychotic to control anger, hostility and brief psychotic episodes • Anticonvulsant, e.g. Carbamazepine.
Histrionic personality disorder	**Definition** According to DSM-IV histrionic personality disorder is characterized by self dramatization, a craving for novelty and excitement and self-centered approach to personal relationships. According to ICD-10, histrionic personality disorder is characterized by a pervasive pattern of excessive emotionality and attention-seeking behavior.

Contd...

Contd...

	Clinical features • Tends to be well liked, successful, popular and sociable • Failure to evoke attention and approval result in anxiety • Highly distractible and flighty by nature • Interpersonal relationships are superficial • Difficulty in maintaining a meaningful and stable relationship • Uncomfortable in situations in which he or she is not the center of attention • Display rapidly shifting and shallow expression of emotions • Consistently use appearances to draw attention to self • Has a style of speech that is excessively impressionistic and lacking in detail • Self-dramatizing attention seeking tendency. **Treatment** • Psychoanalytical psychotherapy • Anxiolytics • Antidepressants • Antipsychotic.
Narcistic personality disorder	**Definitions** According DSM-IV Narcissistic personality is defined as 'An exaggerated sense of self-worth, they lack empathy and are hyper sensitivity to the evaluation of others'. According to ICD-10 Narcissistic personality is defined as pervasive pattern of grandiosity, need for admiration and lack of empathy that begins by early adulthood and present in a variety of context. **Clinical features** • Has a grandiose sense of self importance. • Preoccupied with fantasies of unlimited success, power brilliance and beauty. • Believe that he/she is special and unique. • Require excessive admiration. • Interpersonally exploitative. • Lacks empathy, is unwilling to recognize or identify with feelings and needs for others. • Being overly self centered. • Optimistic, relaxed, cheerful and care free. • Mood can easily change. • Frequently choose a person who will be obedient. • Grandiose sense of self importance. • Impaired interpersonal relationship. • Unable to recognize the desire and feelings of others. • Unwillingness to take risk where defeat is possible. **Treatment** • Individual psychodynamic psychotherapy. • Psychoanalysis. • Antidepressants. • Lithium carbonate to control mood swings.

Box 10.7: Nursing process for cluster 'B' personality disorder

Nursing diagnosis: Risk for violence, directed at others related to inability to tolerate frustration (antisocial character) as evidenced by body language (muscle tension, facial expression, rigid posture); increased motor activity, irritability, agitation, hostile behavior.

Contd...

Contd...

Outcome identification	Nursing intervention
Client will be able to: • Develop and use nonaggressive, socially acceptable behaviors to gratify needs and interact with others. • Demonstrate self-control as evidenced by relaxed posture and manner.	• Convey accepting attitude toward client. Work on development of trust. Be honest, keep all promises, and convey message that the behavior, not the client, is unacceptable. • Maintain low level of stimuli in client's environment (low lighting, few people, simple decor, low noise level). • Provide structured environment, set firm limits (e.g. consistent schedule, ward rules, expectations of the client for cooperating). • Encourage verbalization of feelings and provide outlet for expression • Remove all dangerous objects from client's environment as appropriate. • Remain calm and nonaggressive in communicating with client.
Nursing diagnosis: Risk for self-mutilation related to: Parental emotional deprivation (unresolved fears of abandonment) as evidenced by history of self-inflicted injuries.	
Outcome identification	**Nursing intervention**
Client will not harm self.	• Observe client's behavior frequently. Do this through routine activities and interactions; • Avoid appearing watchful and suspicious. • Secure a verbal contract from client that he or she will seek out staff member when urge for self-mutilation is felt. • If self-mutilation occurs, care for client's wounds in a matter-of-fact manner. • Do not give positive reinforcement to this behavior. • Encourage client to talk about feelings he or she was having just before this behavior occurred. • Act as a role model for appropriate expression of angry feelings, and give positive reinforcement • Remove all dangerous objects from client's environment. • If warranted by high acuity of the situation,
Nursing diagnosis: Chronic low self-esteem related to lack of positive feedback; repeated negative feedback unmet dependency needs; retarded ego development, Dysfunctional family system, evidenced by acting-out behaviors, such as excessive use of alcohol and feelings of inadequacy, diminished self-worth.	
Outcome identification	**Nursing intervention**
Client will be able to: • Verbalize a sense of worth whileness. • Make healthy choices regarding management of/be involved in meeting own care needs.	• Encourage verbalization of feelings of inadequacy, worthlessness, fear of rejection, and need for acceptance from others. • Assist client to identify positive aspects about self related to social skills, work abilities, education, talents, and appearance. • Provide clear, consistent, verbal/nonverbal communication. Be truthful and honest. • Explore the relationship between feelings of inadequacy and aggressive behaviors, use of drugs. • Review ways to improve the quality of interaction with others. • Help client identify positive aspects of the self and develop ways to change the characteristics that are socially unacceptable. • Encourage independence in the performance of personal responsibilities and in decision-making related to own self-care. Offer recognition and praise for accomplishments.

Contd...

Contd...

Nursing diagnosis: Impaired social interaction related to inability to engage in satisfying personal relationships, evidenced by difficulty meeting expectations of others.	
Outcome identification	**Nursing intervention**
Client will be able to: • Express increased sense of self-worth. • Participate willingly in activities/programs without use of manipulation.	• Note expressions of hopelessness/worthlessness (e.g. 'I'm a loser,' 'It's fate.'). • Face and deal with clients expression of powerlessness and inability to control situation. • Encourage client to make requests/ask for what is wanted in a clear, straightforward manner and express feelings clearly to others difference in relationship/commitments. • Have client discuss thoughts/feelings about family, peers, authority figures, opposite sex, violence, and victims. Give feedback on the 'correctness' of thinking process. Describe feelings when someone says 'no.' Review with client feelings regarding authority and violating rights of others. • Help client recognize behaviors that do not get intended response and discuss possible modification. • Involve in group activities, (e.g. occupational/vocational therapy, psychotherapy, outdoor education program, codependency meetings).

Cluster C Personality Disorder: Behavior Regarded as Anxious or Fearful Disorder

(1. Avoidant PD, 2. Dependent PD, 3. Obsessive Compulsive PD)

Avoidant personality disorder	**Definition** DSM-IV defines avoidant social personality as 'A pervasive pattern of social inhibition, feelings of inadequacy, and hypersensitivity to negative evaluation, beginning by early adulthood and present in a variety of contexts'. **Clinical features** • Avoids occupational activities that involve significant interpersonal contact, because of fears of criticism, disapproval, or rejection. • Unwilling to get involved with people unless certain of being liked • Shows restraint within intimate relationships because of a fear of being shamed. • Preoccupied with being criticized or rejected in social situations • Is inhibited in new interpersonal situations because of feelings of inadequacy • Views self as socially inept, personally unappealing, or inferior to others • Is unusually reluctant to take personal risks or to engage in any new activities because they may embarrassing. **Treatment** • Hospitalization • Self-help group • Therapeutic community • Environmental manipulation • Assertiveness • Pharmacotherapy: Psycho stimulants, e.g. methylphenidate for attention deficit/hyperactivity.

Contd...

Contd...

Dependent personality disorder	**Definition** DSM-IV defines Dependent personality disorder as 'A pervasive and excessive need to be taken care of that leads to submissive and clinging behavior and fears of separation, beginning by early adulthood and present in a variety of contexts'. **Clinical features** • Difficulty making everyday decisions without advice and reassurance from others • Needs others to assume responsibility for most major areas of his or her life • Difficulty initiating or doing things on his or her own • Lack of self-confidence in judgment even though has motivation or energy • Goes to any level to obtain nurturance and support from others, to the point of volunteering to do things even though that are unpleasant. • Feels uncomfortable or helpless when alone because of extreme fears of being unable to care for himself or herself. • Urgently seeks another relationship as a source of care and support when a close relationship ends. **Treatment** • Psychotherapy • Group therapy (because it offers an opportunity for the development of supportive peer relations) • Use of antidepressants and anti anxiety drugs (because these patients often experience fatigue, malaise and vague anxiety)
Obsessive compulsive (anankastic) personality disorder **In ICD-10 called as anakastic personality disorder**	**Definition** According to DSM-IV obsessive compulsive personality disorder defines as 'A pervasive pattern of preoccupation with orderliness, perfectionism, and mental and interpersonal control, at the expense of flexibility, openness, and efficiency, beginning by early adulthood and present in a variety of contexts.' **Clinical features** • Preoccupied with details, rules, lists, order, organization, or schedules in one's life. • Excessively devoted to work and productivity to the exclusion of leisure activities and friendships (not accounted for by obvious economic necessity) • Difficulty in personal relationship. • Unable to discard worn-out or worthless objects even when they have no sentimental value • Reluctant to delegate tasks or to work with others unless they submit to exactly his or her way of doing things • Shows rigidity and stubbornness. **Treatment** Medication may be useful as an adjunct to other forms of therapy during crises in which anxiety and depression are prominent.

NURSING MANAGEMENT: CARE PLAN

Box 10.8: Nursing process for cluster 'C' personality disorders

Nursing diagnosis: Self disturbance related to lack of positive feedback.

Outcome identification	Nursing intervention
Client will be able to: • Develop a sense of worthwhileness.	• Encourage client to describe and verbalize feelings about self. • Provide safe, supportive environmental to discuss issue of abuse of behavior.

Contd...

Contd...

	• Encourage client to verbalize feelings of insecurity. • Discuss feelings of worthlessness. • Identify situations in which client pushed others. • Give feedback regarding nonverbal behaviors. • Encourage increased sense of responsibility.
Nursing diagnosis: Ineffective family process related to temporary family disorganization.	
Outcome identification	**Nursing intervention**
Client will be able to: • Express feelings freely and appropriately.	• Identify individual factors that may contribute to difficulty of family in providing needed assistance the client. • Determine information available to understand by family. • Discuss underlying reasons for client's behaviors. • Encourage and assist client to develop problem-solving skills. • Help individuals to look at own behavior in relation to the client's.
Nursing diagnosis: Ineffective role performance related to: need to perform rituals, Evidenced by: inability to fulfil usual patterns of responsibility	
Outcome identification	**Nursing intervention**
Client will be able to resume role related responsibilities	• Determine client's previous role within the family and extent to which this role is altered by the illness. • Discuss client's perception of role expectations. • Encourage client to discuss conflicts evident within the family system. • Identify how client and other family members have responded to this conflict. • Explore available options for changes or adjustments in role. • Give client lots of positive reinforcement for ability to resume role responsibilities by decreasing need for ritualistic behaviors.

COMMON TREATMENT MODALITIES OF PERSONALITY DISORDERS

Interpersonal Psychotherapy

- It may be brief and time-limited or may be long-term, depending on therapeutic goals.
- It suggested for paranoid, schizoid and schizotypal borderline, dependent, narcissistic personality disorder.

Psychoanalytical Psychotherapy

- This therapy specially considered for patient with histrionic personality.
- It focuses on the unconscious motivations for seeking total satisfaction from others.

Group Therapy

- It especially appropriate for antisocial personality disorders.
- It is helpful in overcoming social anxiety and developing interpersonal trust.

Behavior Therapy

- It offers reinforcement for positive change. Social skills training and assertiveness training teach alternative ways to deal with frustration.
- It may useful for client with obsessive-compulsive disorder, antisocial and avoidant personality disorder.

Psychopharmacology

These drugs have no effect in the direct treatment of the disorder itself. Some symptomatic relief can be achieved.

- **Thiothixime:** Useful with schizotypal disorder.
- **Carbamazepine and tranylcypromide:** Decrease level of impulsive self destructive act.
- **Haloperidol:** Improvement in illusion, ideas of reference.
- **Fluxetine, sertaline:** Reduce anger.
- **Lithium carbonate and propranolol:** Useful for violent behavior.

APPLICATION OF NURSING PROCESS

Assessment

- Physical assessment of patients with suspected personality disorders can provide valuable information resulting from behaviors.
- Evidence of self-mutilation or suicide attempts can be observed.
- Physical indicators of substance abuse can also indicate symptoms arising from a personality disorder.
- Laboratory studies can demonstrate substance use, nutritional status, and sexually transmitted diseases that can result from the patient's PD.
- Subjective information taken through history may not provide accurate data with patients suffering from a personality disorder.
- History taking can still offer information into the patient's disorder. Key points include medical history, psychiatric history, family history, work and school history, substance use, nutrition, and established interpersonal relationships.

Diagnosis/Outcome Identification

Nursing diagnoses are formulated from the data gathered during the assessment phase and with background knowledge regarding etiological implications for the disorder. Some common nursing diagnoses for the client with all types of personality disorder are explained with care plan under each clusters of personality disorder.

Planning/Implementation

Based on selected nursing diagnoses client with personality disorder are presented interventions in a plan of care.

Evaluation

Reassessment is conducted to determine if the nursing actions have been successful in achieving the objectives of care. Evaluation of the nursing actions for the client with personality disorder may be facilitated by gathering information using the following types of questions:

- Has the client been able to seek out staff when feeling the desire for self-harm?
- Has the client avoided self-harm?
- Can the client correlate times of desire for self-harm to times of elevation in level of anxiety?

- Can the client discuss feelings with staff (particularly feelings of depression and anger)?
- Can the client identify the true source toward which the anger is directed?
- Can the client able to verbalize understanding of basis for his or her anger.

HABIT AND IMPULSE CONTROL DISORDERS

(Comes under behavioral disorder)

What is Impulse?

A sudden desire to do something without thinking about the consequences.

Definition

Box 10.9: Definition of impulse
Impulse control disorder can be defined as the failure to resist an impulsive act or behavior that may be harmful to self or others.

ICD-10 CLASSIFICATION OF HABIT AND IMPULSE CONTROL DISORDER AND ITS DESCRIPTION

Box 10.10: Classification of impulse control disorder	
F63.0	Pathological gambling
F63.1	Pathological fire-setting [pyromania]
F63.2	Pathological stealing [kleptomania]
F63.3	Trichotillomania
F63.8	Other habit and impulse disorders
F63.9	Habit and impulse disorder, unspecified

(Only 4 important conditions are discussed below)

F63.0 Pathological Gambling

Pathological gambling is characterized by persistent and recurrent maladaptive gambling that causes economic problems and significant disturbances in personal, social, or occupational functioning.

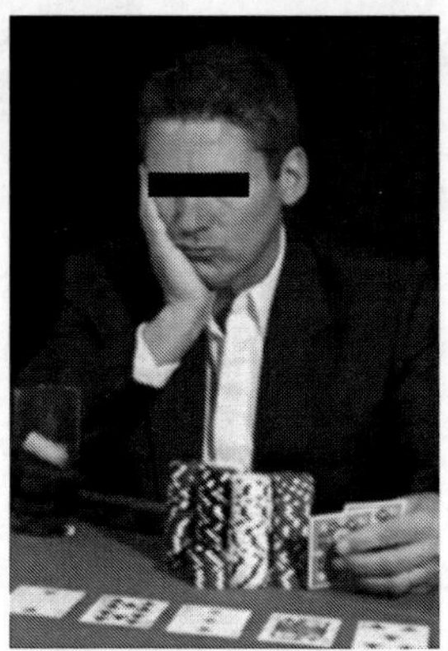

Fig. 10.1: Pathological gambling

F63.1 Pathological Fire Setting [Pyromania]

Pyromania is the recurrent, deliberate, and purposeful setting of fires. Associated features include tension or affective arousal before setting the fires; fascination with, interest in, curiosity about, or attraction to fire and the activities and equipment associated with firefighting; and pleasure, gratification, or relief when setting fires or when witnessing or participating in fire activity.

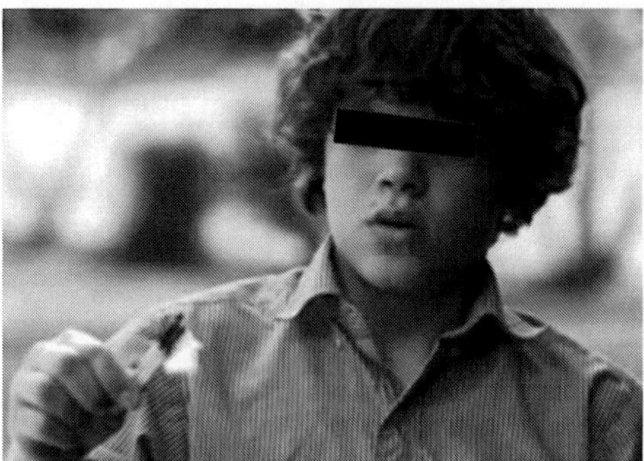

Fig. 10.2: Boy setting fire

F63.2 Pathological Stealing [Kleptomania]

The essential feature of kleptomania is a recurrent failure to resist impulses to steal objects not needed for personal use or for monetary value. The objects taken are often given away, returned surreptitiously, or kept and hidden.

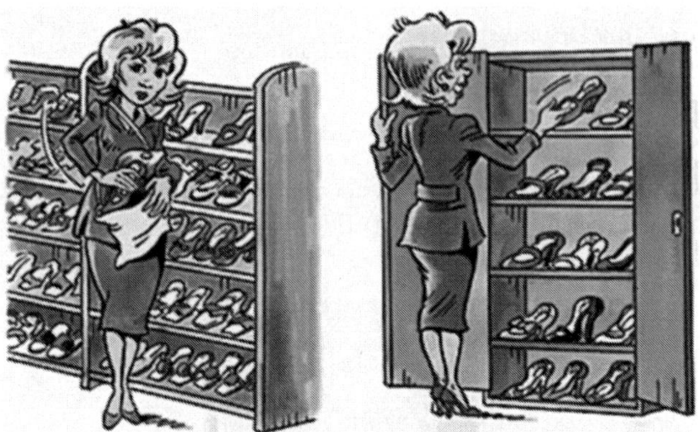

Fig. 10.3: Rich lady stealing sandals

Note: Persons with kleptomania usually have the money to pay for the objects they impulsively steal.

F63.3 Trichotillomania

Trichotillomania is a chronic disorder characterized by repetitive hair pulling, driven by escalating tension and causing variable hair loss that is usually but not always visible to others.

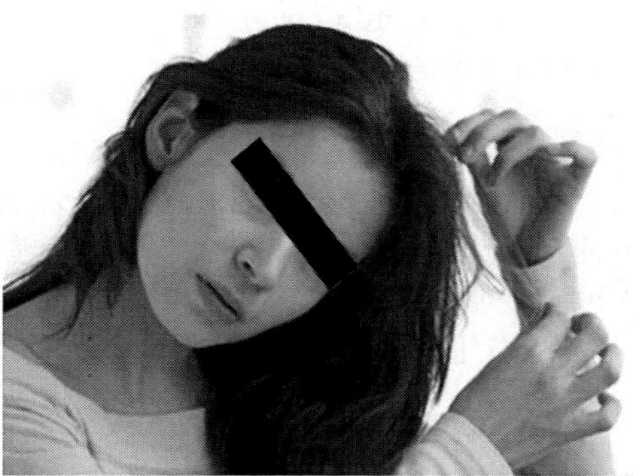

Fig. 10.4: Girl pulling hair driven by tension

ETIOLOGY

Psychodynamic Factors

An impulse is a disposition to act to decrease heightened tension caused by the buildup of instinctual drives or by diminished ego defenses against the drives.

Psychosocial Factors

- Psychosocial factors implicated causally in impulse-control disorders are related to early-life events. The growing child may have had improper models for identification, such as parents who had difficulty controlling impulses.
- Exposure to violence in the home.
- Alcohol abuse.

Biological Factors

Impulsive and violent activity is associated with specific brain regions, such as the limbic system.

- Low cerebrospinal fluid (CSF) levels of 5-hydroxy indole acetic acid (5-HIAA) and impulsive aggression
- Temporal lobe epilepsy and certain impulsive violent behaviors
- Testosterone associated with violent and aggressive behavior.

TREATMENT

Treatment for impulse control disorder may involve any combination of the following:

- Habit reversal
- Medication management.

Habit Reversal

The idea here is to help the person identify the action when it is occurring–and then learn to replace that action with something else that is less harmful.

For example, if patient is having habit of pulling hair, she might be asked to clench fists instead. Therapist might also teach breathing exercises which can use to help relax body soothe tense muscles and control urges.

Medication Management

Medications can play an important role in both treating and preventing the development of an impulse control disorder.

A number of medications commonly used to treat impulse control disorders include:

- **Antidepressants:** While these drugs have been commonly used for treating various impulse disorders, there are mixed findings on the drug's actual effectiveness in treating impulse control disorders.
- **Mood stabilizers/anti-epileptics:** More studies are needed to better determine the effectiveness of these medications in treating impulse control disorders.
- **Opioid antagonists:** Opioid antagonists such as naltrexone have showed the strongest promise for successfully treating impulse control disorders.
- **Atypical neuroleptics:** Atypical neuroleptics such as olanzapine have not shown to provide much benefit to those with an impulse control disorder.
- **Glutamatergic agents:** N-acetyl cysteine (NAC) is a glutamatergic agent that has shown potential benefit in treating impulse control disorder.

SEXUAL DISORDERS

Introduction

Sexuality broadly refers to all aspects of being sexual and is one dimension of personality. Human beings are sexual beings. Sexuality is a basic human need and an innate part of the total personality. It influences our thoughts, actions, and interactions, and it is involved in aspects of physical and mental health.

Sexual Response Cycle

- Desire
- Excitement
- Plateau
- Orgasm
- Resolution

Normal sexuality is difficult to define. But it is easier to define abnormal sexuality. Sexual behavior is diverse and determined by a complex interaction of factors. It is affected by relationships with others, by life circumstances, and by the culture in which a person lives. Humans, like other animals, have always been interested in sexuality and have depicted almost every form of sexual behavior.

Definition

Box 10.11: Sexual disorders

Sexual disorders are characterized by disturbances in sexual desire and in psychophysiological changes that characterize the sexual response cycle and cause marked distress and interpersonal difficulty.

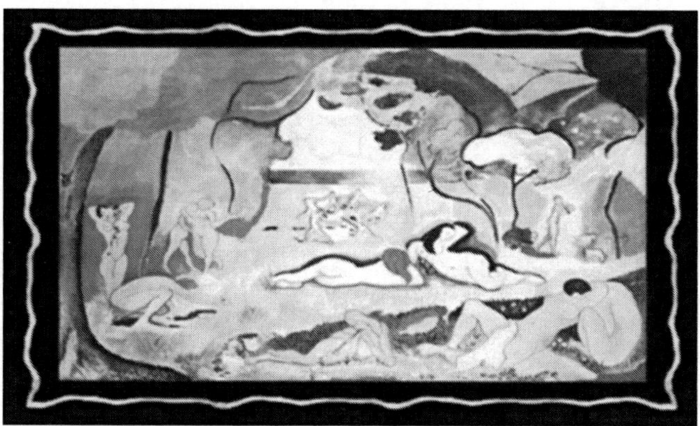

Fig. 10.5: Human sexuality

TYPES OF SEXUAL DISORDERS

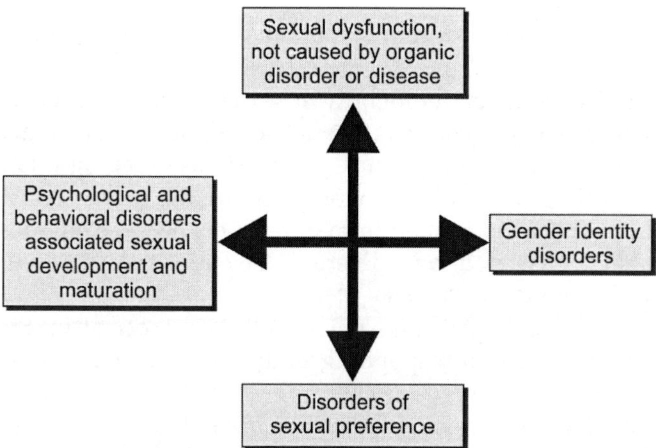

Fig. 10.6: Types of sexual disorder

Box 10.12: Understanding the concept of above mentioned sexual disorders

Sexual dysfunctions	Paraphilia (disorder of sexual preference)	Gender identity disorder	Psychological and behavioral disorders associated sexual development and maturation
Sexual dysfunction is a significant disturbance in the sexual response cycle, which is not due to an underlying organic cause.	A paraphilia is a recurring sexually exciting fantasy, impulse or behavior related to non-human objects, e.g. things, fabrics, designs, the suffering or humiliation of oneself or the partner, children or other non-consenting persons.	It is commonly refered as *transsexuality.* People with this disorder have the subjective feeling that they were born the wrong sex. They may dress as the opposite sex, take sex hormones, or undergo sex change operations.	This disorder usually begins in adolescence and is characterized by uncertainty regarding the gender identity (or) sexual orientation.

ETIOLOGY

In most cases there is not just one cause for a sexual problem; there are often several causes. They are:

Biologic Causes

- Anomalies of the body that cause sexual problems. Examples of this are disorders in hormonal regulation as a result of certain medicines that cause a reduced interest in making love, irritations of the vagina that cause pain when making love or certain operations on the genitals.
- Temporal lobe epilepsy that may cause changes in sexual behavior between seizures.
- Various organic reasons, medication and other drug use, physical illnesses (most notably diabetes mellitus), surgery (such as prostatectomy), and degenerative neural disorders (e.g. multiple sclerosis) may be involved in sexual desire, arousal, and pain disorders.

Psychodynamics

- Individual causes of sexual desire disorders may include religious beliefs, obsessive-compulsive.
- Personality, conflicts with gender identity or sexual preference, sexual phobias, fear of losing control over sexual urges, secret sexual deviations, fear of pregnancy, inadequate grieving following the death of a spouse, depression, and aging-related concerns.
- **Psychoanalytical theories** state that paraphilias are the product of childhood desires that survive into adulthood in their immature forms because emotional development has been inhibited, distorted, and diverted. Deviations arise when these immature forms of libido dominate adult sexual life.
- **Freudian view:** Arrested psychosexual development occur in Freud's oral, anal, and phallic phases when corresponding body parts provide sources of instinctual gratification.
- **Behavioral theorists** believe any paraphilia/sexual dysfunction can be acquired through conditioning, in which an initial pairing of an object is accidentally associated with/then becomes necessary for sexual release.
- **Social factors** may be values and standards that one have received in education, traumatic events or the behavior of the partner. Certain stress factors, e.g. unemployment, a bad financial situation, little knowledge of the body and family quarrels can influence the sexual perception.

ICD-10 CLASSIFICATION OF SEXUAL DISORDERS

F52 Sexual dysfunction
F64 Gender identity disorders
F65 Disorders of sexual preference
F66 Psychological and behavioral disorders associated with sexual development and maturation

Detail description of each sexual disorder according to ICD-10

F52 Sexual Dysfunction not Caused by Organic Disorder

Comes under behavioral syndromes associated with physiological disturbances and physical factors.

Sexual dysfunctions are cognitive, affective, and behavioral problems that prevent an individual or couple from engaging in satisfactory sexual intercourse and orgasm. Sexual dysfunctions are also seen as disturbances in one more of the sexual response cycle's phases, or pain associated with arousal or intercourse.

Subclassification

ICD	Disease name	Discription of condition
F52.0	**Lack or loss of sexual desire (frigidity)**	Sexual desire disorders or decreased Libido **(frigidity)** are characterized by a lack or absence of sexual desire for some period of time or libido for sexual activity or of sexual fantasies.
F52.1	**Sexual aversion and lack of sexual enjoyment**	**Sexual aversion:** This disorder is characterized by a persistent or recurrent extreme aversion to, and avoidance of, all genital sexual contact with a sexual partner. Individuals displaying hypoactive desire are often neutral or indifferent toward sexual interaction. • May cause marked distress or interpersonal difficulty. • Touching and kissing may even be avoided. • Extreme anxiety such as panic attacks may actually occur. **Lack of sexual enjoyment:** Genital response (orgasm or ejaculation) all occur during sexual stimulation, but are not accompanied by pleasurable sensations or feelings of pleasant excitement.
F52.2	**Failure of genital response (Two types)**	• **Female sexual arousal disorder** is described as the inability of a woman to complete sexual activity with adequate lubrication. Often, these women experience pain with intercourse and avoid sexual contact with their partner. • **Male erectile disorder (Impotence; Erectile dysfunction):** This disorder is characterized by an inability to have or sustain penile erection till the completion of satisfactory sexual activity.
F52.3	**Orgasmic dysfunction**	• **Female orgasmic disorder:** It is characterized by persistent or recurrent delay in, or absence of, orgasm following a normal sexual excitement phase. In short, a women's inability to achieve organism by masturbation or coitus. It has two types: – **Primary orgasmic dysfunction:** Never experienced orgasm by any kind of stimulation. – **Secondary orgasmic dysfunction:** Experienced at least one orgasm, regardless of the means of stimulation, but no longer does so. Sometimes referred to as an **anorgasmia.** • **Male orgasmic disorder:** It is characterized by persistent or recurrent delay in, or absence of orgasm following a normal sexual excitement phase. Sometimes called **retarded ejaculation**. – **Primary disorder:** History of never having experienced an orgasm. – **Secondary disorder:** Occasional problems in ejaculation.
F52.4	**Premature ejaculation**	This disorder is defined as ejaculation before the completion of satisfactory sexual activity for both partners. In severe cases, it is characterized by ejaculation either before penile entry into vagina or soon after penetration. It is a very common disorder in the clinical setting. **The causes can be:** Biological (relatively uncommon) or psychological (e.g. performance anxiety).

Contd...

Contd...

ICD	Disease name	Discription of condition
F52.5	**Nonorganic vaginismus**	This disorder is characterized by an involuntary spasm of the lower 1/3rd of vagina, interfering with coitus. Penile entry is either painful or impossible. *(Before a presumption of nonorganic vaginismus, it is important to rule out organic factors (e.g. local pathology causing pain)*
F52.6	**Nonorganic dyspareunia**	Genital pain before, during, or after sexual intercourse; much higher incidence in women than men; often associated with vaginismus.
F52.7	**Excessive sexual drive**	Rarely, both men **(satyriasis)** and women **(nymphomania)** may complain of excessive sexual drive as a problem.

Management

Basic principles of direct treatment of sexual dysfunction (Lopiccolo, 1978)

- Mutual responsibility information and education attitude change
- Eliminating performance anxiety increasing communication and effectiveness of sexual technique
- Changing destructive life styles and sex roles.

Biological Treatment

Pharmacotherapy

- Sildenafil, oral phentolamine, Transurethral alprostadil (erectile disorder) Intravenous methohexital sodium has been used in desensitization therapy.
- Antianxiety agents. Bromocriptive, a dopamine agonist, may improve sexual function impaired by hyperprolocatinemia.
- Dopaminergic agents have been reported to increase libido and improve sex function.

Hormone Therapy

- Androgens increase the sex drive.
- Antiandrogens have been used to treat compulsive sexual behavior in men.
- Antiestrogens increases libido.

Mechanical Treatment Approaches

Vacuum pump: These are mechanical devices that patients without vascular diseases can use to obtain erections. The blood drawn into the penis following the creation of the vacuum is kept there by a ring placed around the base of the penis.

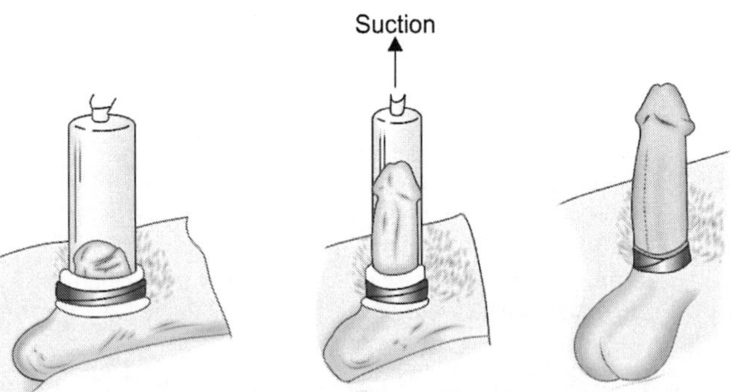

Fig. 10.7 : Vaccum pump device used to obtain erections

- **EROS:** A device developed to create clitoral erections in women. It is a small suction cup that fits over the clitoral region and drawn blood into the clitoris.
- Kegel exercises may also increase blood flow to the vulvar/vaginal tissues, as well as strengthen the muscles involved in orgasm.

Surgical Treatment

Male prostheses vascular surgery hymenectomy for dyspareunia vaginoplasty and release of vaginal adhesions.

Dual Sex Therapy: (William Masters and Virginia Johnson)

Treatment is based on a concept that the couple must be treated when a dysfunctional person is in a relationship both are involved in a sexually distressing situation; both must participate in the therapy program. The keystone of the program is the round table session in which a male and female therapy team clarifies, discusses, and works through problems with the couple.

Treatment is short-term and behaviorally oriented Therapist suggests specific sexual activities. Initially, intercourse is inter directed and the couple learn to give and receive bodily pleasure without the pressure of performance or penetration. The aim of the therapy is to establish an effective communication within the marital unit. Psychotherapy sessions follow each new exercise period, and problems and satisfactions are discussed.

Specific Techniques of Exercises

- **Vaginismus:** Woman is advised to dilate her vaginal opening with her fingers or with dilators.
- **Premature ejaculation:**
  - **Sequeeze technique** is used to raise the threshold of penile excitability. In this exercise the man or the woman stimulates the erect penis until the earliest sensations of impending ejaculation are felt. At this point, the woman forcefully sequeezes the coronal ridge of the gland, the erection is diminished, and ejaculation is inhibited.
  - **Stop start technique** in which the woman stops all stimulation of the penis when the man first senses an impending ejaculation.
- **Erectile disorder:** Sometimes told to masturbate to prove that full erection and ejaculation are possible.
- **Lifelong female orgasmic disorder:** Women are directed to masturbate, sometimes using a vibrator.

Hypnotherapy

Focus specifically on the anxiety producing situation—that is, the sexual interaction that results in dysfunction.

Behavior Therapy

Behavior therapists assume that sexual dysfunction is learned maladaptive behavior, which causes patients to be fearful of sexual interaction. Hierarchy of anxiety provoking situations ranging from least threatening to most threatening systematic desensitization assertiveness training.

Group Therapy

Used to examine both intrapsychic and interpersonal problems in patients with sexual disorders. Groups can be organized in several ways.

Analytically Oriented Sex Therapy

The sex therapy is usually conducted over a longer period than usual, which allows learning or relearning of sexual satisfaction under the realities of patient's day-to-day lives.

F64 GENDER IDENTITY DISORDERS

It is commonly refered as *transsexuality*. People with this disorder have the subjective feeling that they were born with wrong sex. They may dress as the opposite sex, take sex hormones, or undergo sex change operations.

Subclassification and its Description

F64.0	**Transsexualism**	In this, there is persistent and significant sense of discomfort regarding one's own anatomic sex and a feeling that it is inappropriate to one's perceived gender. The person will be preoccupied with the wish to get rid of one's own genitals and secondary sex characteristics and to adopt the sex characteristics of the other sex.
F64.1	**Dual-role transvestism**	It is characterized by wearing of clothes of the opposite sex person in order to enjoy the temporary experience of membership of the opposite sex, but without any desire for a permanent sex change (unlike *Transsexualism*).
F64.2	**Gender identity disorder of childhood**	**For female:** Persistent and intense distress about being a girl, and a strong desire to be a boy which occurs before puberty. **For male:** Persistent and intense distress about being a boy and an intense desire to be a girl or, more rarely, insistence that he is a girl which occurs before reaching puberty.

Management

- **Sex reassignment surgery:** Alter person's sexual anatomy to match internal identity. Genitalia altered to look like those of opposite sex.
  (1 year living as opposite sex before surgery recommended).
- **Behavioral treatment to alter gender identity:** Shaping of more masculine behaviors. May only be effective for individuals who want treatment for GID.

F65 DISORDERS OF SEXUAL PREFERENCE (PARAPHILIAS)

Paraphilias are group of abnormal sexual behaviors characterized by:

- Recurrent intense sexual urges and fantasies involving unusual objects or activities.
- Acts on the urges or is markedly distressed by them.
- The preference has been present for at least six months.

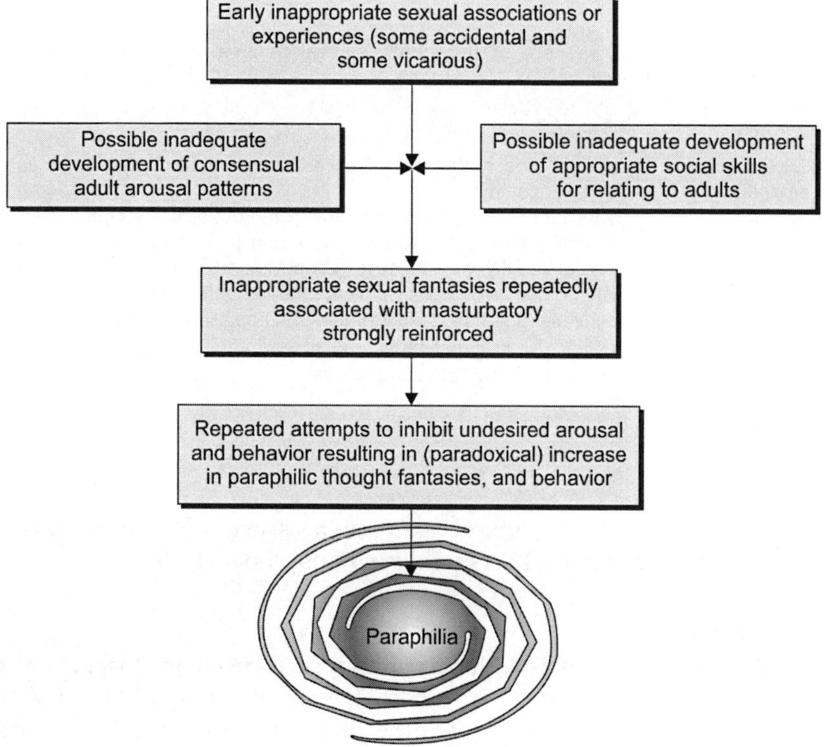

Fig. 10.8: Psychopathology of paraphilias

ICD-10 Subclassification and its Description

F65.0	**Fetishism**	Getting sexually aroused by non-living and generally not sexually arousing objects, e.g shoes, lingerie, soft fabrics, etc.
F65.1	**Fetishistic transvestism**	This is characterized by wearing of articles or clothing of the opposite sex in order to create the appearance and feeling of being a member of the opposite sex. *The cross-dressing is closely associated with sexual arousal. Once orgasm occurs and sexual arousal declines, there is a strong desire to remove the clothing.*
F65.2	**Exhibitionism**	It is characterized by recurrent or a persistent tendency to expose one's genitalia to unsuspecting strangers (usually of the opposite sex), almost invariably associated with sexual arousal and masturbation.
F65.3	**Voyeurism**	This is a persistent (or) recurrent tendency to observe unsuspecting persons, naked (or) engaged in sexual activity.
F65.4	**Pedophilia**	Pedophilia is scientifically defined as getting sexually aroused by a child in pre-puberty or child younger than13 years old. *To be sexually aroused by children in puberty is known under the term 'hebephilia' or 'ephebophilia'*
F65.5	**Sadomasochism**	A preference for sexual activity, either as recipient (masochism), or as provider (sadism), or both, which involves induction of pain and humiliation by self or to opposite sexual partner.

Contd...

Contd...

F65.6	**Multiple disorders of sexual preference**	The likelihood of more than one abnormal sexual preference occurring in one individual.
F65.8	**Other disorders of sexual preference**	A variety of other patterns of sexual preference and activity may occur, each being relatively uncommon. • These include such activities as making obscene telephone calls, rubbing up against people for sexual stimulation in crowded public places (frotteurism), sexual activity with animals (zoophilia), use of strangulation or anoxia for intensifying sexual excitement, and a preference for partners with some particular anatomical abnormality such as an amputated limb. • These also include sexual arousal with urine (urophillia), feces (corprophillia), enemas (klismaphilia) and others.

MANAGEMENT

Drug Therapy

Antipsychotic have been used for severe aggression associated with paraphilias. *Other therapy includes:* Behavior therapy, aversion therapy, psychoanalysis.

Biological Treatment

Biological treatment of individuals with paraphilias has focused on blocking or decreasing the level of circulating androgens. The most extensively used of the antiandrogenic medications are the *progestin*. It decreases the libido and thus breaks the individual's pattern of compulsive deviant sexual behavior.

Psychoanalytical Therapy

In this type of therapy, the therapist helps the client to identify unresolved conflicts and traumas from early childhood. The therapy focuses on helping the individual resolve these early conflicts, thus relieving the anxiety that prevents him or her from forming appropriate sexual relationships. In turn the individual has no further need for paraphilic fantasies.

Behavioral Therapy

Aversion therapy has been used to modify undesirable behavior. Aversion methods of treatment of paraphilias involve paring noxious stimuli, such as electric shocks and bad odors, with the impulse which then diminishes. Behavioral therapy also includes skills training and cognitive restructuring in an effort to change the individual's maladaptive beliefs.

PSYCHOLOGICAL AND BEHAVIORAL DISORDERS ASSOCIATED WITH SEXUAL DEVELOPMENT AND MATURATION

Sexual Maturational Disorder

The individual suffers from uncertainty about one's gender identity or sexual orientation (heterosexual, homosexual, or bisexual), which causes anxiety or depression usually begins in adolescence.

Egodystonic Sexual Orientation

In this disorder, the sexual orientation is clear. However, the individual wishes to change the orientation because of the associated distress or psychological symptoms. This disorder is seen most commonly in homosexuality.

What is homosexuality
It is a sexual or romantic desire for people of the same sex. It is a normal variant of sexual orientation. It occurs in 3 to 10% of men and 1 to 5% of women.

Sexual Relationship Disorder

The gender identity disorder or disorder of sexual preference leads to difficulties in establishing and/or maintaining sexual relationships. In such a case both diagnosis should be made.

Management

- **For seeking a change in sexual orientation:** Behavior therapy, aversion therapy (rarely used), covert sensitization, supportive psychotherapy, etc.
- **For seeking removal of distress only:** Antidepressants and benzodiazepine.

Nursing Management

Box 10.13: Nursing process for sexual disorders

Outcome identification	Nursing intervention
Nursing diagnosis: Sexual dysfunction related to depression and conflict in relationship, biological or psychological contributing factors to the disorder evidenced by loss of sexual desire or function.	
Outcome identification	**Nursing intervention**
Client will be able to come out from depression and maintain good relationship with partner.	• Assess the client's sexual history and previous level of satisfaction in sexual relationships. • Assess client's perception of the problem. • Help client determine time dimension associated with the onset of the problem and discuss what was happening in life situation at that time. • Assess clients level of energy • Review medication regimen; observe for side effects • Provide information regarding sexuality and sexual functioning. • Refer for additional counseling or sex therapy if required.
Nursing diagnosis: Ineffective sexuality patterns related to conflicts with orientation or variant preferences evidenced by expressed dissatisfaction with sexual behaviors (e.g. voyeurism, trasvestism).	
Outcome identification	**Nursing intervention**
Client will able to develop normal sexual behavior	• Take sexual history, noting clients expression of areas of dissatisfaction with sexual pattern. • Assess clients stress life and relationship with sexual partner. • Note cultural, social, ethnic, racial, and religious factors that may contribute to conflict regarding sexual practices. • Be accepting and nonjudgmental • Assist therapist in plan of behavior modification to decrease variant behaviors. • Teach the client that sexuality is a normal human response and is not synonymous with any one sexual act.

Contd...

Contd...

Nursing diagnosis: Disturbed personal identity related to parenting patterns that encourage culturally unacceptable behaviors for assigned gender evidenced by statements of desiring to be of the opposite gender; exhibiting behaviors culturally associated with the opposite gender.	
Outcome identification	**Nursing intervention**
Client will be able to: • Verbalize to have normal personal identity	• Spend time with client and show positive regard • Be aware of own feelings and attitudes toward this client and his or her behavior. • Allow client to describe his or her perception of the problem. • Discuss with client type of behaviors that are most culturally acceptable. Practice these behaviors through role playing or with play therapy strategies.
Nursing diagnosis: Impaired social interaction related to social and culturally unacceptable behaviors evidenced by peer rejection and identification with members of the opposite gender.	
Outcome identification	**Nursing intervention**
Client will be able to: • Engage in satisfying relationship with others	• Once the client feels comfortable with the new behaviors in role playing or one nurse client interactions, they may be tried in group situations. • If possible remain with the patients during interactions with the others.

EATING DISORDERS

Eating disorders are a group of conditions characterized by abnormal eating habits that may involve either insufficient or excessive food intake to the detriment of an individual's physical and emotional health.

Definition

Eating disorders are syndromes characterized by severe disturbances in eating behavior and by distress or excessive concern about body shape or weight.

ICD-10 Classification of Eating Disorder

(It comes under F50–F59 behavioral syndromes associated with physiological disturbances and physical factors)

Box 10.14: Eating disorders
F50.0 Anorexia nervosa
F50.1 Atypical anorexia nervosa
F50.2 Bulimia nervosa
F50.3 Atypical bulimia nervosa
F50.4 Overeating associated with other psychological disturbances
F50.5 Vomiting associated with other psychological disturbances
F50.8 Other eating disorders
F50.9 Eating disorder, unspecified

As above mentioned conditions, there are two main types of eating disorder:

1. Anorexia nervosa, 2. Bulimia nervosa

Box 10.15: Core concepts

Anorexia nervosa	Bulimia nervosa
Anorexia nervosa (AN) is a serious, chronic illness of starvation, brought on by severe disturbance of body image and a morbid fear of obesity.	A maladaptive eating pattern characterized by recurrent binge eating that is taking large amount of food in short period of time followed by compensatory behaviors.

Definitions

Box 10.16: Definition of anorexia nervosa and bulemia nervosa

Anorexia nervosa	Bulimia nervosa
Anorexia nervosa (AN), in which a person maintains a low body weight due to a preoccupation with body weight and shape. This is achieved by drastically reducing calorie intake, and sometimes by excessive exercise, self-induced vomiting or laxative abuse. The patients often have a greatly distorted body image, and a strong conviction that weight loss is desirable. **Subtypes** • **Restricting type**: During the current episode of anorexia nervosa, the person *has not* regularly engaged in binge-eating or purging behavior (self-induced vomiting or misuse of laxatives, diuretics, or enemas). • **Binge-eating-purging type:** In current episode of anorexia nervosa, the person *has* regularly engaged in binge-eating or purging behavior.	Bulimia nervosa (BN), characterized by repeated periods of binge eating, followed by compensatory behavior such as purging, fasting or excessive exercise. Purging can take the form of self-induced vomiting, or misuse of laxatives or other drugs. During a binge, the person has a sense of loss of control over eating, and both bingeing and purging are often accompanied by feelings of guilt or shame. People with BN are often secretive about this behavior. **Subtypes** • **Purging:** – Bulimics self-induce vomiting. – Rapidly remove the food from the body before it can be digested, or use laxatives, diuretics, or enemas. • **Nonpurging:** – Exercise or fast excessively after a binge to offset the caloric intake after eating. – Purging-type may also exercise or fast, but as a secondary form of weight control.

Etiologic Theories

Psychodynamics

The individual reflects a developmental arrest in the very early childhood years. The tasks of trust, autonomy, and separation-individuation are unfulfilled, and the individual remains in the dependent position.

Symptoms are often associated with a perceived loss of control in some aspect of life and may center on fears of sexual maturity/intimacy. Additionally, eating disorders are often associated with depression, anxiety, phobias, and cognitive problems.

Biological Causes

First-degree female relatives and monozygotic twin offspring of patients with anorexia nervosa have higher rates of anorexia nervosa and bulimia nervosa. Children of patients with anorexia nervosa have a lifetime risk for anorexia nervosa that is ten fold that of the general population (5%).

Families of patients with bulimia nervosa have higher rates of substance abuse, particularly alcoholism, affective disorders, and obesity.

These disorders may be caused by due to neuroendocrine abnormalities within the hypothalamus. Biologic influences in BN may be associated with the neurotransmitters serotonin and norepinephrine.

Psychosocial Factors

High levels of hostility, chaos, and isolation and low levels of nurturance and empathy are reported in families of children presenting with eating disorders.

Family Dynamics

Issues of control become the overriding factors in the family of the client with an eating disorder. These theories suggest that eating disorders result from very early and profound disturbances in mother-infant interactions.

There is a high value placed on perfectionism in this family, and the child believes she or he must please others and satisfy these standards. Behaviors associated with food and eating provide feelings of control over one's life.

Box 10.17: Clinical features

Anorexia nervosa	Bulimia nervosa
• Weight loss, or in children a lack of weight gain, leading to a body weight below 15% than normal. • A self-perception of being too fat, with an intrusive dread of fatness, which leads to a self-imposed low weight threshold. • A widespread endocrine disorder involving the hypothalamic-pituitary-gonadal axis, manifest in the female as amenorrhea, and in the male as a loss of sexual interest and potency. **Additional features** • Intense fear of becoming obese • Fear does not decrease even if the body becomes thin and underweight • No known medical illness **The following features support the diagnosis, but are not necessary to be present** • Self-induced vomiting • Self-induced purging • Excessive exercise • Use of appetite suppressants and/or diuretics **Physical symptoms due to starvation** • Pale conjunctiva and mucous membranes • Poor skin turgor/muscle tone • Edema • Excessive loss of hair; increased growth of hair on body (lanugo) • Hypothermia • Bradycardia; cardiac irregularities; hypotension	• Recurrent episodes of overeating in which large amounts of food are consumed in short periods of time. • Persistent preoccupation with eating and a strong desire or a sense of compulsion to eat (craving). • The patient attempts to counteract the fattening effects of food by one or more of the following: – Self-induced vomiting – Self-induced purging – Alternating periods of starvation – Use of drugs such as appetite suppressants or diuretics. • A self-perception of being too fat, with dread of fatness (usually leading to underweight). **Additional features** • Rapid and out-of-control eating. • Controlled when interrupted by another person. • Cycle may be repeated several times a week or, in more serious cases, several times a day. **Physical symptoms due to overeating:** • Chronic gastric reflux after eating. • Dehydration and hypokalemia. • Esophagitis, oral trauma, laceration • Peptic ulcers. • Calluses or scars on back of hands due to repeated trauma from incisor. • Constant weight fluctuations. • The frequent contact between teeth and gastric acid, in particular, may cause: – Severe dental caries – Perimolysis or the erosion of tooth enamel. – Swollen salivary glands

Management

Box 10.18: Medical management

Anorexia nervosa	Bulimia nervosa
• Nutrition therapy—Zinc helps in increasing body weight • Drug therapy—Olanzepine brings obsession condition regarding intake of food and increasing the body weight to the considerable level. • Serotonin and histamine antagonist, e.g. cypropheptadine (Periactin).	• Selective serotonin reuptake inhibitors (SSRIs), e.g. fluoxetine (Prozac) • Other antidepressants, e.g. tricyclic antidepressants, e.g. amitriptyline (Elavil), imipramine (Tofranil). • Dopamine reuptake blocker, e.g. bupropion. • Monoamine oxidase inhibitors (MAOIs), e.g. phenelzine (Nardil), tranylcypromine sulfate (Parnate) • Antipsychotic drugs, e.g. risperadone (Risperdal), olanzapine (Zyprexa) • Anti convulsant drugs—Phenytoin, Valporic acid.

Therapies for Treating Eating Disorders

- **Cognitive analytic therapy:** The aim of this short-term therapy is for the patient to recognize problematic patterns of behavior and understand their origins, as well as how coping mechanisms they have developed over time might be worsening these problems.
- **Cognitive behavior therapy (CBT):** This is a structured therapy based on the idea that our thoughts, feelings, behaviors and physical sensations interact. It involves challenging unhelpful thoughts and beliefs, thus reducing the negative emotions and problematic behaviors that accompany them.
- A specific form of CBT for eating disorders focuses on modifying unhealthy eating and weight control behaviors, and unhelpful ideas related to weight, shape and appearance.
- **Interpersonal psychotherapy:** This focuses on interpersonal problems such as disputes or conflicts, difficulties with role transitions, complicated grief or interpersonal skills deficits, that may trigger or maintain an eating disorder. There is no specific focus on eating disorder symptoms.
- **Focal psychodynamic therapy:** This is concerned with how a person's relationships with others may mirror the relationships they had during childhood and how this links with eating disorder symptoms.
- **Family therapy:** This highlights the family as being the key resource in a person's recovery. Family therapy for an is symptom oriented, emphasising the family's role in the restoration of normal weight and eating.

Nursing Management

Box 10.19: Nursing process for eating disorders

Nursing diagnosis: Imbalanced Nutrition: less than body requirements related to inadequate food intake; self-induced vomiting, excessive laxative use, body weight 15% (or more) below expected; evidenced by pale conjunctiva and mucous membranes; poor skin turgor/muscle tone.

Contd...

Contd...

Outcome identification	Nursing intervention
Client will be able to: • Verbalize understanding of nutritional needs. • Establish a dietary pattern with caloric intake adequate to regain/maintain appropriate weight.	• Establish a minimum weight goal and daily nutritional requirements. • Contract with client regarding commitment to therapeutic program and meeting specific dietary needs and goals. • Use a consistent approach. Sit with client while eating; present and remove food without persuasion and/or comment. Promote pleasant environment and record intake. • Provide small, frequent, and nutritionally dense meals and supplemental snacks, as appropriate. • Be alert to choices of low-calorie foods/beverages; hoarding food, disposing of food in various places, such as pockets or wastebaskets. • Maintain a regular weighing schedule, such as Monday/Friday before breakfast in same attire, and graph results. • Monitor exercise program and set limits on physical activities. • Avoid giving laxatives.
Nursing diagnosis: Actual or risk for deficient fluid volume related to Inadequate intake of food and liquids, consistent self-induced vomiting, evidenced by dry skin and mucous membranes, decreased skin turgor, output greater than input (diuretic use),dehydration and weakness.	
Outcome identification	**Nursing intervention**
Client will be able to: • Verbalize understanding of causative factors and behaviors necessary to correct fluid • Maintain/demonstrate improved fluid balance	• Monitor vital signs, capillary refill, status of mucous membranes, skin turgor. • Monitor amount and types of fluid intake. Measure urine output accurately. • Discuss strategies to stop vomiting and laxative/diuretic use. • Identify actions necessary to regain/maintain optimal fluid balance (e.g. specific fluid intake schedule). • Administer/monitor intravenous (IV) fluids and electrolytes as indicated.
Nursing diagnosis: Disturbed body image/chronic low self esteem related to morbid fear of obesity, perceived loss of control in some aspect of life as evidenced by distorted body image (views self as fat even in the presence of normal body weight or severe).	
Outcome identification	**Nursing intervention**
Client will be able to: • Acknowledge self as an individual. • Accept responsibility for own actions.	• Have client draw picture of self. • Involve in personal development program, preferably in a group setting. Provide information about proper application of makeup and grooming. • Recommend consultation with an image consultant. • Suggest disposing of 'thin' clothes as weight gain occurs. • Assist client to confront changes associated with puberty/sexual fears. Provide sex education as necessary. • Establish a therapeutic nurse/client relationship. • Promote self-concept without moral judgment. • State rules clearly regarding weighing schedule, • Assist client to learn strategies other than eating for dealing with feelings. • Use cognitive-behavioral or interpersonal psychotherapy approach, rather than interpretive therapy. • Involve in group therapy. • Refer to occupational/recreational therapy.

SLEEPING DISORDERS

Definition

Sleep can be defined as a normal state of altered consciousness during which the body rests, it is characterized by decreased responsiveness to the environment, and a person can be aroused from it by external stimuli.

Stages of Sleep

Stages of sleep can be identified behaviorally, functionally and electrophysiologically.

Electrophysiologic monitoring of sleep is called *Polysomnography* which shows that sleep can be divided into REM and NREM. NREM sleep can be further divided into 4 stages.

Non-rapid Eye Movement (NREM) Sleep

NREM sleep is characterized as follows:

Stage 1

- Includes lightest level of sleep
- Stage lasts a few minutes
- Decreased physiological activity begins with gradual fall in vital signs and metabolism
- Sensory stimuli such as noise, easily arouse sleeper.

Stage 2

- Includes period of sound sleep
- Relaxation progresses
- Arousal is still relatively easy
- Stage lasts 10–20 mts
- Body functions continue to slow
- The brain waves are frequently mixed and low voltage in pattern, with bursts of activity can be monitored.

Stage 3

- It involves initial stages of deep sleep
- Sleeper is difficult to arouse and rarely moves
- Oxygen consumption
- Muscles are completely relaxed
- Vital signs decline, but remain regular
- Stage lasts 15–30 mts.

Stage 4

- It is deepest stage of sleep
- It is very difficult to arouse sleeper
- If sleep loss has occurred, sleeper will spend considerable portion of night in this stage
- Vital signs are significantly lower than during walking hours
- Stage lasts approximately 15–30 mts
- Sleep walking and enuresis may sometimes occur in this stage.

Rapid Eye Movement (REM) Sleep

- Vivid, full-color dreaming occurs
- Stage usually begins about 90 mts after sleep has begun
- Stage typified by autonomic responses of rapidly moving eyes, fluctuating heart and respiratory rates, and increased or fluctuating blood pressure
- Loss of skeletal muscle tone occurs
- Gastric secretion increase
- It is very difficult to arouse sleeper
- Duration of REM sleep increases with each cycle and averages 20 mts
- Stage is characterized by low voltage, random fast waves, as in stage 1 NREM.

Sleep Cycle

Once person falls asleep, then he passes through 4–6 complete sleep cycles; each consists of 4 stages of NREM sleep and a period of REM sleep. The cyclical pattern usually progresses from stage 1 through stage 4 of NREM, followed by a reversal from stage 4 to 3 to 2, ending with a period of REM sleep.

Flow chart 10.1: Shows sleep cycle

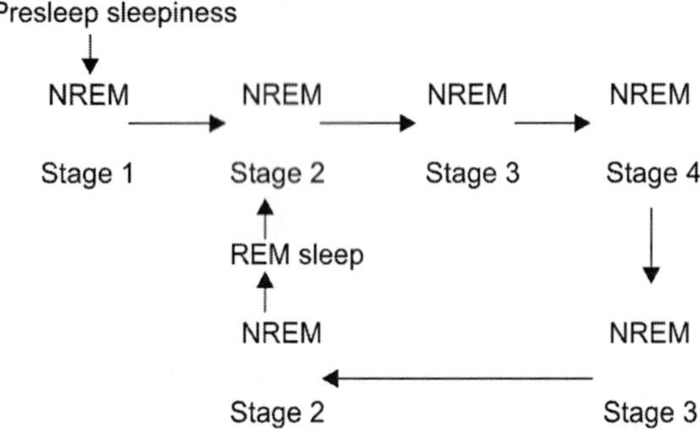

With each successive cycle, stages 3 and 4 of NREM sleep shorten and the period of REM lengthens. REM sleep lasts up to 60 mts during the last sleep cycle. The number of sleep cycle depends on the amount of time that the person spends sleeping usually average of 90 mts per cycle.

Normal Sleep Requirements and Patterns

Sleep duration and quality vary among persons of all age groups and as follows:

- Infants : 16 hours/day
- Toddlers : 12 hours/day
- Preschoolers : 11 hours/day
- Schoolers : 9–10 hours/day
- Adolescents : 8–9 hours/day
- Adults : 6–8 hours/day

Factors Affecting Sleep

A number of factors affect the quality and quantity of sleep. Often more than one factor combined to cause a sleep problem.

- Physical illness (e.g. nausea, mood disorders, breathing difficulty, pain)
- Drugs and substances use
- Lifestyle
- Usual sleep patterns and excessive daytime sleepiness
- Emotional stress
- Environment (ventilation)
- Sound
- Exercise and fatigue
- Food and caloric intake.

SLEEP DISORDERS

Definition

Sleep disorders is defined as inability to fall asleep or to stay asleep as long as desired.

There are several nonorganic sleep disorder in which few important among them are explained below.

Dyssomnias

The dyssomnias include sleep disorders characterized by difficulty in initiating or maintaining sleep (insomnia) or by excessive sleepiness. These disorders may arise predominantly from within the body (intrinsic), from external sources (extrinsic), or from disruption of circadian rhythm.

Intrinsic Sleep Disorders

- **Insomnia:** It is the persistent difficulty in initiating or maintaining sleep.
  - **Idiopathic insomnia** is a rare disorder characterized by a lifelong history of inability to obtain adequate sleep. Its cause is thought to be an abnormality in the neurologic control of sleep.
  - **Psychophysiologic insomnia** is more common and is characterized by learned sleep and heightened physiologic response to stress. The total sleep time is often within normal range but is felt to be inadequate. They will fall asleep unintentionally in low stimulus situations, such as watching TV, but feel increased arousal when they go to bed. It is difficult to get sleep in places , other than their usual bedroom.

  Management of insomnia is complex. Sleep should be restricted by curtailing time bed to the minimum believed necessary with a consistent rising time. Relaxation exercises can be helpful, but they should initially be practiced at times other than bedtime so that by the time they are introduced at bedtime, they are effective. Referral to a sleep specialist or mental health professional who can work with the client over a period of time should be considered.
- **Narcolepsy:** Narcolepsy is one of the disorders characterized by excessive daytime sleepiness. The client also experiences disturbed nocturnal sleep and repeated episodes

of almost irresistible daytime drowsiness followed by brief periods of sleep, especially when engaged in monotonous activities.

Many narcoleptic clients also experience *cataplexy*, a sudden loss of muscle tone at times of unexpected emotion (e.g. Fright). Malfunctioning of the mechanism controlling REM sleep leads to *sleep paralysis* for one to several minutes, and *hypnagogic hallucinations*, i.e. Hallucinatory experiences that occur at sleep onset or awakening.

- **Sleep apnea syndrome:** Sleep apnea is characterized by cessation of breathing for 10 seconds or longer occurring at least 5 times/hour. Sleep apnea can be classified as obstructive and central nervous system apnea.
- **Periodic limb movement disorder:** It may also contribute to daytime sleepiness and frequent nocturnal wakening. Originally described as nocturnal myoclonus, it is characterized by periodic episodes of repetitive, stereotypic leg movements that occur during sleep, causing partial arousals. It is common in the elderly population. Clonazepam, a benzodiazepine, or baclofen, a skeletal muscle relaxant, may be ordered to diminish the magnitude of the movement and frequency of arousals.
- **Restless leg syndrome:** Restless leg syndrome involves anything 'crawling', itching or tingling sensations of the leg while at rest and causes an almost irresistible urge to move. The syndrome is often most severe before sleep onset. Clients always have periodic limb movements during sleep. Treatment is similar to that of periodic limb movement disorder.

Extrinsic Sleep Disorders

It encompasses a range of factors, from environmentally to chemically induced. Some environmental factors temporarily present during hospitalization.

Circadian Rhythm Sleep Disorders

In the general population, the circadian rhythm sleep disorders, such as **time zonechange syndrome and shift work sleep disorder** are not uncommon. Elderly and chronically ill clients who live alone may be vulnerable to irregular sleep-wake patterns.

In this disorder, prolonged ignoring or absence of external cues to time, such as regular meal timings, work periods and daylight leads to erratic periods of sleeping and wakefulness. Internal circadian cues may also be damped as a result of ageing or diffuse brain disease.

Parasomnias

The parasomnias are disorders that occur during sleep but that usually do not produce insomnia or excessive sleepiness. It may be due to partial arousal or abnormalities in sleep-wake transition.

- **Arousal disorders:** Partial arousal occur during slow- wave sleep. **Sleepwalking**, also known as **somnambulism**, may include semi purposeful behavior, such as dressing. However the behavior may be lacking in coordination and appropriateness, such as voiding in the closet. The occurrence of sleep walking in adults is associated with anxiety.

Sleep terrors are sudden arousals from slow wave sleep accompanied by screaming, tachycardia, tachypnea, diaphoresis, and other manifestations of fear. If awakened, the person is often disoriented and has little recall of the nature of the dream image. Sleep terrors usually occurs in young children.

- **Sleep-wake transition disorders:** Sleep-wake transition disorders are common in the general population. **Sleep starts** refers to the sudden jerking movement of the legs that often occurs as a person is falling asleep. Nocturnal leg cramps also common. The frequency and intensity may be greater with high caffeine intake, stress, or intense physical activity before going to bed. **Sleep talking** also may occur during times of stress.
- **Parasomnias usually associated with REM sleep: Nightmares** are frightening dreams that arise in REM sleep and are often vividly recalled on awakening. **Sleep paralysis** is one of the classic signs of narcolepsy, but can occur in isolation. This effect may be an extension of the normal state of low muscle tone during REM sleep.
- **Other parasomnias:** Other parasomnias are not specifically associated with particular sleep stage. **Sleepbruxism** refers to grinding of the teeth during sleep and may lead to dental damage. **Sleep enuresis**, or bed wetting, may occur in adult in association with other disorders, such as Obstructive Sleep apnea syndrome. **Primary snoring** is distinguished from Obstructive Sleep apnea syndrome by its rhythmic nature without episodes of apnea or hypoventilation.

Assessment and Management

Diagnostic Assessment

- Polysomnography
- Electroencephalogram
- Multiple sleep latency test (MSLT)

MSLT is performed to assess the impairment of daytime alertness. It is performed a day after a standard polysomnogram. The time required for clients to fall asleep when in a relaxed state is evaluated at 2 hour intervals, with each nap limited to 20 minutes. The type of sleep also is assessed.

Nursing Process

Assessment

Assess client's usual sleep habits and recent sleep quality as part of the initial nursing history. If sleep quality is reported to be poor, explore the nature of disturbances by noting the following:

- Usual activities in the hour before retrieving
- Number and perceived cause of awakenings
- Frequency and duration of naps
- Events associated with initial onset of sleep disturbances
- Ease of falling asleep in places other than the usual bedroom
- Use of alcohol, sleeping pills, and other medications
- Incidence of morning headaches
- Frequency of snoring, apparent pauses in breathing, and kicking movements

- Objective data may include visible signs of fatigue and lack of sleep, such as circles under the eyes, lack of coordination, drowsiness and irritability.

Nursing Care Plan

Box 10.20: Nursing process sleep disorder

Nursing diagnosis: Disturbed sleep pattern related to lack of cues for day-night schedule, manifested by erratic sleep schedule, frequent naps and nocturnal wandering.

Outcome identification	Nursing intervention
Client increases nocturnal sleep time by 20% over next 2 weeks.	• Offer meals at regular times, corresponding to client's previous pattern • Provide active meaningful activities during daytime hours, including exposure to natural light, and an outdoor environment when possible • Monitor frequency and duration of naps • Create an individualized bedtime ritual that includes a quieting activity, a light carbohydrate snack, going to the bathroom and settling a routine • Do not waken even if incontinent. Change and assist the client to the bathroom when he or she spontaneously awakens • If turning or other care is necessary, try to provide for periods up to 2 hours of undisturbed sleep time whenever possible.

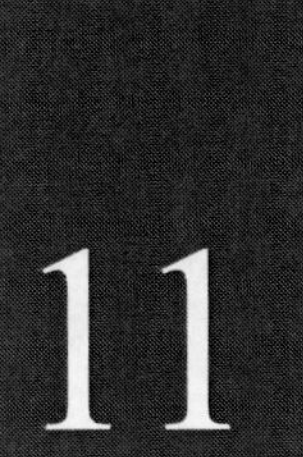

Nursing Management of Childhood and Adolescent Disorders Including Mental Deficiency

Child psychiatry is concerned with the assessment and treatment of children's emotional, behavioral and relationship problems. Children are not small adults, but immature and developing individuals. Childhood is a period of life characterized by change and the necessity for adaptation.

During childhood, the child undergoes a remarkable transformation from a helpless, dependent infant to an independent, self-sufficient individual with his own views and outlook capable of living separately from his family. In order to judge whether any observed emotional, social or intellectual functioning is abnormal, it has to be compared with the corresponding normal range for the age group.

Differences of Child psychiatry from adult psychiatry:

- The child's existence and emotional development depends on the family or care givers; cooperation with family members; sometimes written consent.
- The developmental stages are very important assessment of the diagnosis.
- Use of psychopharmacotherapy is less common in comparison to adult psychiatry.
- Children are less able to express themselves in words.
- The child who suffers by psychiatric problems in childhood can be an emotionally stable person in adulthood, but some of the psychic disturbances can change a whole life of the child and his family.

The common disorders of childhood and adolescent disorders including mental deficiency are discussed in this chapter.

CLASSIFICATION OF CHILDHOOD DISORDERS (ICD-10)

Mental Retardation (F70–F79)

F70 Mild mental retardation
F71 Moderate mental retardation
F72 Severe mental retardation
F73 Profound mental retardation.

Disorders of Psychological Development (F80–F89)

F80 Specific developmental disorders of speech and language
F81 Specific developmental disorders of scholastic skills
F82 Specific developmental disorders of motor function
F83 Mixed specific developmental disorders

F84 Pervasive developmental disorders
F88 Other disorders of psychological development
F89 Unspecified disorder of psychological development.

Behavioral and Emotional Disorders with Onset Usually Occurring in Childhood and Adolescence (F90–F98)

F90 Hyperkinetic disorders
F91 Conduct disorders
F92 Mixed disorders of conduct and emotions
F93 Emotional disorders with onset specific to childhood
F94 Disorders of social functioning with onset specific to childhood and adolescence
F95 Tic disorders
F98 Other behavioral and emotional disorders with onset usually occurring in childhood and adolescence.

MENTAL RETARDATION (F70–F79)

Internationally, the definition of mental retardation has moved away from a medical model to that of an educational model which is functional and support-based and emphasizes the rights of the individual.

Mental retardation is a developmental disability that is marked by lower-than-normal intelligence and limited daily living skills. It is normally present at birth or develops early in life.

Definition

Mental retardation means a 'condition of arrested or incomplete development of mind of a person which is specially characterized by sub-normality of intelligence'.

Mental retardation refers to significantly subaverage general intellectual functioning, existing concurrently with deficits in adaptive behavior and manifested during the developmental period.

Prevalence

About 3% of world population is estimated to be mentally ill. In India, about 5 per 1000 children are mentally retarded and more than 20 million children are estimated to be mentally retarded. The incidence is increasing at the age of 5 with the number of cases identified at the age of 15.

Box 11.1: Classification of mental disorder

		IQ Range		
S. No.	**Classification**	**Stanford-Binet and Cattell tests**	**Wechsler scales**	**Approximate percentage (%)**
1	Mild	52 – 67	55 – 69	89
2	Moderate	36 – 51	40 – 54	7
3	Severe	20 – 35	25 – 39	3
4	Profound	0 – 19	0 – 24	1

Etiology

The etiology of mental retardation may be primarily biological or primarily psychosocial, or some combination of both. In approximately 30–40% of individuals seen in clinical settings, the etiology cannot be determined. Five major predisposing factors have been identified are:

1. Genetic and hereditary factors
2. Early alterations in embryonic development
3. Pregnancy and prenatal factors
4. General medical conditions acquired in infancy or childhood
5. Environmental influences and other mental disorders.

Genetic and Hereditary Factors

Hereditary factors are implicated as the cause in approximately 5% of the cases. These factors include inborn errors of metabolism, such as Tay-Sachs disease, phenylketonuria, and hyperglycinemia. Also included are chromosomal disorders, such as Down syndrome and Klinefelter's syndrome, and single-gene abnormalities, such as tuberous sclerosis and neurofibromatosis.

Early Alterations in Embryonic Development

Prenatal factors that result in early alterations in embryonic development account for approximately 30% of mental retardation cases. Damages may occur in response to toxicity associated with maternal ingestion of alcohol or other drugs. Maternal illnesses and infections during pregnancy (e.g. rubella, cytomegalovirus) and complications of pregnancy (e.g. toxemia, uncontrolled diabetes), etc. can also lead to mental retardation.

Pregnancy and Perinatal Factors

Approximately, 10% of cases of mental retardation are the result of factors that occur during pregnancy (e.g. fetal malnutrition, viral and other infections, and prematurity) or during the birth process.

General Medical Conditions Acquired in Infancy or Childhood

General medical conditions acquired during infancy or childhood account for approximately 5% of cases of mental retardation. They include infections, such as meningitis and encephalitis; poisonings, such as from insecticides, medications, and lead; physical trauma, such as head injuries, asphyxiation, and hyperpyrexia.

Environmental Influences and Other Mental Disorders

Between 15 and 20% of cases of mental retardation are attributed to deprivation of nurturance and social, linguistic and other stimulation, and to severe mental disorders, such as autistic disorder.

Classification of Mental Retardation

- **Mild Mental Retardation:** This is the most common type of mental retardation, accounting for 85–90% of all cases. In the preschool period, these children often develop

like other normal children, with very little deficit. Later, they often progress up to the 6th class in school and can achieve vocational and social self-sufficiency with a little support. This group has been referred as 'educable'.
- **Moderate mental retardation:** About 10% of all persons with mental retardation have an IQ between 35 and 50. This group is 'trainable', although many of these persons can also be educated. They drop out school after the 2nd class (grade). They can be trained to support themselves by performing semiskilled or unskilled work under supervision.
- **Severe mental retardation:** Severe mental retardation is often recognized early in life with poor motor development and absent or markedly delayed speech and other communication skills. Later in life, elementary training in personal health care can be given and they can be taught to talk. This group is termed as 'dependent'.
- **Profound mental retardation:** This group accounts for about 1–2% of all persons with mental retardation. The achievement of developmental milestone is markedly delayed. They often need nursing care or 'life support' under a carefully planned and structured environment.

Signs and Symptoms

- Delayed developmental milestones
- Inability to follow commands or directions
- Reduced ability to learn
- Expressive language problems
- Psychomotor skill deficits
- Difficulty in performing self-care activities
- Neurological impairments
- Medical problems such as seizures can complicate
- Liable mood and low self-esteem
- Irritability
- Acting out behavior
- Lack of curiosity.

Diagnosis

The diagnosis is made by the following steps:
- History
- Physical examination
- Neurological examination
- Mental status examination, for the assessment of associated psychiatric disorders and the clinical assessment of the level of intelligence.
- Investigations
  - Urine and blood tests to rule out metabolic causes
  - Electroencephalogram (EEG), especially in presence of seizures
  - Chromosomal studies, e.g. in Down's syndrome, prenatal (by amniocentesis or chorionic villi biopsy) and postnatal
  - Computed tomography (CT) scan or Magnetic resonance imaging (MRI) scan of brain

- Thyroid function tests (TFTs)
- Liver function tests (LFTs).
- Psychological tests—the commonly used tests for measurement of intelligence include:
  - Stanford-Binet, Binet-Simon or Binet-Kamat tests
  - Wechsler Intelligence Scale for Children (WISC) for 6½–16 years of age
  - Wechsler's Preschool and Primary Scale of Intelligence (WPPSI) for 4 – 6½ years of age
  - Bhatia's battery of performance tests, etc.

Treatment

- There is no specific treatment for mental retardation
- Behavioral modification
- Environmental supervision
- Speech therapy
- Family therapy and support
- Vocational training
- Treatment of associated psychiatric symptoms.

Preventive Measures of Mental Retardation

Primary Prevention

This consists of:

- Improvement in socioeconomic condition of society at large, aiming at elimination of under-stimulation, malnutrition, prematurity and perinatal factors.
- Education of lay public, aiming at removal of the misconceptions about mental retardation.
- Medical measures for good perinatal medical care to prevent infections, trauma, excessive use of medications, malnutrition, obstetric complications, and diseases of pregnancy.
- Universal immunization of children with Bacillus Calmette-Guerin (BCG), polio, diphtheria, pertussis (whooping cough) and tetanus (DPT), and measles, mumps, and rubella (MMR).
- Facilitating research activities to study the causes of mental retardation and their treatment.
- Genetic counseling in at-risk parents, e.g. in phenylketonuria, Down's syndrome.

Secondary Prevention

- Early detection and treatment of preventable disorders, e.g. phenylketonuria.
- Early detection of handicaps in sensory, motor or behavioral areas with early remedial measures and treatment.
- Early recognition of presence of mental retardation. A delay in diagnosis may cause unfortunate delay in rehabilitation.
- Treat associated psychiatric features.

Tertiary Prevention

- Adequate treatment of psychological and behavioral problems.
- Behavior modification, using the principles of positive and negative reinforcement.
- Rehabilitation in vocational, physical, and social areas.
- Parental counseling is important to lessen the levels of stress, and encouraging formation of parents' or carers' organization(s) and self-help groups.
- Institutionalization or residential care may be needed for individuals with profound mental retardation.

Nursing Management

Nursing Process

Nursing care plan for a child with mental retardation is given in the box below.

Box 11.2: Nursing care plan for mental retardation

Nursing diagnosis: Risk for injury related to altered physical mobility or aggressive behavior.

Outcome identification	Nursing intervention
Client will not experience injury.	• Create a safe environment for the client. • Ensure that small items are removed from area where client will be ambulating and that sharp items are out of reach. • Store items that client uses frequently within easy reach. • Pad side rails and headboard of client with history of seizures. • Prevent physical aggression and acting out behaviors by learning to recognize signs that client is becoming agitated.

Nursing diagnosis: Self-care deficit related to impaired physical mobility or lack of maturity.

Outcome identification	Nursing intervention
Client will be able to participate in self-care activities.	• Assess the ability to do self-care activities. • Work on one aspect of self-care at a time. • Provide simple, concrete explanations. • Offer positive feedback for efforts. • Encourage independence but intervene when client is unable to perform.

Nursing diagnosis: Impaired verbal communication related to developmental delay.

Outcome identification	Nursing intervention
Client will be able to communicate with their needs and desires.	• Assess the level of communication pattern. • Maintain consistency of staff assignment. • Anticipate and fulfill client's needs until satisfactory communication patterns are established. • Learn (from family, if possible) special words client uses that are different from the norm. • Identify nonverbal gestures or signals that client may use to convey needs if verbal communication is absent. • Practice these communications skills repeatedly.

Nursing diagnosis: Impaired social interaction related to speech deficiencies or difficulty adhering to conventional social behavior.

Contd...

Contd...

Outcome identification	Nursing intervention
Client will be able to interact with others.	• Assess the socialization of the client. • Remain with client during initial interactions with others on the unit. • Explain to other clients the meaning behind some of the client's nonverbal gestures and signals. • Use simple language to explain to client which behaviors are acceptable and which is not. • Establish a procedure for behavior modification by positive reinforcement and aversive techniques.

DISORDERS OF PSYCHOLOGICAL DEVELOPMENT (F80–F89)

Specific developmental disorders are characterized by an inadequate development in usually one specific area of functioning. These may include reading (developmental reading disorder), language (developmental language disorder), arithmetic or mathematics (developmental arithmetic or mathematics disorder), articulation (developmental articulation disorder or phonological disorder), or coordination (developmental coordination disorder). Sometimes, more than one developmental disorder is present.

Before making a diagnosis of specific developmental disorder, it is important to keep in mind the mental age, IQ, sociocultural background, schooling, impairment in vision and hearing, or any neurological deficit.

Specific Developmental Disorders of Speech and Language (F80)

It is also called as developmental language disorder, developmental communication disorder, or dysphasia. This is a specific developmental disorder in which the child's use of speech sounds which is below the appropriate level for its mental age, but in which there is a normal level of language skills.

The articulation abnormalities are not caused by a neurological abnormality and nonverbal intelligence is within normal range. There are three main types:

1. **Phonological disorder:** Also called as *dyslalia*, it is characterized by below par accuracy in the use of speech sounds despite normal language skills. The problems include severe articulation errors that make it difficult for others to understand the speech. Speech sounds or phonemes are omitted, distorted or substituted (e.g. wabbit for rabbit, ca for car, bu for blue).
2. **Expressive language disorder:** It is characterized by a below par ability of using expressive speech. The problems include restricted vocabulary, difficulty in selecting appropriate words, and immature grammatical usage. Cluttering of speech may also be present.
3. **Receptive language disorder:** The disorder often presents as a receptive-expressive language disorder and both receptive and expressive impairments are present together. The disorder is characterized by a below par understanding of language. Problems include failure to respond to simple instructions.

Acquired Aphasia with Epilepsy (Landau-Kleffner): In this disorder, child loses receptive and expressive language skills after previous period of normal language development. The paroxysmal abnormalities on the EEG are present and in the majority of cases epileptic seizures occur as well.

Some children become mute in a period of few months. Usually, the onset is between the ages of three and seven years, with skills being lost over days or weeks. An inflammatory encephalitic process has been suggested as a possible cause of this disorder.

Specific Developmental Disorders of Scholastic Skills (F81)

Specific Reading Disorder

It is also called as developmental reading disorder or *dyslexia*. It refers to a difficulty in learning to read in a person who has good intelligence, strong motivation, and who has received appropriate teaching. The child presents with a serious delay in learning to read which is evident from the early years. The problems may include omissions, distortions, or substitutions of words, long hesitations, reversal of words, or simply slow reading.

Specific Arithmetic Disorder

It is also called as developmental arithmetic disorder or developmental mathematic disorder or *dyscalculia*.

The arithmetical performance is significantly below the level of the general intelligence, reading and spelling skills are within normal range. The deficit concerns mastery of basic computational skills of addition, subtraction, multiplication, and division rather than of the more abstract mathematical skills involved in algebra, trigonometry, geometry, or calculus.

Specific Developmental Disorder of Motor Function (F82)

It is also called as motor skills disorder, developmental coordination disorder, clumsy child syndrome or motor dyspraxia. It is characterized by poor coordination in daily activities of life, e.g. in dressing, walking, feeding, and playing. There is an inability to perform fine or gross motor tasks.

Treatment

- The treatment is based on learning theory principles and is behavioral in approach (use of special remedial teaching).
- Cooperation of neurologist and speech therapist is very important.
- Psychiatric treatment is necessary if the child has secondary psychic problems, for example in relationship with other children or family.
- Nootropic drugs, psychotherapy and special education are useful.
- Parental education and counseling are also important.

Pervasive Developmental Disorders (PDD) (F84)

Disorders characterized by qualitative abnormalities in reciprocal social interactions and in patterns of communication, and by a restricted, stereotyped, repetitive repertoire of interests and activities. These disorders include:

- Childhood autism
- Atypical autism

- Rett's syndrome
- Asperger's syndrome
- Others.

Childhood Autism

Infantile autism was described for the first time by *Leo Kanner* in 1943 as 'autistic disturbance of affective contact'. This syndrome has variously been described as autistic disorder, pervasive developmental disorder, childhood autism, childhood psychosis and pseudodefective psychosis.

Autisms are severe impairment of developmental disorder which presents before age of 3 years. The abnormal functioning manifests in the areas of social interaction, communication and repetitive behavior. In causes an unknown organic brain insult is suggested.

Incidence

This syndrome is more common (3–4 times) in males and 30–40 cases per 100,000 children. Although, earlier it was thought to be commoner in upper socioeconomic classes.

Onset

Typically, the onset occurs before the age of 2½ years though in some cases, the onset may occur later in childhood. Such cases are called as childhood onset autism or childhood onset pervasive developmental disorder. Autism occurring before or after 2½ years of age is not clinically very different.

Clinical Features

1. Inability to relate

- No emotional interaction with people
- Emotional responses to parents, strangers and inanimate objects are the same
- Absent social smile
- Lack of eye-to-eye-contact
- Gaze avoidance is a characteristics feature
- No or abnormal social play; prefers solitary games
- Marked impairment in making friends
- Lack of imitative behavior
- Absence of fear in presence of danger.

2. Language impairment

- Interpersonal verbal communication is markedly affected
- Absent or delayed speech
- In infancy, absence of communicative sounds.

3. Preoccupation with certain objects and rituals with resistance to change (e.g. the same food).

4. Other features

- Labile mood and nonspecific anger and fear
- Overactivity and distractibility

- Disturbed sleep
- Mannerisms and stereotyped behaviors
- Attachment may develop to inanimate objects
- Hyperkinesis is commonly associated
- Varying degrees of mental retardation are present in 75% of cases
- Epilepsy may develop in adolescence in 20–25% of severe cases
- Enuresis and encopresis may occur.

Treatment

Specific treatment is unknown for autistic disorders. Autistic children usually require special schooling or residential schooling although attempts of integrations are also started. Special techniques for teaching autistic children and special psychotherapeutic approaches were developed.

Psychotherapy

Psychotherapy is not effective in treatment of infantile autism. However, patient at counseling and supportive psychotherapy are very useful in allaying parental anxiety and guilt and overstimulation of the child should be avoided during treatment.

Behavior Therapy

- Development of a regular routine.
- Increase new positive behaviors.
- Structured class room training, aiming at learning new material and maintenance of acquired learning.
- Teach new skills.
- Speech therapy and/or sign language teaching.
- Encourage interpersonal interactions.

Psychopharmacotherapy

Sometimes antipsychotic drugs and antidepressants are used to cope with aggressive behavior and depression. The commonly using drugs may be;

Haloperidol decreases hyperactivity and behavioral symptoms. Risperidone, an atypical antipsychotic, is helpful in children of aged 5 and above. The starting dose for Risperidone is usually 0.25–0.5 mg (based on body weight), with a dose range of 0.02–0.06 mg/kg/day.

Other drugs such as SSRIs, chlorpromazine, amphetamines, imipramine, multivitamins and triiodothyronine have been tried with limited success and should be used only by the experts in the field.

Anticonvulsant medication is used for the treatment of generalized or other seizures, if present.

Nursing Management

Box 11.3: Nursing process for autistic disorder

Outcome identification	Nursing intervention
Nursing diagnosis: Risk for self-mutilation related to neurological changes.	
Outcome identification	**Nursing intervention**
Client will not harm self.	• Work with the child on a one-to-one basis. • Try to determine the reason for self-mutilate behavior. • Try to intervene with diversional activities. • Protect the child when self-mutilate behaviors occur, e.g. padded hand mitts, or arm covers may provide protection when the risk for self-harm exists.
Nursing diagnosis: Impaired social interaction related to inability to trust, neurological changes.	
Outcome identification	**Nursing intervention**
Client will establish social interactions with others.	• Assign a limited number of caregivers to the child. • Ensure that warmth, acceptance, and availability are conveyed. • Provide child with familiar objects, such as familiar toys or a blanket. • Support child's attempts to interact with others. • Give positive reinforcement for eye contact with something acceptable to the child (e.g. food, familiar object). Gradually replace with social reinforcement (e.g. touch, smiling, and hugging).
Nursing diagnosis: Disturbed personal identity related to inadequate sensory stimulation, neurological changes.	
Outcome identification	**Nursing intervention**
Client will name own body parts as separate and individual from those of others.	• Assist child to recognize separateness during self-care activities, such as dressing and feeding. • Assist the child in learning to name own body parts. This can be facilitated by the use of mirrors, drawings, and pictures of the child. • Encourage appropriate touching of, and being touched by, others.

Atypical Autism

It is a type of pervasive developmental disorder that differs from childhood autism either in age of onset or in failing to fulfill all diagnostic criteria.

Abnormal and impaired development manifests after age 3 years or there are impairments in communication and stereotyped behavior is present, but emotional response to caregivers is not affected.

Atypical autism is diagnosed often in profoundly retarded individuals.

Rett's Syndrome

This is described by *Rett* in the year 1964. The syndrome is reported only in girls. Normal early development is followed by partial or complete loss of speech and of skills in locomotion and use of hands, together with deceleration in head growth.

Onset: In most cases, onset is between 7 and 24 months of age.

Features

- Loss of purposive hand movements, hand-wringing stereotypes, and hyperventilation.
- Social interaction is poor in early childhood, but can develop later.

- Motor functioning is more affected in middle childhood, muscles are hypotonic, kyphoscoliosis and rigid spasticity in the lower limbs occurs in majority of cases.
- Aggressive behavior and self-injury are rather rare, the antipsychotic drugs for the control of challenging behavior is not often needed.

Asperger's Syndrome

This is described by *Asperger* as autistic psychopathy in 1944, characterized by the same kind of impairment of social activities and stereotyped features of behavior as is described in autistic children. There is no delay of speech and cognitive development. The condition occurs predominantly in boys (8:1).

Often associated with marked clumsiness. There is a strong tendency for the abnormalities to persist into adolescence and adult life. Psychotic episodes occasionally occur in early adult life.

Other Childhood Disintegrative Disorder

These are very rare developmental disorders with a short period of normal development before onset. The child loses his acquired skills within few months.

The common features include general loss of interest in the environment, stereotyped, repetitive motor mannerisms, and autistic-like abnormalities in social interaction and communication.

These children usually remain without speech and unable to lead independent lives.

BEHAVIORAL AND EMOTIONAL DISORDERS WITH ONSET USUALLY OCCURRING IN CHILDHOOD AND ADOLESCENCE (F90–F98)

Hyperkinetic Disorders/Attention Deficit Disorder (ADD) (F90)

Hyperkinetic disorder (F90) is first described by *Heinrich Hoff* in 1854. Since, then this disorder known by a variety of names such as minimal brain dysfunction (MBD), hyperkinetic syndrome, Strauss syndrome, organic drivenness and minimal brain damage.

Hyperkinetic disorders occur mostly in first five years of life, and they are several times more frequent in boys than in girls. IQ ranges from subnormal to high intelligence. Specific learning disabilities often coexist with hyperkinetic syndrome. The main marks of the syndrome are:

- Inattention
- Impulsivity
- Hyperactivity.

Prevalence is from 3–10% of elementary-school children.

Etiology

- Genetic predisposition
- Maternal deprivation
- Environmental toxins(For example, Lead)
- Intrauterine or postnatal brain damage
- Neurological dysfunction.

Types

There are four types of ADD, they are as follows:

1. **Attention deficit disorder with hyperactivity (ADHD):** This is the most common type. The characteristic clinical features are:

- *Poor attention span with distractibility*
  - Fails to finish the things started
  - Shifts from one uncompleted activity to another
  - Easily distracted by external stimuli
  - Often loses things.
- *Hyperactivity*
  - Fidget and squirm in their seats
  - Difficulty in sitting still at one place for long
  - Moving about here and there
  - Talks excessively
  - Interference in other people's activities.
- *Impulsivity*
  - Impatient
  - Acts before thinking, on the spur of the moment
  - Difficulty in waiting for turn at work or play.

2. **Attention deficit disorder without hyperactivity:** It is a rare disorder with similar clinical features, except hyperactivity.
3. **Residual type:** It is usually diagnosed in a patient in adulthood, with a past history of ADD and presence of a few residual features in adult life.
4. **Hyperkinetic disorder with conduct disorder (Hyperkinetic conduct disorder):** In this, the hyperkinetic disorder may be associated with conduct disorders.

Treatment

- Parents and teachers have to be advised how to cope with hyperactive children.
- Behavioral modification
- Counseling and supportive psychotherapy
- Mild doses of antipsychotics are sometimes prescribed
- **Stimulant medication:** Dextroamphetamine or dexamphetamine (2.5–20 mg/day) and methylphenidate (5–60 mg/day) have been traditionally used. Currently, methylphenidate is the drug of choice in the treatment of ADD, with a high response rate.

Course

A large majority (about 80%) of patients improve on their own by the time of puberty, though a few (15–20%) may have persistent symptoms even in adulthood. Impulsivity and inattention are usually the most common residual features after puberty while hyperactivity often tends to remit.

ADD can also present in adulthood. This includes graduates of childhood onset ADD which continue to have symptoms in adulthood and those who begin with symptoms for the first time in adulthood.

Nursing Management

Box 11.4: Nursing process for hyperkinetic disorder

Nursing diagnosis: Risk for injury related to impulsive and accident prone behavior and the inability to perceive self-harm.	
Outcome identification	**Nursing intervention**
Client will be free of injury.	• Ensure a safe environment for the child • Identify and limit behaviors that put child at risk for injury • Provide necessary supervision to prevent injury during therapeutic activities • Parental counseling.
Nursing diagnosis: Impaired social interaction related to intrusive and immature behavior.	
Outcome identification	**Nursing intervention**
Client will demonstrate ability to interact appropriate with others.	• Develop a trusting relationship • Discuss with client which behaviors are and are not acceptable • Behavioral modifications by reinforcement • Employ consequences for unacceptable behavior • Provide group situations for client.
Nursing diagnosis: Low self-esteem related to dysfunctional family system and negative feedback.	
Outcome identification	**Nursing intervention**
Client will demonstrate increased feelings of self-worth.	• Ensure that goals are realistic • Plan activities that provide opportunities for success • Convey unconditional acceptance and positive regard • Give positive reinforcement for achievements.

Conduct Disorder (F91)

Conduct disorder is characterized by a persistent and significant pattern of conduct, in which the basic rights of others are violated or rules of society are not followed.

Conduct disorders are diagnosed when the child is showing persistent and serious dissocial or aggressive behavior patterns. The onset occurs much before 18 years of age, usually even before puberty.

Etiology

- Early maternal rejection
- Parental separation
- Family neglect
- Abuse or violence
- Large family size
- Broken family/dysfunctional family.

Types

- **Conduct disorder confined to the family context:** The dissocial or aggressive behavior is intent on family members and occurs mostly at home. Social relationships outside the family are within the normal range.
- **Unsocialized conduct disorder:** Aggressive and dissocial behavior is connected with the child's poor relationships with other children and peers groups.

- **Socialized conduct disorder:** The diagnosis is applied when the child is showing aggressive and dissocial behavior, but relationship with children of the same age is adequate.
- **Oppositional defiant disorder (ODD):** Children under age of 9–10 years, showing persistently negativistic, provocative and disruptive behavior. This type of behavior is often directed towards a new member of the family, i.e. step father or mother.

Features

The typical features include the following:

- Frequent lying
- Stealing or robbery
- Running away from home and school
- Truancy
- Physical violence such as rape, fire-setting, assault or breaking-in, use of weapons
- Cruelty towards other people and animals.

In addition to this the secondary complications often develop such as:

- Substance abuse
- Unwanted pregnancies
- Sexually transmitted diseases (STDs)
- Criminal record
- Suicidal and homicidal behavior.

Treatment

The treatment of conduct disorder is usually difficult.

- Family situation should be consider and its relation to the child's disorder. The family therapy is necessary to enhance emotional support and understanding.
- In the cases of dysfunctional families, abused or neglected children, an adoptive homes, foster care or supervised residence is recommended.
- Behavioral modification.
- Drug treatment may be needed in presence of epilepsy (anticonvulsants), hyperactivity (stimulant medication), impulse control disorder and episodic aggressive behavior (lithium, carbamazepine), and psychotic symptoms (antipsychotics).

Nursing Management

Box 11.5: Nursing process for conduct disorder

Nursing diagnosis: Risk for other-directed violence related to characteristics of temperament, peer rejection, negative parental role models, dysfunctional family dynamics.

Outcome identification	Nursing intervention
Client will not harm others or others' property.	• Observe client's behavior frequently through routine activities and interactions. • Redirect violent behavior with physical outlets for suppressed anger and frustration. • Encourage client to express anger. • Ensure that a sufficient number of staff is available to indicate a show of strength if necessary. • Administer tranquilizing medication as per doctor's order.

Contd...

Contd...

Nursing diagnosis: Impaired social interaction related to negative parental role models; impaired peer relations leading to inappropriate social behavior.	
Outcome identification	**Nursing intervention**
Client will be able to interact with others.	• Develop a trusting relationship with the client. • Convey acceptance of the person separate from the unacceptable behavior. • Discuss with client which behaviors are and are not acceptable. • Describe the consequence of unacceptable behavior. • Provide group situations for client.
Nursing diagnosis: Defensive coping related to low self-esteem and dysfunctional family system.	
Outcome identification	**Nursing intervention**
Client will accept responsibility for own behaviors and interact with others without becoming defensive.	• Explain to client the correlation between feelings of inadequacy and the need for acceptance from others. • Provide immediate nonthreatening feedback for unacceptable behaviors. • Help identify situations that provoke defensiveness and practice through role-play more appropriate responses. • Provide immediate positive feedback for acceptable behaviors.

Mixed Disorders of Conduct and Emotions (F92)

A group of disorders characterized by the combination of persistently aggressive, dissocial or defiant behavior with overt and marked symptoms of depression, anxiety or other emotional upsets. Mood disorders in children are often expressed by a challenging behavior or somatic symptoms. For example, depressive conduct disorder.

Separation Anxiety Disorder of Childhood (F93.0)

The child is showing anxiety when being separated from persons who are for him emotionally important (parents, family members). School refusal is often a symptom of separation anxiety disorders.

Treatment

- In the case of school, refusal the child should be returned to school immediately and strict limits should be established.
- The treatment is focused on family structure and recommendation in the ways of upbringing.
- In severe cases, use of antidepressants is necessary.

Phobic Anxiety Disorder of Childhood (F93.1)

The phobic states most commonly encountered in children involve fear of animals, insects, dark and school. Animal and insect phobias usually start at the age of 5 years and almost none start in adult life. Some phobias start in the late adolescence, i.e. agoraphobia.

Treatment

- Psychotherapy and a sensible parental handling
- The anxiety reducing techniques are useful, i.e. desensitization.

Social Anxiety Disorder of Childhood (F93.2)

There is a social apprehension or anxiety when encountering new, strange, or socially threatening situations. A fear of social encounters is associated with avoidance behavior, which produces problems in functioning in a peer group and in the school performance as well. The social acceptance of the child can be very difficult and can have impact on his or her further personal development.

Treatment

- Psychotherapy
- Anxiolytic drugs.

Sibling Rivalry Disorder (F93.3)

Some degree of emotional disturbance usually following the birth of an immediately younger sibling is shown by a majority of young children.

Sibling rivalry disorder should be diagnosed only if the degree or persistence of the disturbance is unusual and associated with abnormalities of social interaction.

The children with sibling rivalry disorder are acting with serious hatred to the newborn; in severe cases, they are showing physical harming behavior and persistent competition to gain parents attention.

Treatment

- Psychotherapy dealing with family structure
- Prevention.

Elective Mutism (F94.0)

It is characterized by a marked, emotionally determined selectivity in speaking, such that the child demonstrates a language competence in some situations but fails to speak in other (definable) situations.

These children show specific personality features as social anxiety and oversensitivity.

Treatment

- Psychotherapy
- In severe cases, anxiolytic drugs.

Tic Disorders (F95)

A tic is an abnormal involuntary, rapid, recurrent, non rhythmic motor movement (usually involving circumscribed muscle groups) or vocal production that is of sudden onset and that serves no apparent purpose.

Tic disorder may be transient or chronic. Transient form is more common in boys and can occur in 5–20% of children. Tics are experienced as irresistible, but can be suppressed for shorter periods of time.

Types of Tic Disorders

- Transient tic disorder
- Combined vocal and multiple motor tic disorder (*de la Tourette*)
- Other tic disorders

A special type of chronic tic disorder is *de la Tourette's syndrome* or *Tourette's disorder*.

Tourette's Disorder

The essential feature of Tourette's disorder is the presence of multiple motor tics and one or more vocal tics. They may appear simultaneously or at different periods during the illness.

The disturbance causes marked distress or interferes with social, occupational, or other important areas of functioning.

- **Motor Tics:** The motor tics in Tourette's disorder can be simple or complex.
  - **Simple motor tics:** These may include eye blinking, grimacing, and shrugging of shoulders, tongue protrusion.
  - **Complex motor tics:** These are facial gestures, stamping, jumping, hitting self, squatting, twirling, echopraxia (repetition of observed acts), and copropraxia (obscene acts).

Motor tics are often the earliest to appear, beginning in the head region and then progressing downwards. These are later followed by the vocal tics.

- **Vocal Tics:** The vocal tics in Tourette's disorder can also be simple or complex.
  - **Simple vocal tics:** Simple vocal tics include coughing, barking, throat-clearing, sniffing, and clicking.
  - **Complex vocal tics:** Includes repetition of particular words or sentences, and sometimes the use of socially unacceptable (often obscene) words (coprolalia), and the repetition of one's own sounds or words (palilalia).

Etiology

The etiology of Tourette syndrome is not known. Abnormalities in levels of dopamine, serotonin, gamma-aminobutyric acid (GABA), acetylcholine, and norepinephrine have been associated with Tourette's disorder.

Complications of pregnancy (e.g. severe nausea and vomiting or excessive stress), low birth weight (LBW), head trauma, carbon monoxide poisoning, and encephalitis are thought to be associated with the onset of non-genetic Tourette's disorder. There is some evidence to suggest that Tourette syndrome may be inherited as autosomal dominant disorder.

Treatment

- **Pharmacotherapy:** Antipsychotics are often helpful in small doses and several drugs have been tried including haloperidol, risperidone, olanzapine, aripiprazole, ziprasidone, quetiapine, and sulpiride.
- Behavioral modification and cognitive therapy.
- Cooperation with the family is important.

Other Behavioral and Emotional Disorders with Onset Usually Occurring in Childhood and Adolescence (F98)

Nonorganic Enuresis (F98.0)

Enuresis is repetitive voiding of urine; the child is not able of voluntary bladder control during the day (*enuresis diurnal*) or during the night (*enuresis nocturnal*). This is normal in infancy.

Most children achieve bladder control by the age of three years. By the age of 5 years, there are still about 7% of children who wet their bed. Technically, enuresis is diagnosed only after 5 years of age.

The enuresis may be present from birth (*enuresis primaria*), or it may occur after a period of time of acquired bladder control (*enuresis secundaria*). Nonorganic enuresis is more common (about two times) in males.

Etiology

The exact cause of enuresis is unknown. The following may be the causes of nonorganic enuresis like emotional disturbances, insecurity, sibling rivalry, death of a parent.

The organic causes are present in about 5% of cases and include worm infestation spina bifida, neurogenic bladder, urinary tract infection (UTI), diabetes mellitus, and seizure disorder.

In secondary enuresis, the age of onset is usually 5–8 years. Enuresis tends to remit spontaneously and only 1% of children with enuresis continue to have the disorder in adulthood.

Management

- Restriction of fluid after 8 PM, in nocturnal enuresis.
- Bladder training for increasing the holding-time of bladder. It can be done by positive reinforcements.
- Interruption of sleep before the expected time of bed wetting.
- Conditioning devices, which cause an alarm to sound as soon as the voided urine touches the bed sheet. The alarm causes inhibition of further micturition and the child awakens. If properly used, it is an effective method of therapy.
- Supportive psychotherapy for the child, parents and the whole family is often needed.
- **Pharmacotherapy:** Antidepressant drug may be useful usually imipramine (25–75 mg/day).

It should never be used for children under the age of 6 years. Intranasal desmopressin has been found useful in some patients and is a good alternative.

Nonorganic Encopresis (F98.1)

This involves repeated intended or unintended passage of feces in places not appropriate for that purpose after bowel control is physiologically possible.

Normally, toilet training is achieved between the ages of 2 and 3. Encopresis is diagnosed after the age of 4 years. Encopresis can be either of:

- **Primary type**, where toilet training has never been achieved, or
- **Secondary type**, where encopresis emerges after a period of bowel control. This type typically occurs between the ages of 4 and 8.

Etiology

- Inappropriate toilet training
- Sibling rivalry
- Maturational lag
- Underlying hyperkinetic disorder
- Emotional disturbances
- Mental retardation
- Childhood schizophrenia
- Autistic disorder.

Management

- Teach the child to establish more normal bowel habit, for example by sitting on the toilet regularly after the meals.
- Behavioral modification by positive reinforcement.
- The family environment should be warm and understanding.
- The emotional disturbances of the child should not be ignored and should be dealt with at the earliest.
- Anxiolytics or antidepressants.

Feeding Disorder of Infancy and Childhood (F98.2)

Feeding disorder generally involves food refusal and extreme faddiness in the presence of an adequate food supply, a reasonably competent caregiver, and the absence of organic disease. It can be associated with rumination (repeated regurgitation without nausea). Occurs often in children in institutional care or mentally retarded.

Pica of Infancy and Childhood (F98.3)

Persistent eating of non-nutritive substances (soil, wall paint, etc.) is termed as *pica*. It is common in mentally retarded children or very young children with normal intelligence level.

Stereotyped Movement Disorder (F98.4)

This includes voluntary, repetitive, stereotyped, nonfunctional (and often rhythmic) movements that do not form part of any recognized psychiatric or neurological condition. It is of the following types:

- The non-self-injurious movements:
  - Body-rocking
  - Head-rocking
  - Hair-plucking (trichotillomania)
  - Hair-twisting
  - Finger-flicking mannerisms
  - Hand-flapping

- Stereotyped self-injurious behavior:
  - Repetitive head-banging
  - Face-slapping
  - Eye-poking
  - Biting of hands, lips or other body parts.

This is common among mentally retarded children, or in some children with visual impairment.

Stuttering (Stammering, F98.5)

Stuttering is the frequent repetition of prolongation of sounds or syllables or words. It could be transient phase in early childhood or persistent speech failure until adult life. The disorder is a fairly common one, affecting 2–5% of all children and 0.5–1% of all adults. Males are more commonly affected.

Cluttering (F98.6)

Cluttering is a rapid rate of speech with breakdown in fluency, but no repetitions or hesitations, of a severity to give rise to diminished speech intelligibility.

Speech is erratic and dysrhythmic, with rapid jerky spurts that usually involve faulty phrasing patterns.

Other Disorders

Other childhood disorders include the following:

- **Gratification habits:** They have been considered by some as masturbatory equivalents.
- **Schizophrenic disorders with early onset** in childhood occur, but they are very rare and the prognosis is poor, because of influence on psychic development. Treatment quite often includes antipsychotic drugs and residential care.
- **Manic-depressive disorder** is rare before puberty, but increases in incidence during adolescence. Treatment resembles that of adults, only electroconvulsive therapy (ECT) is not applied before adolescence.

12 Nursing Management of Patient with Organic Mental Disorders

All psychological and behavioral processes, whether normal or abnormal are a result of normal or deranged brain function. Organic psychiatric disorders are those with demonstrable pathology or etiology, or which arise directly from a medical disorder.

Organic psychiatric disorders cause psychological dysfunctions in cognitive, the sensorium, thinking, perception and/or emotion/mood. In order to exclude an organic psychiatric disorder a detailed history, mental state examination, physical examination and appropriate investigations should be carried out.

CLASSIFICATION (ICD 10)

Box 12.1: F00–09 Organic, including symptomatic, mental disorders

- F00 Dementia in Alzheimer's disease
- F01 Vascular dementia
- F02 Dementia in other diseases classified elsewhere
- F03 Unspecified dementia
- F04 Organic amnesic syndrome, not induced by alcohol and other psychoactive substances
- F05 Delirium, not induced by alcohol and other psychoactive substances
- F06 Other mental disorders due to brain damage and dysfunction and to physical disease
- F07 Personality and behavioral disorders due to brain disease, damage and dysfunction
- F09 Unspecified organic or symptomatic mental disorder

DELIRIUM (F05)

The word delirium comes from the Latin ***delirare*** means to become crazy or to rave. Delirium is the common type of organic mental disorders seen in clinical practice. It is otherwise known as acute confusional state, acute brain syndrome, acute organic reaction, toxic psychosis, and metabolic encephalopathies.

Definition

Delirium is an acute reversible global cognitive impairment with fluctuating disturbance in consciousness.

Epidemiology

- It is the commonest problem in all health care facilities.
- 5–15% of medical and surgical inpatients are estimated with delirium.

- This is higher in postoperative cases.
- The prevalence is 0.4% in general population, 1.1% in general population aged > 55 years.
- 9–30% in general hospital admissions and 5–55% in elderly general hospital admissions.
- Severely burned patients: approximately 20%.

Predisposing Factors

- Previous history of delirium
- Chronic medical illness
- Very young and old persons
- Drug dependency
- Cerebral lesions
- Treatment with psychotropic medicines
- Present or past history of head injury
- Surgical interventions.

Etiology

Any factor which can disturb the brain metabolism can cause delirium and they are endless. This will be varied from individual to individual. The common etiologies are given in box 12.2.

Types

- Delirium due to general medical condition
- Substance induced delirium
- Delirium due to multiple etiologies
- Delirium not otherwise specified.

Box 12.2: Common causes of delirium

Infection	Systemic infections, meningitis, encephalitis, septicemia, etc.
Trauma	Head injury, postoperative conditions
Neoplasm	Primary and secondary neoplasms of brain
Metabolic	Water and fluid imbalances, hypoxia, uremia, hepatic failure
Vascular	Circulatory disturbances
Drugs	Alcohol, barbiturates, digitalis, anticonvulsants, opiates, cannabis, etc.
Others	Vitamin deficiency (especially B_1, B_{12}, heavy metal ingestion, epilepsy, aneurism, sensory deprivation

Clinical Features

Delirium is characterized by the following features;

- ***Clouding of consciousness*** is the most important diagnostic sign. It refers to drowsiness, decreased awareness of surroundings, disorientation in time and place, and distractibility. At its most severe the patient may be unresponsive, but more commonly the impaired consciousness is quite subtle.
- Relatively acute in onset, fluctuating course, worse at night.

- Marked perceptual disturbances such as illusions, hallucinations also occur (most commonly visual hallucinations).
- Transient persecutory delusions.
- Irritability and agitation, or somnolence and decreased activity.
- Impaired concentration and memory.
- Disturbance in sleep wake cycle.
- Diurnal variation is marked, usually with worsening of symptoms in the evening and night (called ***sun downing***).
- Generalized autonomic dysfunction, speech and thought disturbances are often present.

Diagnosis

Delirium is one of the medical emergency and investigations to be done without any delay. Guided by thoroughly taken history, physical examination and mental status examination.

A neurological examination may give the reliable cues. Laboratory tests include a full or a complete hemogram and urinalysis, serum electrolytes, Cerobrospinal Fluid (CSF) analysis. Liver function Test (LFT) may be done. An Eletro encephalogram (EEG) is valuable and will show changes in rhythm and slowing.

According to ICD-10, for a definite diagnosis of delirium symptoms in each of the following should be there:

- Impairment of consciousness
- Global cognitive disturbances
- Psychomotor disturbances
- Disturbance in sleep wake cycle
- Mood disturbances.

The onset is usually rapid and the total duration of the condition is much less than 6 months.

Management

Delirium is managed where it occurs usually in general hospitals. Psychiatrists may be asked to assess the patient, make the diagnosis and give advice. Treatment is directed both at the symptoms and at the cause, and includes both medical and environmental interventions.

Box 12.3: Management of delirium

Environmental components
- Quiet surroundings, constant lighting, clock, calendar, regular routine
- Clear simple communications
- Limit numbers of staff
- Involve family

Medical components
- Monitor vital signs
- Investigate and treat underlying cause (e.g. antibiotics, oxygen, stop drug)
- Control agitation or psychotic symptoms with antipsychotics

Identify the various causes and manage it immediately like:

- 50 mg of 50% dextrose IV for hypoglycemia
- O_2 for hypoxia

- 100 mg of B_1 IV for vitamin deficiency
- IV fluids for fluid imbalances
- Benzodiazepines
  - Diazepam 10 mg
- Antipsychotics
  - Haloperidol 5 mg
  - Chlorpromazine 50 mg.

(Nursing management is discussed later in this chapter)

DEMENTIA

The word ***dementia*** is derived from two Latin word ***de*** (apart/away) and ***mens*** (mind) and is the progressive decline in cognitive function due to damage or disease in the brain beyond what must be expected from normal aging. It is also known as chronic organic brain syndrome.

Definition

Dementia is defined as a progressive, generalized impairment of intellectual functions and memory without impairment of consciousness.

Dementia is an acquired global impairment of intellectual, memory and personality but without impairment of consciousness.

Epidemiology

- Estimated prevalence of dementia is 1.03% of the population.
- It is a disorder of old age and 5% of persons over 65 years of age
- Over 85 years of age it is four to five times more common
- Concordance rate among twins is high
- In some families dementia of Alzheimer's type runs with an autosomal recessive type of inheritance.

Etiology

Like delirium, dementia is a symptom complex and arises from a multitude of causes.

Box 12.4: Causes of dementia

Alzheimer's disease (50–60% of cases)
Vascular dementia (20–25%)
Dementia with Lewy bodies (10–15%)
Other causes (<10%)

Degenerative disorders
- Frontotemporal dementia
- Pick's disease
- Huntington's disease
- Prion disease
- Progressive supranuclear palsy

Metabolic disorders
- Alcoholic dementia
- Vitamin B_{12} deficiency

Contd...

Contd...

Infections
- HIV
- Syphilis

Other causes
- Normal pressure hydrocephalus
- Intracranial tumors
- Subdural hematoma
- Head injury

Clinical Features

- Progressive worsening of memory
- Recent memory is affected at first with difficulty to learn new material
- Later even remote memory is affected
- Confusion with performing simple tasks
- Poor concentration
- Emotional liability
- Easily distracted and concentration is hard to sustain
- Disorientation of time, place and person
- Inability to recognize familiar faces in late stages
- Anxious, irritable and depressed in early stages
- Deterioration of personality with lack of personal care
- Hallucinations(visual type) and delusions (usually persecutory) may be present
- Catastrophic reaction–when confronted with tasks which are beyond his control, there are flashes of anger and tearfulness
- Inappropriate sexual behavior
- Impaired thinking and judgment
- Confabulation is common
- Delirium may be superimposed with already existing dementia
- Dementia increases the risk for delirium from systemic infections.

Classification

According to ICD-10 dementias are classified as:
- Dementia of Alzheimer's Type (DAT)
- Vascular dementias like
  - Acute onset
  - Multi-infarct dementia
  - Subcortical vascular dementia
- Dementia in other diseases like
  - Lewy body dementia
  - Pick's disease
  - Creutzfeldt–Jakob
  - Huntington's disease
  - Parkinson's disease

- HIV disease
- Hypothyroid dementia
• Dementia unspecified.

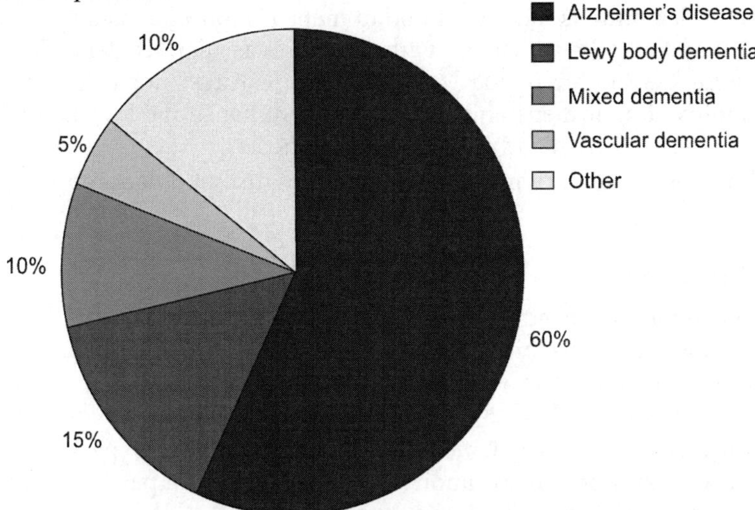

Fig 12.1: Percentage distribution of dementia

Alzheimer's Dementia

Dementia of Alzheimer's Type **(DAT)** is the most frequent type of dementia seen in about 60–70% of all dementias. It is a primary degenerative cerebral disease of unknown etiology. It is more commonly seen in women. DAT is characterized with marked reduction of neurons, appearance of neurofibrillary tangles and senile plaques (beta-amyloid), especially cholinergic system is affected.

The same pathological changes take place in both the senile (onset over the age of 65) and the presenile form (onset under the age of 65). A 39–43 amino acid fragment of—amyloid precursor protein (APP)—amyloid protein (Abeta), accumulates in the brain parenchyma to form the typical lesions associated with Alzheimer's disease.

Alzheimer's dementia is characterized by memory loss, especially short-term dysphasia and dyspraxia sense of smell impaired early behavioral changes, e.g. wandering, psychotic symptoms at some stage, relentlessly progressive. Survival of persons with DAT is 5–8 years.

At present DAT is not considered as a treatable disorder. However, cholinesterase inhibitors such as rivastigmine (1.5–6 mg/bd), donepezil (5–10 mg/day) have been used in moderate type of DAT.

Vascular Dementia

In practice the term vascular dementia usually applies to multiinfarct dementia. Multi-infarct dementia is also known as arteriosclerotic dementia and is an ischemic disorder caused by multiple cerebral infarcts, with the extent of cerebral infarction being related to the degree of cognitive impairment. It is associated with chronic hypertension and arteriosclerosis.

Macroscopically there are multiple cerebral infarcts, local or general atrophy of the brain with secondary ventricular dilatation and evidence of arteriosclerotic changes in major arteries.

Multi-infarct dementia is more common in men. The onset is usually acute, peaks in the 60s and 70s, and may be associated with a cerebrovascular accident. Clinical features include: stepwise deterioration; focal neurological features; nocturnal confusion; fits; fluctuating cognitive impairment; and emotional incontinence and low mood. Death tends to occur on average between 4 and 5 years after diagnosis.

The treatment of the underlying cause can prevent further deterioration by preventing further infarctions

Lewy Body Dementia

This type of dementia is believed to be the second most common cause of the degenerative dementias. A Lewy body is an intracytoplasmic concentrically laminated round to elongated eosinophilic inclusion which often has a dense central core surrounded by a paler peripheral rim. Classically, Lewy bodies are found in idiopathic Parkinson's disease.

This is fluctuating type of dementia; delirium-like phases parkinsonism, visual hallucinations. Antipsychotics medication should be avoided in patients with Lewy body dementia, because it can worsen the symptoms.

Dementia in Pick's Disease

Pick's disease is slightly more common in women, with a peak age of onset between 50 and 60. Clinical features include: personality deterioration, with features of frontal lobe dysfunction; nominal aphasia; memory impairment; perseveration. Macroscopically there is selective asymmetrical atrophy of the frontal and temporal lobes which, because of its severity, causes the gyri to become very thin this is known as knife-blade atrophy of the gyri.

Dementia in Creutzfeldt-Jakob Disease

Creutzfeldt–Jakob disease (CJD) is a rare progressive dementia over 1–2 months, which is believed to be transmitted by infection with a prion—a glycoprotein viral sub particle lacking ribonucleic acid. Multiple neurological signs (pyramidal + extra pyramidal, ataxia).

Dementia in Huntington's Disease

This occurs in persons having a strong family history of Huntington's disease. Onset occurs at a relatively young age, i.e. 20–40s. The symptoms include schizophrenia like psychosis, depression and irritability. Involuntary choreiform movements; dementia occurs later.

Dementia in HIV Disease

About 50–70% of patients suffering from AIDS exhibits a triad of cognitive, behavioral and motoric deficits of sub cortical dementia type and is known as AIDS-dementia complex (ADC). Symptoms include forgetfulness, slowness and poor concentration, difficulties with problem-solving and reading, apathy, social withdrawal, and affective disorder. Neurological signs (tremor, ataxia, hyperreflexia, etc).

Hypothyroid Dementia

This is one of the treatable and reversible types of dementia. It accounts for less than 1% of dementias. Since, clinical diagnosis of hypothyroid dementia may be difficult, laboratory tests should be used for correct diagnosis. Prompt treatment can reverse this type of dementia.

Investigations

The diagnostic tests are of great importance in finding the cause. The common investigations include:

- Complete blood count
- Urinalysis
- Blood glucose, serum electrolytes
- Renal function test
- Thyroid function test
- Serum B_{12} and folate level
- X-ray, ECG, X-ray skull
- EEG, lumbar puncture
- CT/MRI of brain
- Neuropsychological tests.

Management

- Hospitalization for the treatment of medical complications if any.
- Symptomatic treatment.
- Maximizing patients' opportunities for social interaction and participating in activities such as walking, singing, dancing, etc.
- Environmental manipulation and focus on coping skills to reduce stress.
- Caring for the caregiver is an essential element of managing the patient with Alzheimer's disease.
- The 3R's—***Repeat, Reassure, and Redirect***—can help caregivers reduce troublesome behaviors and limit the use of medications.

Box 12.5: Comparison of delirium and dementia

Feature	Delirium	Dementia
Onset	Acute	Insidious, progressive
Course	Reversible; usually recover in 1 week may take up to one month	Irreversible
Clinical features	Disorientation, bewilderment, anxiety, poor attention, clouding of consciousness.	Clear consciousness
	Perceptual abnormalities (illusions, hallucinations)	Global impairment of cerebral functions (e.g., recent memory, intellectual impairment and personality deterioration with secondary behavior abnormalities)
	Paranoid ideas/delusions	Hallucinations may occur
	Fluctuating course with lucid intervals	Progressive course

- Anxiety can be treated with low doses of benzodiazepines (lorazepam and oxazepam).
- For depression mild doses of SSRI's such as citalopram or sertraline can be administered.
- Psychotic symptoms can be treated with low doses of antipsychotics such as haloperidol and risperidone. It should be avoided in Lewy body type.

NURSING MANAGEMENT

Assessment

Nursing assessment of the client with organic brain disorder is based on knowledge of the symptomatology associated with the various disorders. Nurses play a significant role in acquiring the client history. From the client history, nurses should assess the following:

- Type, frequency, and severity of mood swings, personality and behavioral changes
- Cognitive changes, such as problems with attention span, thinking process, problem-solving, and memory
- Language difficulties
- Disorientation
- Appropriateness of social behavior.

The nurse also should obtain information regarding current and past medication usage, history of other drug and alcohol use, and possible exposure to toxins.

Assessment of physical systems should emphases:

- Signs of damage to the nervous system
- Evidence of diseases of other organs that could affect mental function.

Nursing Diagnosis

Appropriate nursing diagnoses are drawn from client's data base. The possible nursing diagnoses are:

- Risk for trauma related to impairments in cognitive and psychomotor functioning.
- Risk for other-directed violence related to impairment of impulse control; hallucinations.
- Disturbed thought processes related to cerebral degeneration evidenced by disorientation, confusion, memory deficits, and inaccurate interpretation of the environment.
- Low self-esteem related to loss of independent functioning evidenced by expressions of shame and self-degradation and progressive social isolation.
- Self-care deficit related to disorientation, confusion, memory deficits evidenced by inability to fulfill activites of daliy living (ADLs).

Planning

The nursing care for organic mental disorders is given in **box.** The selected nursing diagnoses with outcome identification and intervention are given in the box 12.6.

Evaluation

In the final step of the nursing process, reassessment occurs to determine if the nursing interventions have been effective in achieving the intended goals of care. Evaluation of the client with cognitive disorders is based on a series of short-term rather than on long-term goals.

Resolution of identified problems is unrealistic for this client. Instead, outcomes must be measured in terms of slowing down the process rather than stopping or curing the problem.

Box 12.6: Nursing process for organic brain disorders

Nursing diagnosis: Risk for trauma related to impairments in cognitive and psychomotor functioning.

Outcome identification	Nursing intervention
Client will not experience injury.	• Arrange furniture and other items in the room to accommodate client's disabilities • Store frequently used items within easy access • Do not keep bed in an elevated position. Pad side rails and head board if client has history of seizures • Assign room near nurses' station; observe frequently • Assist client with ambulation • Keep a dim light on at night • Frequently orient client to place, time, and situation • If client is prone to wander, provide an area within which wandering can be carried out safely • Soft restraints may be required if client is very disoriented and hyperactive

Nursing diagnosis: Disturbed thought processes related to cerebral degeneration evidenced by disorientation, confusion, memory deficits, and inaccurate interpretation of the environment.

Outcome identification	Nursing intervention
Client will interpret the environment accurately and maintain reality orientation to the best of his or her cognitive ability.	• Frequently orient client to reality • Use clocks and calendars with large numbers that are easy to read. Notes and large, bold signs may be useful as reminders • Allow client to have personal belongings • Keep explanations simple • Use face-to-face interaction and speak slowly and do not shout • Discourage rumination of delusional thinking. Talk about real events and real people • Monitor for medication side effects

Nursing diagnosis: Self-care deficit related to disorientation, confusion, memory deficits evidenced by inability to fulfill ADLs

Outcome identification	Nursing intervention
Client will accomplish ADLs to the best of his or her ability. Unfulfilled needs will be met by caregivers.	• Provide a simple, structured environment: – Identify self-care deficits and provide assistance as required – Allow plenty of time for client to perform tasks – Provide guidance and support for independent actions by talking the client through the task one step at a time – Provide a structured schedule of activities that does not change from day-to-day – ADLs should follow usual routine as closely as possible • Perform ongoing assessment of client's ability to fulfill nutritional needs, ensure personal safety, follow medication regimen, and communicate need for assistance with activities that he or she cannot accomplish independently • Assess prospective caregivers' ability to anticipate and fulfill client's unmet needs

Contd...

Contd...

Outcome identification	Nursing intervention
	• Provide information to assist caregivers with this responsibility • Ensure that caregivers are aware of available community support systems from which they may seek assistance when required. Examples include adult day care centers, housekeeping and homemaker services, local or national support organization, etc.

Client and Family Education

Educate the family members regarding the following aspects:

- Nature of the illness
  - Possible causes
  - Symptoms
- Management of the illness
  - Client safety and nutrition
  - How to maintain reality orientation
  - Providing assistance with ADLs
  - Difficult behaviors
  - Medications
- Support services
  - Caregiver support groups
  - Home health care
  - National and international organizations like Alzheimer's society, etc.

ORGANIC AMNESTIC SYNDROME

Amnesic (or *amnestic*) syndrome completes the triad of conditions (with dementia and delirium) which affect memory and which always have an organic cause. Its features are

- Selective loss of recent memory.
- Confabulation: The unconscious fabrication of recent events to cover gaps in memory.
- Time disorientation.
- Attention and immediate recall intact.
- Long-term memory and other intellectual faculties intact

Amnesic syndrome is rare, and in practice difficult to distinguish from some dementias.

Etiology

- It is due to damage to the mammillary bodies, hippocampus or thalamus
- The usual cause is alcohol induced thiamine deficiency (*Korsakoff's syndrome*), which is treated with thiamine and abstinence
- Herpes simplex encephalitis
- Severe hypoxia
- Head injury
- Surgical procedures (e.g. bilateral temporal lobectomy)
- Neoplasms in brain.

Clinical Features

Two types of amnesia may occur.

1. ***Retrograde amnesia:*** Pathological inability to recall events that occurred prior to the onset of the illness.
2. ***Anterograde amnesia:*** Pathological inability to lay down new memories after the onset of the illness.

The features includes:

- Impairment of memory is characterized by a severe impairment of recent memory (short term memory).
- This is associated with impaired remote memory (long-term memory).
- Confabulation is common and with the progression of the disease it often disappears.

Management

- Treatment of the underlying causes (like thiamine deficiency)
- Usually treatment doesn't help in reducing the disease but the further complications can be prevented
- Supportive therapy and treatment of the associated medical illnesses.

OTHER ORGANIC MENTAL DISORDERS (DUE TO BRAIN DAMAGE AND DYSFUNCTION, DUE TO PHYSICAL DISEASE)

This group of disorders are related to brain dysfunction due to primary cerebral disease, systemic disease (secondary) or toxic substances. The common clinical conditions in this group includes epilepsy, limbic encephalitis, Huntington's disease, head injury.

Brain neoplasms, vascular cerebral disease, cerebral malformations, collagen diseases (e.g. Systemic lupns erythematosus (SLE)), hyper and hypothyroidism, metabolic disorders.

Drugs like steroids, propranolol, levodopa, methyldopa, alcohol and other psycho active substances are also comes in this group.

Organic Hallucinosis

Organic hallucinosis is defined as being a disorder of persistent or recurrent hallucinations, in any modality but usually visual or auditory, which occurs in clear consciousness without any significant intellectual decline.

Delusional elaboration of the hallucinations may occur, but often insight is preserved. Usually the patients realize that the hallucinations are not real.

Box 12.7: Causes of organic hallucinosis

S. No.	Cause	Example
1	Psychoactive substance use	Alcohol abuse (alcoholic hallucinosis), amphetamines, cocaine, LSD Flashback phenomena—following the use of hallucinogens
2	Intoxication	Drugs – amantadine, bromocriptine, ephedrine, levodopa, etc.
3	Intracranial	Brain tumors, head Injury, migraine, infections, e.g. neurosyphilis Epilepsy—particularly temporal lobe epilepsy
4	Sensory deprivation	Deafness, poor vision, torture (in prisoners of war)
	Endocrine	Hypothyroidism—'myxoedematous madness'

Organic Catatonia

ICD-10 defines organic catatonic disorder as a disorder of diminished (stupor) or increased (excitement) psychomotor activity associated with catatonic symptoms; the extremes of psychomotor disturbance may alternate.

The stuporous symptoms may include complete mutism, negativism and rigid posturing. Excitement manifests as gross hypermotility. Other catatonic symptoms that may occur include stereotypes and waxy flexibility.

The most important causes are encephalitis and carbon monoxide poisoning. Treatment of the underlying cause and symptomatic treatment with low dose of short acting benzodiazepines, or Electro convulsive therapy (ECT) if needed can be given.

Organic Delusional (Schizophrenia Like) Disorder

Organic delusional or schizophrenia like disorder is defined as persistent or recurrent delusions, with or without hallucinations.

The delusions are most often persecutory type, but grandiose delusions or delusions of bodily change, jealousy, disease or death may occur. Memory and consciousness are not affected.

The most common cause is psychoactive substance use, particularly amphetamine and related substances, cocaine and hallucinogens.

Intracranial causes, such as tumors and epilepsy, Huntington's disease.

Symptomatic treatment can be done and low dose of an antipsychotic medication such as Risperidone, haloperidol, Olanzapine can be administered.

Organic Mood Disorders

Organic mood disorder is characterized by a change in mood (depressive or hypomanic), usually accompanied by a change in the overall level of activity, which is caused by organic pathology.

The causes of organic mood disorders include psychoactive substances, medications (such as corticosteroids, levodopa, cycloserine) endocrine factors, intracranial, systemic disorders like hepatic failure, renal failure, etc.

Organic Anxiety Disorder

Organic anxiety disorder is characterized by the features of generalized anxiety disorder and/or panic disorder caused by organic pathology.

The symptoms include tremor, paresthesia, choking, palpitations, chest pain, dry mouth, nausea, abdominal pain ('butterflies'), loose motions and increased frequency of micturition.

There may be secondary cognitive impairment, for example poor concentration. The causes of this condition are manifold. The most important conditions to exclude in clinical practice are hyperthyroidism, pheochromocytoma and hypoglycemia.

Organic Personality Disorder

Organic personality disorder is characterized by a significant alteration in the premorbid personality. Such alteration always involves more profoundly the expression of emotions, needs and impulses. Cognition may be defective, mostly or exclusively in the areas of planning actions and anticipating their likely consequences.

The most common cause is head injury. Other intracranial causes include brain tumors, brain abscesses, subarachnoid hemorrhage, neurosyphilis and epilepsy, particularly when the frontal or temporal lobes are involved. For example, temporal lobe epilepsy may result in aggressive behavior, hyposexuality or hypersexuality. Other causes of organic personality disorder include Huntington's disease, Wilson's disease, and medication such as corticosteroids, psychoactive substance use and endocrinopathies.

Miscellaneous Organic Mental Dsiorders

Other organic mental disorders include organic dissociative disorder, organic emotionally liable disorder and mild cognitive disorder.

13 Psychiatric Emergencies and Crisis Intervention

INTRODUCTION

A psychiatric emergency is an acute disturbance of behavior, thought or mood of a patient which if untreated may lead to harm, either to the individual or to others in the environment. So, time is one of essence in a psychiatric emergency.

In other terms, psychiatric emergency is the clinical application of psychiatry in emergency settings. Conditions requiring psychiatric interventions may include attempted suicide, substance abuse, depression, psychosis, violence and other rapid changes in behavior. Psychiatric emergency services are rendered by professionals in the field of medicine, nursing, psychology and social work.

Individuals may arrive in psychiatric emergency services settings through their own voluntary request, a referral from another health professional, or through involuntary commitment.

Definition of Psychiatric Emergency

It is defined as a disturbance in one own thought, mood and action which causes sudden distress to the individual himself or others and sudden disability which requires immediate management.

Key Words

Reason for psychiatric emergency:

- Mental illness
- Substance abuse
- Medical conditions like:
  - Low blood sugar related to diabetes
  - Hypoxia
  - Traumatic brain injury
  - Reduced blood flow to brain
- Central nervous system (CNS) infection such as meningitis.

ASSESSMENT REQUIRED IN PSYCHIATRIC EMERGENCY

Immediate Assessment

Assessment of the condition and the dangerous of the patient's behaviors like loud, agitated angry and threatening behavior.

Note How the Patient Brought Casualty

Tied, handcuffed or restrained requires cautious assessment despite calm or withdrawal behavior.

Reports About Behavior

The reports of dangerousness or violent behaviors from the informants must be thoroughly investigated.

Patient's History

Chief complaints—onset with progression.
Any precipitant—economical loss, marital disharmony, drugs, physical illness, etc.
Previous psychiatric illness.
Medical history (drugs, alcoholic).
Family history of psychiatric illness.

Physical Examination

It should be through with particular emphasis on drug intoxication, withdrawal symptoms and acute or chronic.

Laboratory Tests

These are selected on the basis of the findings of examination and the differerential diagnosis.

Psychiatric Emergencies May Occur

A. In hospitals:
- Emergency departments
- Medical or surgical units
- Psychiatric wards or clinics
- Others.

B. Outside hospitals:
- Homes
- Streets
- Markets
- Others.

Types of Psychiatric Emergency

- Suicide and parasuicide
- Voilent or agressive behavior or excitement
- Stupor
- Panic attack
- Delirium tremens
- Withdrawl symptoms of drug dependence
- Alcohol or drug overdose
- Epilepsy or status epileptics
- Hysterical attack.

SUICIDE OR DELIBERATE SELF-HARM AND PARASUICIDE

Definition

'Suicide is the act of deliberately killing oneself'.

—World Health Organization (WHO)

'Suicide is a type of deliberate self-harm and is defined as an intentional human act of killing oneself.

—Kaplan, 2006

Classification of Suicide

Durkheim described three different social categories:

1. **Egoistic:** Due to loss of integration, leads to a sense of isolation and morbid individualism.
2. **Altruistic:** As seen in war, army men dying for the country.
3. **Anomic:** When there is disturbances in the balance of the individual's aspiration on the hand and the values of society on the other.

Epidemiology

- In India, 150–200 people commit suicide everyday.
- Suicide rate in India was 11.2 per 100,000 in 2002. The rates vary across the country with states such as Kerala having the highest suicide rate.
- Rates are higher in urban than in rural settings. Studies of completed suicides show that 90–94% of the patients are mentally ill while committing the act. Depression accounts for nearly half the number of patients committing suicide followed by alcohol abuse (34%) and schizophrenia (13%). (Maithry, 2007)
- Women attempt suicide more times than men, but what interesting is men are successful in committing suicide compared to women.

Etiology

- **Genetic:** Genetic abnormalities in the serotonergic neurotransmitter system may be responsible for the heightened familial risk for suicide (Mann, Brent, and Arango, 2001). 18 % evident in monozygotic twins.
- **Physiologic stress responsiveness:** Excessive stress causes neurochemical changes directly contribute to suicidal behavior.
- **Mental illness:** Depression, alcoholism, drug abuse, schizophrenia, personality disorders, etc.
- **Physical illness:** Chronic medical illness, epileptics the risk is four times more.
- **Psychological mechanisms:** Suicide is a displaced form of autoplastic aggression by a dependent or helpless person.
- **Neurotransmitter depletion:** Those who complete suicide have extremely low levels of the neurotransmitter serotonin, or 5-hydroxytryptamine (5-HT).

Risk Factors

- **Sex:** Men commit suicide more than four times as often as women.
- **Age:** Suicide rates increase with age among men. Suicides peak after the age of 45; among women, the greatest number of completed suicides occurs after age 55. The suicide rate, however, is rising most rapidly among young persons, particularly males 15–24 year old.
- **Occupation:** The higher a person's social status, die of suicide, but a fall in social status also increases the risk.
- **Depression:** About 25 times more than normal individual.

Other Risk Factors

- Previous history of suicidal attempt.
- No spouse, widowed, divorced, separated.
- Social isolation.

Common methods of committing suicide:

- Hanging
- Shooting
- Rushing in front of running vehicles
- Jumping from high places
- Burning
- Poisoning.

Management of Suicidal Patient

Assessing Suicidal Risk

Assess for following:

- **Seriousness of suicidal attempt:** The more lethal attempt, the greater suicide risk. For example, a patient who cuts his wrist or attempts to hang or shoot himself has more severe suicide risk than that someone who has taken an overdose of 10 aspirin tablets.
- **Evaluation of intentions:** Asking about suicidal intentions is very important. It will not make suicidal more likely.

  Systemic enquires about:
  - Thoughts life is worth living
  - Wishes to die
  - Suicidal ideation
  - Suicidal intent
  - Suicidal specific preparatory acts (e.g. planning with precautions against discovery)
  - Actual suicidal trial.
- **Family and personal history:** If the patient has a past history of suicide attempts, or a family history of suicide attempts, the risk of suicide increases.

- **History of intentional self-harm:**
  - Serious deliberate self-harm
  - Repeated dangerous attempts
  - Continuing wish to kill or harm self
  - Writing a farewell suicidal note.
- **Presence of mental disorders:**
  - Severe depression with guilt feelings hopelessness and helplessness. Depressed patient may not be able to plan and commit suicide while severely depressed. However, it was found that suicide may occur during recovery from severe depression.
  - Schizophrenia (on recovery from acute phase or in chronic—schizophrenic illness).
  - Substance abuse with psychiatric and physical complications.
  - Personality disorders (e.g. borderline personality disorder; these patients have poor impulse control and chronic emotional instability).
- **Presence of adverse social and medical conditions:**
  - Social factors (e.g. home, work, finances, etc.) need to be assessed.
  - Medical problems (especially if they are painful disabling or rapidly deteriorating in spite of medical interventions).
- **Presence of homicidal ideation:** To kill a spouse, children or parents, in order to spare them intolerable suffering after committing suicide (some severely depressed suicidal patients have homicidal ideas).

Interviewing the Patient: Guidelines

- Show willingness to talk and show interest
- Make an introductory statement followed by specific statement
- Ask about onset, duration and lethality and furtherance of plans
- Should be interviewed alone as long as their capability
- Get the consent of the patient for interviewing the family members
- Identifying associated symptoms like hopelessness that appears to be necessary for development of suicidal intent – by mental health examination (MSE) and history
- Identify the risk factors associated with suicide.

Box 13.1: Kubler-Ross's statges of grief

Extent of suicidal ideation	Plans for furtherance and lethality
• When you begin to have the thoughts? • Event precipitating? • How often? Do you feel life isn't worth? • What makes you feel better? • What makes you feel worse? • Any plan to end life? • How much control do you have? • What stops you from killing yourself?	• Do you have any access? • Have you imagined your funeral? • Have you 'practiced'? • Have you changed your will or life insurance policy or given away your possessions?

C) Management of Suicidal Ideation Patient

Flowchart 13.1: Management of suicidal ideation

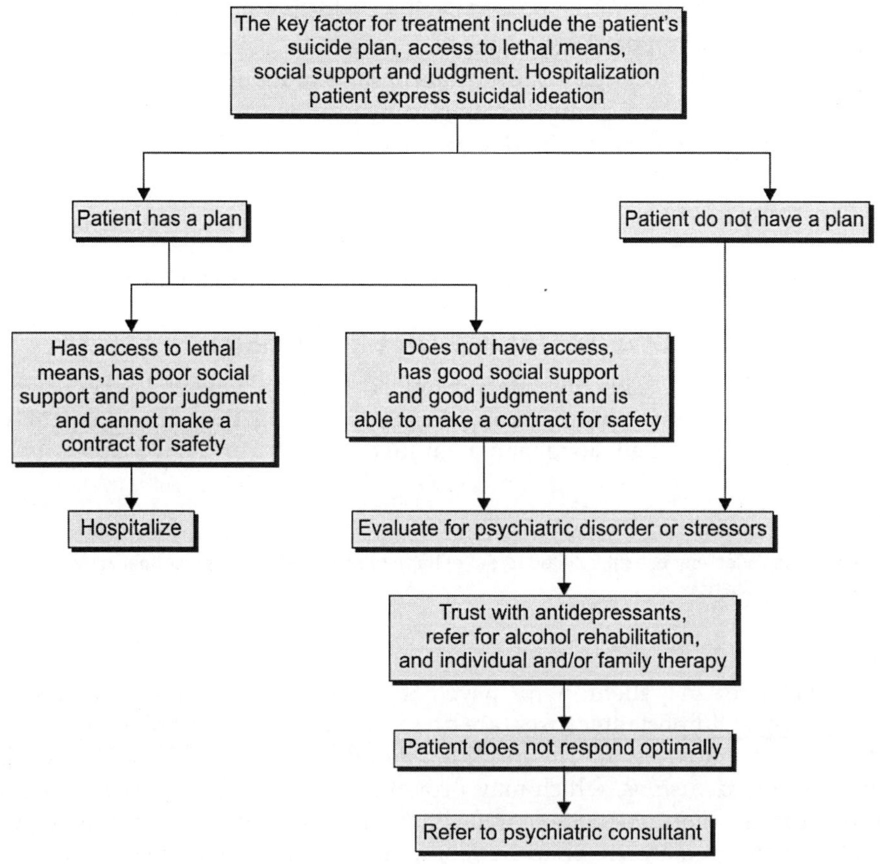

Precautions

- If the patient is admitted, the following steps are to be followed.
- Continuous observation of patient (even he is going to bathroom).
- Place hospital gown without ties, belts, shoe laces, sharp instruments, stockings, etc.
- Sedated the agitated patient and place the restraints if necessary.
- Evaluate precautions regularly.

Nursing Interventions

- Has one to one relationship
- Have staff member with the patient all the time
- Assess suicidal risks daily
- Ask the suicide plan
- Explain suicide precautions

- Remove all sharp objects and potentially dangerous items from patient's possession
- Keep the window locked, so that the patient cannot open
- Stay with the client when he or she is meeting the personal hygiene
- Be alert to the possibility of the patient saving up his/her medications
- Observe record and report if any changes
- Talk about his or her feelings, relationships or life situation
- Be alert about decreased communication, conversations about death, low frustration tolerance and dissatisfaction with dependency
- Do not joke about death
- Refer to spiritual source
- Encourage and support the client's expression of anger/emotions
- Teach problem solving approach, social skills, and self-care activities.

VIOLENT OR AGRESSIVE BEHAVIOR OR EXCITEMENT

Violent is physical aggression by one person on another, violent is most commonly associated with psychotic features, and disorders. During this stage, patient will be irrational, uncooperative, delusional and assaultive.

Definition

Violent behavior includes any patient initiated threat of harm to self, health care personnel, or others in the patient's sphere of influence.

Causes

Aggressive behavior in patients with psychiatric disorders has many possible causes. Probably the most important causes are the presence of comorbid substance abuse, dependence, and intoxication. In addition, the disease process itself may produce hallucinations and delusions, which may provoke violence. Often, poor impulse control related to neuropsychiatric deficits may facilitate the discharge of aggressive tendencies. Finally, underlying personality characteristics, such as antisocial personality traits, also may influence the use of violent acts as a means to achieve certain goals.

Environmental factors that are associated with aggressive behavior include a chaotic or unstable home or hospital situation, which may encourage maladaptive aggressive behaviors. Individuals may become aggressive for different reasons at different times.

Biological Factors

- Neurotransmitter—lower 5HT1
- Limbic system—partial complex seizures
- Chromosomal abnormalities—XXY.

Endocrine

- Increased androgens—males
- Premenstrual syndrome—females
- Alcohol and drug—it decreased the control impulse and impairs judgment.

Psychosocial Features

- Development—child abuse
- Accessibility—easy accessibility to guns
- Poverty, unemployment.

Box 13.2: Engel's stages of grief

- Schizophrenia especially paranoid
- Mania
- Paranoid psychosis
- Personality disorder especially antisocial type
- Alcohol intoxication or withdrawal
- Substance intoxication with cocaine, amphetamines, anabolic steroids, phencyclidine
- Substance withdrawal
- Post-traumatic stress disorder
- Dementia.

Box 13.3: Martocchio's clusters of grief

- Scars or wounds on the face, arms, or torso suggesting past violent altercations.
- Jailhouse tattoos (e.g. primitive figures, crosses, 'LOVE' printed across the knuckles).
- Abnormal pupil size (either increased or decreased), suggesting substance intoxication or withdrawal.
- Speech that is threatening, loud, or profane.
- Increased muscle tension, such as sitting on the edge of the chair or gripping the arms.
- Tremor.
- Hyperactivity, such as pacing.
- Slamming doors or knocking over furniture.

Management

An excited patient is usually brought tied up with a rope or in chains. The first step should be to remove the chains. A large proportion of aggression and violence is due to the patient feeling humiliated at being tied up in this manner.

Initial Management

Talk: Talk to the patient and see if he responds. Firm and kind approach by the nurse is essential.

Food: If talking does not defuse the situation, and then offer the patient, sometimes to eat or drink. Food may have a calming effect on the patient's anxiety and tension.

Medication:

- Chlorpromazine, 50–150 mg (IM).
- Haloperidol, 5–10 mg (Single IM/IV dose).
- To sedate the patient—diazepam, 10–40 mg (IV slowly).
- Other drugs—carbamazepine, phenytoin.

Physical restraints: Call for need of physical restrain—an agitated patient, cannot establish rapport, who not complies with the request to take medications.

Nursing Management

- Keep environmental stimuli, such as lighting and noise levels to a minimum, assign a single room, limit interactions with others.
- Remove hazardous objects and substances; caution the patient when there is possibility of an accident.
  - Stay with the patient as hyperactivity increases to reduce anxiety levels and foster a feeling of security.
  - Following application of restraints, observe patient every 15 minute to ensure that nutritional and elimination needs are met.

Box 13.4: Sander's phases of bereavement

- Never see a potentially violent person alone.
- Keep a comfortable distance away from the patient (arm length).
- Be prepared to move, a violent patient can strike out suddenly.
- Maintain a clear exit route for both the staff and patient.
- Give prescribed antipsychotic medications.

STUPOR AND CATATONIC STUPOR

Definition

- Stupor is defined as a state of diminished consciousness in which the patient remains mute and still although the eyes remain open and may follow external objects. *(A state of reduced sensibility or consciousness).*
- 'Catatonic stupor is a marked decrease in response to the environment with reduction in spontaneous movement characterized by negativism, catalepsy mutism, verbigeration, echolalia, echopraxia and excitement.'

Causes

- Functional psychiatric disorder
- Affective illness
- Neurological disorders
- Basal ganglia—Parkinsonism
- Limbic system—viral encephalitis
- Diencephalon—tumors
- Brain lesions
- Metabolic disorders
- Toxic agents.

Management

- Maintaining the hydration
- Check the vital signs every one hour
- Keep airway patency
- Provide ventilate support if necessary
- Taking care of skin, nutrition, elimination and personal hygiene is required.

PANIC ATTACKS

Episodes of acute anxiety and panic can occur as a part of psychotic or neurotic illness.

The patient will experience palpitations, sweating, tremors, and feelings of choking, chest pain, nausea, abdominal distress, and fear of dying, paresthesia, chills or hot flashes.

Management

Emergency

- Give reassurance first
- Restraint the patient if it is needed
- Diazepam 10 mg or lorazepam 2 mg may be administered as prescribed.

Physical

- Search for causes
- Monitor vital signs
- Provide comfortable position
- Respiratory support should be given if the patient is in choking or chest pain.

Psychological

- Assess patient's anxiety level
- Teach the patient for coping skill and problem-solving technique
- Encourage the patient to ventilate his or her feelings
- Be supportive to the patient
- Remove all the sharp weapons.

(***Refer Chapter 8 for more details about panic attack***)

DELIRIUM TREMENS

It is a severe form of alcohol withdrawal. It involves sudden and severe mental or nervous system changes.

Causes

- It can occur when person stop drinking alcohol after a period of heavy drinking, especially when enough food is not taken.
- It may also be caused by head injury, infection, or illness in people with a history of heavy alcohol use.
- It is especially common in those who drink 4–5 pints of wine, 7–8 pints of beer, or 1 pint of 'hard' alcohol every day for several months.

Symptoms

Symptoms most often occur within 48–96 hours after the last drink. But, they can occur 7–10 days after the last drink. Symptoms may get worse quickly, and can include:

- Body tremors
- Agitation, irritability

- Confusion, disorientation
- Decreased attention span
- Delirium
- Fear
- Hallucinations (seeing or feeling things that are not really there)
- Quick mood changes
- Restlessness, excitement
- Sensitivity to light, sound, touch
- Stupor, sleepiness, fatigue.

Treatment

The goals of treatment are to:

- Save the person's life
- Relieve symptoms
- Prevent complications.

A hospital stay is needed. The health care team will regularly check and treat:

- Blood chemistry results, such as electrolyte level
- Vital signs (temperature, pulse, breathing rate, blood pressure)
- To stay calm and relaxed (sedate the patient) until the delirium tremens (DTs) are finished.

Outlook (Prognosis)

Delirium tremens is serious and may be life-threatening. Some symptoms related to alcohol withdrawal may last for a year or more, including emotional mood swings, feeling tired, sleeplessness.

Possible Complications

- Injury from falls during seizures
- Injury to self or others caused by mental state (confusion/delirium)
- Irregular heartbeat, may be life-threatening
- Seizures.

Nursing Management

- Keep patient in quiet and safe environment
- Sedative with injection diazepam 10 mg IV
- Maintain fluid-balance
- Maintain nutritional balance
- Reassure patient and family.

WITHDRAWAL SYMPTOMS OR DRUG DEPENDENCE

If a person becomes physically dependent on a substance, substance abuse may continue simply to avoid withdrawal symptoms.

If heavy drinking occurs over a long time, a decrease in blood alcohol level may cause symptoms of withdrawal.

Most abused drug interacts with specific nerve cell receptors, either imitating or blocking the actions of normally working neurotransmitters in the brain.

Nursing Management

- Keep the patient in quiet and safe environment
- Avoid arguments and long explanations
- Maintain calm and firm approach
- Give injection diazepam 10 mg IM/IV, tablet clonidine 1 mg.

ALCOHOL OR DRUG OVERDOSE

An alcohol overdose, or alcohol poisoning, is a psychiatric emergency that can result from too much of alcohol consumption at one time.

Definition

Alcohol poisoning is a serious and sometimes deadly consequence of drinking large amounts of alcohol in a short period of time. Drinking too much too quickly can affect your breathing heart rate, body temperature and gag reflex and potentially lead to coma and death.

Signs and Symptoms

- Changes in mental state, including confusion
- Vomiting
- Pale or blue skin
- A decrease in body temperature (hypothermia)
- Passing out (unconsciousness).

Alcohol depresses nervous system, and causes serious complications if person drink at a rate that is much faster than liver can process the alcohol. These include:

- Slowing or stopping breathing, heart rate, and gag reflex, all of which are controlled by nervous system.
- Cardiac arrest following a decrease in body temperature (hypothermia).
- Seizures as a result of low blood sugar levels.

(If any one of the above symptoms appears, the patient should be immediately transferred to emergency department).

Management

Alcohol poisoning treatment usually involves supportive care. This typically includes:

- Careful monitoring
- Prevention of breathing or choking problems
- Oxygen therapy
- Fluids given through a vein (intravenously) to prevent dehydration
- Use of vitamins and glucose to help prevent serious complications of alcohol poisoning.

Drug Overdose

Drug overdoses can be accidental or intentional. They occur when a person takes more than the medically recommended dose.

Signs and Symptoms

- Severe alteration in vital signs and can be life-threatening.
- Sleepiness, confusion, and coma can be dangerous if the person breathes vomit into the lungs (aspirated).
- Skin can be cool and sweaty, or hot and dry.
- Chest pain, shortness of breath.
- Abdominal pain, nausea, vomiting, and diarrhea are possible.
- Vomiting blood, or blood in bowel movements, can be life-threatening.
- Specific drugs can damage specific organs, depending on the drug.

Drug Overdose Treatment

Treatment will be dictated by the specific drug taken in the overdose. Information provided about amount, time and underlying medical problems will be very helpful.

- The stomach may be washed out by gastric lavage (stomach pumping) to mechanically remove unabsorbed drugs from the stomach.
- Activated charcoal may be given to help bind drugs and keep them in the stomach and intestines. This reduces the amount absorbed into the blood. The drug, bound to the charcoal, is then expelled in the stool.
- Agitated or violent people need physical restraint and sometimes sedating medications in the emergency department until the effects of the drugs wear off.
- For certain overdoses, other medicine is given to serve as an antidote to reverse the effects of what was taken.

STATUS EPILEPTICS (SE)

A dangerous condition in which epileptic fits follow one another without recovery of consciousness between them. (*Status epilepticus* is usually defined as 30 minutes of uninterrupted seizure activity).

Death or brain damage from status seizures (as opposed to death from the underlying cause) is most likely to result from:

- Direct damage to the brain caused by the injury that causes the seizures
- Stress on the system from repeated generalized tonic-clonic seizures
- Injury from repeated electrical discharge in the brain.

Management

Box 13.5: Treatment guidelines

American Epilepsy Society (AES) in 2016 issued new guidelines to provide a time-dependent treatment for SE which includes 4 phases.

1. In the stabilization phase, standard first-aid for seizures should be initiated.
2. In the initial therapy phase, a benzodiazepine (specifically IM midazolam, IV lorazepam or IV diazepam) is recommended as initial therapy.
3. In the second phase options include IV fosphenytoin, valproic acid or levetiracetam. If none of these is available IV phenobarbital is a reasonable alternative.
4. In the third phase, if a patient experiences 40+ minutes of seizure activity treatment considerations should include repeating second-line therapy or anesthetic doses of thiopental, midazolam, or pentobarbital.

Emergency Management

Goals: (Aggressive supportive care and prompt termination of electrical seizure activity are the goals).

- Provide a comfortable environment
- Remove the injured objects
- Maintain airway, remove the secretions
- Provide oxygen if necessary
- Establish IV access, ideally in a large vein
- Begin cardiac and other hemodynamic monitoring
- Administer a 50 mL bolus of 50% dextrose IV and 100 mg of thiamine
- If seizure activity does not terminate within 4–5 minutes, start anticonvulsant medication
- In some settings where drug intoxication might be likely, consider also adding naloxone at 0.4–2.0 mg IV to the dextrose bag
- Administer diazepam (0.15 mg/kg) or lorazepam (0.1 mg/kg) IV over 5 minutes, followed by phenytoin. The dose of phenytoin is 18–20 mg/kg, at a rate not to exceed 50 mg/min)
- Ensure airway control
- Correct any metabolic imbalances
- Control hyperthermia.

HYSTERICAL ATTACK

A hysteric may mimic abnormality of any function, which is under voluntary control. The common modes of presentation may be:

- Hysterical fits
- Hysterical ataxia
- Hysterical paraplegia.

(All presentations are marked by a dramatic quality and sadness of mood).

Box 13.6: Difference between epileptic fits and hysterical fit

Epileptic fit: (Characteristic features)	Hysteric or dissociative fit: (Characteristic features)
• It is spontaneous and has sudden onset. • Patient falls down abruptly and may get injury. • He becomes abruptly pale till cyanosis. • Reaction at external stimuli, reflex, and pain sensation are absent. • There can be urinary incontinence and tongue biting during a fit (tonic and clonic). • Facial expression is absent. • Stereotype recurrent characteristic of the fit is noticed.	• It occurs after a psychotrauma. • The patient falls not suddenly, sometimes even slowly not to get hurt. • To be remembered the patient during falling looks downwards. • Any type of convulsive reaction in the face is absent. • Urinary incontinence and tongue biting during a fit is absent. • Joint and pupil reflexes are secured. • Convulsion is atypical (gesticulation, sweeping, tremor, twitching, etc.) • Facial expression is present (suffering, fear, happiness, etc.) • Fits are not similar to each other. Rather fit changes according to situations and circumstances.

Contd...

Contd...

Epileptic fit: (Characteristic features)	Hysteric or dissociative fit: (Characteristic features)
• Duration of the fit is 30 sec to 2 min, total amnesia is followed.	• Duration of the fit is long in order to get more attention (from few minutes to few hours). • There can be partial amnesia. With the help of hypnosis, memory can be brought back.

Management

Emergency

- Reassure the patient
- Administration of mild sedatives
- Suggestion therapy with IV Pentothal.

Physical

- Take a history of physical complaints
- Organic pathology should be clearly ruled out
- Fulfil clients for most urgent dependency needs
- Assess client's level of knowledge regarding effects of psychological problems on the body
- Discus results of laboratory tests and physical examination with client.

Psychological

- Assess client's level of anxiety
- Identify stressors that cause anxiety level to rise
- Demonstrate adaptive coping strategies
- Verbalizes understanding of correlation between times of increased anxiety and onset of physical symptoms
- Counseling by an understanding professional.

NEUROLEPTIC MALIGNANT SYNDROME

It is a hyper-metabolic reaction to dopamine antagonists, primarily antipsychotic drugs, such as phenol-thiazines and butyrophenones. It usually occurs early in treatment and rarely during maintenance treatment.

(Its pathophysiologic basis which is believed to be blockade of central dopamine receptors).

Clinical Features

- Muscle rigidity, hyperpyrexia
- Tachycardia, hypertension, tachypnea
- Change in mental status and autonomic dysfunction.

Laboratory abnormalities include:

- Respiratory and metabolic acidosis
- Myoglobinuria
- Elevated creatine kinase (CK) and leukocytosis.

Mortality rates are between 10 and 20%.

Treatment

- Cessation of antipsychotic drugs
- Supportive care and aggressive treatment of myoglobinuria, fever, and acidosis
- The dopamine agonist bromocriptine 2.5–20 mg tid or dantrolene up to 10 mg/kg IV may be used as a muscle relaxant
- Treatment is usually in an intensive care unit (ICU).

STRESS AND STRESSOR: STRESS ADAPTATION MODEL, COPING RESOURCES AND MECHANISM

Introduction

Stress is a universal experience. Modern life is full of frustrations, deadlines, and demands. Stress is a person environment interaction. Right from the time of birth till the last breath drawn, an individual is invariably exposed to various stressful situations. The modern world, which is said to be a world of achievements is also world of stress and called as **'age of anxiety and stress'.**

Stress is not always bad, because stress with in comfort zone will motivate to achieve things in life and even keep safe when danger looms. But when stress becomes overwhelming, it can damage individual's health, mood, relationships, and quality of life.

Basic Concepts of Stress

- When person feel threatened, the nervous system responds by releasing a flood of stress hormones, including adrenaline and cortisol, which rouse the body for emergency action to focus on forecoming danger.
- This is known as the 'fight or flight' stress response to protect the body. When working properly, stress helps you to stay focused, energetic, and alert. In emergency situations, stress can save your life. For example, sudden response to slam on the brakes to avoid an accident.
- Stress reactions are purposeful and initially protective.
- Stress, on positive side helps to maintain equilibrium, to increase motivation, learning, creativity, development, productivity, and satisfaction.
- On negative side, stress is noxious or unpleasant.
- Complete freedom from stress is death or a nonexistent state.

Definitions of Stress

In simple—stress is a body's response to any kind of demand or threat.

'Stress is a physical or emotional state always present in the person as a result of living. It is intensified in a non-specific response to an internal and external environmental change or threat.'

—Ruth, Murrey, Bectmen

'Stress is a condition in which human system responds to changes in its normal balanced state.'

—Taylor Lemone, 1989

Types of Stress

- **Eustress:** The optimal amount of stress, which helps to promote health and growth. For example, praise from a teacher for a well-written assignment. (Eustress is pleasant and desirable).
- **Neutral stress**: Here, the subject neither feels good nor bad about the stress. Equilibrium or homeostasis is maintained.
- **Distress:** Stress due to an excess of adaptive demands placed upon us. The demands are so great that they lead to bodily and mental damage. For example, UN expected death of a loved person. (Distress is unpleasant, objectionable).

Box 13.7: Stress and stressor

What is stress?	What is stressor?
Stress is defined as 'any process, either in the external environment or within an individual that demands a response from the individual'. Engel, 1962	A factor which promotes the stressful reaction is called a stressor. E.g: Biological, psychological, social or chemical factor that causes physical or emotional tension.

Box 13.8: Causes of stress

Common external causes of stress	Common internal causes of stress
• Major life changes	• Chronic worry
• Work or school	• Pessimism
• Relationship difficulties	• Negative self-talk
• Financial problems	• Unrealistic expectations/perfectionism
• Being too busy	• Rigid thinking, lack of flexibility
• Children and family.	• All-or-nothing attitude.

Following box lists common symptoms of stress. The more symptoms in person indicate more closure to stress overload.

Box 13.9: Signs and symptoms of stress overload

Cognitive symptoms	Emotional symptoms
• Memory impairment	• Sad mood
• Inability to concentrate	• Irritability or short temper
• Impaired judgment	• Agitation, inability to relax
• Seeing only the negative	• Feeling overwhelmed
• Anxious or racing thoughts	• Sense of loneliness and isolation
• Constant worrying	• General unhappiness
Physical symptoms	**Behavioral symptoms**
• Aches and pains	• Eating more or less
• Diarrhea or constipation	• Sleeping too much or too little
• Nausea, dizziness	• Isolating from others
• Chest pain, rapid heartbeat	• Using alcohol, cigarettes, or drugs
• Loss of sex drive.	• Nervous habits (e.g. nail biting, pacing).

Stress Adaptation Model: General Adaptation Syndrome (GAS)

Hans Selye (1907–1982) was a Hungarian endocrinologist, first to give a scientific explanation for biological stress.

Hans Selye developed a framework to describe how people respond to stress. He said that the entire body responds to stress in an attempt to maintain or adapt to the circumstances of the event creating stress. He also recognized that each person has a limited amount of energy to use in dealing with stress. When stress is continuous, the adaptive capacity of the body may be exceeded and disease may result. Unrelenting stress may result in death.

Physiological responses occur in three stages:

1. **Alarm reaction:** Stage 1 is the arousal of the CNS. Catecholamine is excreted, heart rate increases, the strength of heart contraction increases, the blood glucose level increases, this is commonly called the **'flight or fight response'.** Cortisol is also released to increase glucose levels from the stored glucose. If the stressor remains, the body cannot stay in stage 1 without experiencing pathologic changes. Changes occur in thymus, spleen and lymph nodes, and gastric ulcers develop. The thymus, spleen and lymph nodes atrophy in response to the cortisol.

Flowchart 13.2: Flight or fight response

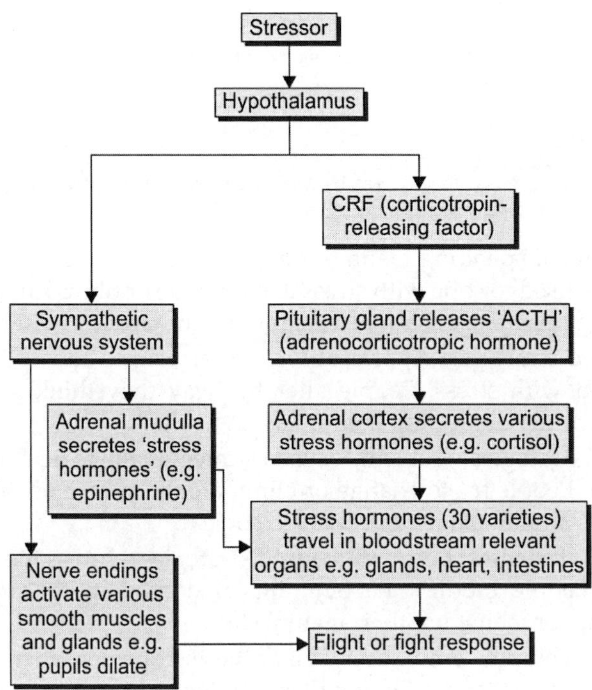

2. **Stage of resistance:** Maximum adaptation occurs in this stage. This bodily signs characteristic of the alarm reaction disappear. Resistance increases to levels above normal; if the stressor is halted in this stage, the body should be able to return to a normal state.
3. **Stage of exhaustion:** This stage occurs when the stressor continues and the body cannot continue to produce hormones as in stage 1 or when damage has occurred to other organs. In this stage, the body has run out of its reserve of body energy and immunity. Mental, physical and emotional resources suffer heavily. The body experiences 'adrenal

exhaustion'. The blood sugar levels decrease as the adrenals becomes depleted, leading to decreased stress tolerance, progressive mental and physical exhaustion, illness and collapse.

Diagrammatic Representation of Stress Adaptation Model

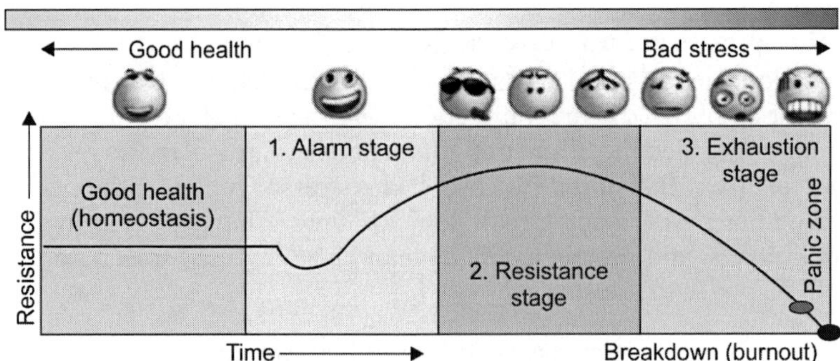

Fig. 13.1: Representation of resistance reaction

Coping with Stress

Core concept: Coping with stress is the process by which a person consciously attempts to master, minimize or tolerate stressors and problems in life.

Coping is the process of spending mental, conscious energy on dealing with problems in life. Mechanisms are used to cope with stress to overcome or diminish the amount of stress experienced. Coping mechanisms can be categorized into three broad types:

1. Appraisal-focused strategies: Appraisal-focused strategies attempt to modify thought processes associated with stress. People alter the way they think about a problem by approaching it differently or altering their goals and values.

2. Problem-focused strategies: Problem-focused strategies aim to deal with the cause of the problem or stressor. People try to change or eliminate the source of stress by researching the problem and learning management skills to solve it.

3. Emotion-focused strategies: Emotion-focused strategies address the feelings associated with the stressor. People modify the emotions that accompany stress perception by releasing, distracting, or managing their mental state.

(A typical person will employ a mixture of all of these strategies when attempting to cope with stress. Skill or prowess at employing these strategies changes over time).

Techniques of Stress Management

There are several ways of coping with stress. Some techniques may help a person to control stress.

- **Autogenic training** is a relaxation technique developed by Johannes Schultz in 1932. The technique involves a set of visualization that induces a state of relaxation for 15 minutes a day. (e.g. lying down, sitting meditation, sitting like a rag doll, etc.). The technique can be used to alleviate many stress-induced psychosomatic disorders.

- **Cognitive therapy** seeks to help the client to overcome difficulties by identifying and changing dysfunctional thinking, behavior, and emotional responses.
- **Physical exercise** is any bodily activity that enhances or maintains physical fitness and gives relaxation to mind.
- **Meditation** is a mental discipline by which one attempts to get beyond the conditioned, 'thinking' mind into a deeper state of relaxation or awareness which gives peace of mind.
- **Diaphragmatic breathing, abdominal breathing, belly breathing** or **deep breathing.**
- **Memory enhancers or smart drugs like** *nootropics:* This improves cognitive abilities including drugs, nutrients and herbs.
- **Relaxation technique** (also known as **relaxation training**) is any method, process, procedure, or activity that helps a person to relax.
- **Fractional relaxation** is a method of releasing muscular tension in one small part of the body at a time, such as relaxing one finger, then relaxing another, then adding another. Then the whole hand is relaxed, followed by the forearm, and then the upper arm. The other arm is relaxed next and continues until the entire body is relaxed.
- **Progressive muscle relaxation** (or PMR) developed by American physician Edmund Jacobson in 1920s. It is a technique of stress management by progressively relaxing each parts of muscles in the body.
- **Stress ball** is a malleable toy, usually not more than 7cm in diameter. It is squeezed in the hand and manipulated by the fingers which helps to relieve stress.
- **Naturopathic medicine:** It is a complementary and alternative medicine like using herbs and foods rather than surgery or synthetic drugs to relieve stress.
- **Time management** refers to a range of skills, tools, and techniques utilized to accomplish specific tasks, projects and goals.
- Listening to certain types of relaxing music, particularly:
  - **New age music** is peaceful music of various styles, which is intended to create relaxation.
  - Listening to classical music.

GRIEF: THEORIES OF GRIEVING PROCESS, PRINCIPLES AND TECHNIQUES OF COUNSELING

Introduction

Grief is a natural response to loss. It is the emotional suffering of one's own feel when something or someone loved is taken away. The more significant the loss, the more intense the grief will be.

Do you know?

'Grief' derived from the latin word '*gravare*', means to burden or cause distress.

Definition

- 'Grief is a great sadness caused by trouble or loss and a heavy sorrow.'
- 'Grief is defined as one's experiences after a loss (Worden, 2005).'

Concepts of Grief

- Grief is the physical, emotional, somatic, cognitive and spiritual response to actual or threatened loss of a person.
- Although everyone experiences grief when they lose someone, grieving affects people in different ways.
- Losing someone suddenly can be extremely traumatic, though, no matter how old that person is.
- Each individual will grieve in his own unique way for the unique loss. There is no right or wrong way to grieve.

Box 13.10: Causes of grief

- Death of a loved ones, cause most intense type of grief
- Divorce or relationship breakup
- Loss of health
- Losing a job
- Loss of financial stability
- A miscarriage
- Retirement
- Death of a pet
- Loss of a cherished dream
- A loved one's serious illness
- Loss of a friendship
- Loss of safety after a trauma
- Selling the family home.

Grief and Loss

Types of Loss

- **Personal loss:** Any significant loss of someone or something that can no longer be seen or felt, heard. (Perceived beauty, pleasure, satisfaction with life).
- **Perceived loss:** Loss that is uniquely defined or experienced by one person but cannot be verified by others. (loss of confidence, prestige).
- **Maturational loss:** Loss that occur on the process of normal development. (Retirement from a career, death of aged parents).
- **Situational loss:** Any sudden, unexpected and definable event that is not predictable (loss of one's job, death of a child, loss, hurricane, flooding).
- **Actual loss:** It can be identified by others and can arise either in response to or in anticipation of a situation.

Symptoms of Grief

While loss affects people in different ways, many experience the following symptoms when they are grieving.

- **Shock and disbelief:** After a loss, it is very hard to accept what happened and denying the truth.
- **Sadness**: Profound sadness is probably the most universally experienced symptom of grief.
- **Anger:** Even if the loss was nobody's fault, person feel angry on himself, or others because of valued loss.

- **Fear**: A significant loss can trigger a host of worries and fears leads to anxious, helpless, or insecure.
- **Physical symptoms**: Even though grief is a strictly emotional process, but often involves physical problems, including fatigue, nausea, weight loss or weight gain, aches and pains, and insomnia.

Theories of Grieving Process

There are mainly 4 theories which explains the process of grieving of an individual at various stages.

What is Grieving process?
It is a sequence of affective, cognitive, and physiological states through which the person responds to and finally accepts an irretrievable loss.

Box 13.11: List of theories of grieving process

- Kübler-Ross's stages of grieving
- Engel's stages of grieving
- Martocchio clusters of grief
- Sander's phases of bereavement.

Kübler-Ross's Stages of Grieving

In 1969, psychiatrist Elisabeth Kübler-Ross introduced what became known as the 'five stages of grief.' These stages of grief were based on her studies of the feelings of patients facing terminal illness, but many people have generalized them to other types of negative life changes and losses, such as the death of a loved one or a breakup.

Table 13.1: Five stages of grief

Stage	Behavioral responses	Nursing implications
1. Denial	'This can't be happening to me.'	• Verbally support client's
2. Anger	'Why is this happening? Who is to blame?'	• Help client to understand that anger is a normal response to feelings of loss and powerlessness.
3. Bargaining	'Make this not happen, and in return I will ____.'	• Listen attentively, and encourage client to talk to relieve guilt and irrational fear; if appropriate, offer spiritual support.
4. Depression	'I'm too sad to do anything.'	• Allow client to express sadness; communicate nonverbally by sitting quietly without expecting conversation; convey caring by touch.
5. Acceptance	'I'm at peace with what happened.'	• Help family and friends to understand client's decreased need to socialize and need for short, quiet visits; encourage client to participate as much as possible in the treatment program.

Engel's Stages of Grieving

Table 13.2: Engel's stages

Stages	Behavioral responses
1. Shock and disbelief	• Refusal to accept loss, stunned feeling
2. Developing awareness	• Anger may be directed at hospital, nurses, etc. • Crying and self-blame

Contd...

Contd...

Stages	Behavioral responses
3. Restitution	• Rituals of mourning (funeral)
4. Resolving the loss	• Still unable to accept new love object to replace lost person • Thinks over and talks about memories of the dead person
5. Idealization	• Produces image of dead person that is almost devoid of undesirable features • Reminders of deceased evoke fewer feelings of sadness • Reinvests feelings in others
6. Outcome	• Behavior influenced by several factors: – Importance of lost object as source of support – Degree of dependence on relationship – Degree of ambivalence toward deceased.

Martocchio Clusters of Grief

Table 13.3: Martocchio clusters

Stage	Behavior responses
1. Shock and disbelief	• Feeling of numbness immediately following the death of a loved one. • Disbelief and denial may persist even though the loss has been accepted intellectually.
2. Yearning and protest	• Anger may be directed at others whose loved ones are still alive, or at the caregivers or God.
3. Anguish, disorganization and despair	• When reality of the loss is genuinely admitted, depression can set in. • Weeping is common at this time. • Activities that were once enjoyed with the deceased are now without attraction.
4. Bereavement	• Bereaved may take on the behavior, personal traits, habits and ambitions of the deceased.
5. Reorganization and restitution	• Achieving stability and a sense of reintegration can take a period of time that ranges widely, from less than a year to several years. • Bereaveds are able to experience a sense of well being and can resume most normal patterns of functioning.

Sander's Phases of Bereavement

Table 13.4: Sander's phase

Phase	Description
1. Shock	• Survivors are left with feelings of confusion, unreality, and disbelief that the loss has occurred.
2. Awareness of loss	• After the funeral, friends and family resume normal activities. The bereaved experience the full significance of their loss.
3. Conservation/ withdrawal	• Survivors feel a need to be alone to conserve and replenish both physical and emotional energy. The social support available to the bereaved has decreased, and they may experience despair and helplessness.
4. Healing: The turning point	• The bereaved move from distress about living without their loved ones to learning to live more independently.
5. Renewal	• Survivors move on to a new self-awareness, an acceptance of responsibility for self, and learning to live without the deceased.

Table 13.5: Summaries of the theories of grieving process

Kübler-Ross	Sander's	Engel's	Martocchio
1. Denial	1. Shock	1. Shock and disbelief	1. Shock and disbelief
2. Anger	2. Awareness of loss	2. Developing awareness	2. Yearning and protest
3. Bargaining	3. Conservation and withdrawal	3. Restitution	3. Anguish, despair and disorganization
4. Depression	4. Healing: The turning point	4. Resolving the loss	4. Identification in bereavement
5. Acceptance	5. Renewal	5. Idealization	5. Reorganization and restitution
		6. Outcome	

Box 13.12: More to know!

In Memory: Elisabeth Kübler-Ross, MD

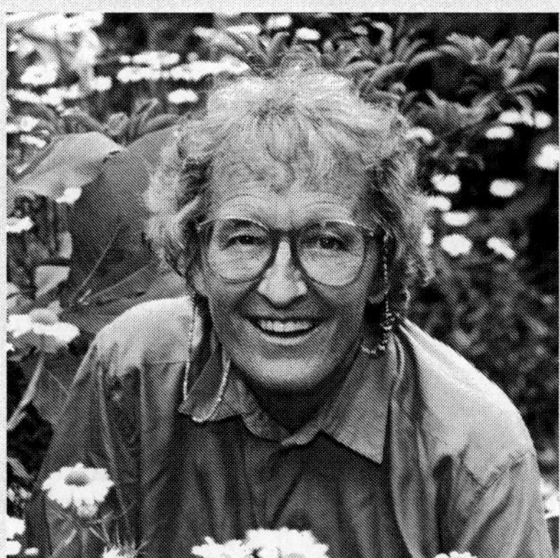

Courtesy: www.marketguy.ca

Elisabeth Kübler-Ross, MD was a psychiatrist and the author of the groundbreaking book *On Death and Dying (1969)*. She spent most of her life working with the dying. She was born in Zurich, Switzerland and she graduated her medicals in 1957. She came to the United States in 1958 and she was appalled by the standard treatment of dying patients where she practiced. 'They were shunned and abused, nobody was honest with them'. Unlike her colleagues, she made it a point to sit with terminal patients, listening as they poured out their hearts to her. She began giving lectures featuring dying patients about what they were going through. Her first book On Death and Dying in 1969 made her an internationally renowned author. She spent many years speaking to room only audiences and writing over twenty books.

In 1995, she suffered a series of major strokes, which left her paralyzed and facing her own death. At the time she said, 'I am like a plane that has left the gate and not taken off. I would rather go back to the gate or fly away.' During this time that she and David Kessler wrote first book together, 'Life Lessons: Two experts on death and dying teach us about the mysteries of life and living.

Elisabeth Kübler-Ross passed away on August 24, 2004. Elisabeth's last book, co-written with David Kessler, 'On Grief and Grieving' was completed one month before her death which was her final legacy.

What if Grief Does not Get Away?

When sadness of loss of loved one does not goes away completely within normal period of grief, it is called dysfunctional grief/pathologic grief.

Characteristics

- Withdrawal from usual task or activities that previously gave pleasure
- Delusion
- Hallucination
- Suicidal ideation
- Phobias
- Obsession
- Loss of control over environment
- Isolation
- Agitated depression
- Restriction of pleasure.

Treatment of Grief

Complicated grief needs treatment like:

- Complicated grief treatment (CGT) is a type of grief therapy that was helpful in a clinical trial.
- Cognitive behavioral therapy (CBT).
- Depression related to grief is sometimes treated with drugs.

Normal grief may not need to be treated. Most bereaved people go through grief and recover within the first 6 months to 2 years. For people who have serious grief reaction, treatment may be helpful. (Treatment methods include discussion, listening, and counseling).

- **Complicated grief treatment (CGT):** It has three phases:
  - **I phase:** Talking about the loss and setting goals toward recovery. The bereaved are taught to work on these two things.
  - **II phase:** The second phase which includes coping with the loss by retelling the story of the death. This helps bereaved people who try not to think about their loss.
  - **III phase:** The last phase looks at progress that has been made toward recovery and helps the bereaved make future plans.
- **Cognitive behavioral therapy (CBT):** It works with the way a person's thoughts and behaviors are connected. CBT helps the patient learn skills that change attitudes and behaviors by replacing negative thoughts and changing the rewards of certain behaviors.
- **Depression related to grief is treated with drugs:** Some health care professionals think depression is a normal part of grief and does not need to be treated. Whether to treat grief-related depression with drugs is up to the patient and the health care professional to decide.

Clinical trials of antidepressants like imipramine, desipramine for depression related to grief have found that the drugs can help relieve depression. However, they give less relief and take longer to work than they do when used for depression that is not related to grief.

Box 13.13: Myths and facts about grief

MYTH: The pain will go away faster if you ignore it.
Fact: Trying to ignore your pain or keep it from surfacing will only make it worse in the long run. For real healing, it is necessary to face your grief and actively deal with it.
MYTH: It's important to be 'be strong' in the face of loss.
Fact: Feeling sad, frightened, or lonely is a normal reaction to loss. Crying doesn't mean you are weak. You don't need to 'protect' your family or friends by putting on a brave front. Showing your true feelings can help them and you.
MYTH: If you don't cry, it means you aren't sorry about the loss.
Fact: Crying is a normal response to sadness, but it's not the only one. Those who don't cry may feel the pain just as deeply as others. They may simply have other ways of showing it.
MYTH: Grief should last about a year.
Fact: There is no right or wrong time frame for grieving. How long it takes can differ from person to person.

CRISIS: TYPES OF CRISIS, CRISIS INTERVENTION—PRINCIPLES, TECHNIQUES AND PROCESS

Introduction

It is easy to think that there are various events that can easily be defined as crisis, like earthquakes, fires, murders, rapes, and disasters. While this is certainly true and we should expect people to react intensely to these life-events, we really need a more sophisticated means for understanding the 'nature of crisis' and the ways in which people react to them.

Any life-event can take on crisis proportions if it is experienced as sudden, intense, unexpected, or emotionally super-charged. Individual do not know what to do to control the situation. Wave after wave of emotion sweeps over individual and unable to predict when situation is going to end.

Thus, any event can be a crisis if it wipes out ability to make sense out of what is happening.

Do you know?
The word crisis derives from Greek word (κρίσις) krisis, which means 'critical'.

Definition

Box 13.14: How do different experts define crisis?

- A state of disequilibrium resulting from the interaction of an event with the individual or family's coping mechanisms, which are inadequate to meet the demands of the situation, combined with the individual or family's perception of the meaning of the event.

  —Taylor, 1982
- 'An upset in equilibrium at the failure of one's traditional problem-solving approach which results in disorganization, hopelessness, sadness, confusion, and panic.'

  —Lillibridge and Klukken, 1978
- 'Crisis is a perception or experience of an event or situation as an intolerable difficulty that exceeds the person's current resources and coping mechanisms.'

  —James and Gilliland, 2001

Key Words Related to Crisis

- **Stress:** It is a body's response to any kind of demand or threat.
- **Coping:** Refers to the things people do to deal with stress and distress.

- **Crisis intervention:** Refers to the methods used to offer immediate short-term help to individual who experience an event that produces emotional, mental, physical and behavioral distress or problems.
- **Ventilation:** It is a technique in which a person airs out their feeling and put problems into words.
- **Catharsis:** One curative factor of group therapy, in which members in a group can express both positive and negative feelings in a nonthreatened atmosphere.

Characteristics of Crisis

- Crisis occurs in all individual at one time or another.
- Crises are personal by nature. What may be considered as crisis situation by one individual may not be so for another.
- Crises are precipitated by specific identifiable events.
- Crises are acute, not chronic and will be resolved in one way or another with a brief period.
- A crisis situation contains the potential for psychological growth or deterioration.

Situation Which can Lead to a Crisis

- **Family situation:** Any family disruption or family disturbance.
- **Economic situation:** Economic changes—loss of a job, medical bills, theft of a purse or cash, or utilities being shut off
- **Community situation:** A lack of housing resources, food resources, or inadequate crime protection.
- **Significant life events:** Life events—the birth of a child, loss of a loved one, a child moving out, an irrational child, or any disturbance to daily activities.
- **Natural elements:** Natural disasters—flooding, tornadoes, weather-related incidents, fire, or any incident that is created by a weather disaster.
- **Suicide:** When a person threatens suicide or plans to commit suicide.

Phases in Development of a Crisis

Caplan was the first to describe the main stages of a crisis reaction. The contributions of later theorists have been based on Caplan's work and have basically consisted on a restatement of his phases. According to Caplan (1964) most crisis reactions follow four distinct phases:

- **Phase-1:** The individual is exposed to a precipitating stressor, anxiety, previous problem-solving technique are employed.
- **Phase-2**: When previous problem-solving technique do not relieve the stressor, anxiety increase further.
- **Phase-3:** All possible resources internal and external are called to resolve the problem and relieve discomfort.
- **Phase-4:** If resolution does not occur in previous phases, Caplan states that 'the tension mounts beyond a further threshold or its burden increases over time to a breaking point, major disorganization of the individual with the drastic results often occurs.'

These phases are congruent with the concept of 'balancing factors' as described by Aguilera (1998). These factors affect the way in which an individual perceives and responds to a precipitating stressor.

Paradigm of Balancing Factors

Every attempt is made to stabilize and regain equilibrium. Various factors can influence an individual's ability to resolve a crisis. Aguilera (1997) describes a paradigm of balancing factors that whether or not an individual experiences a crisis in response to a stressful situation depends on the following three factors. A schematic pattern of balancing factors is given in Flowchart 13.3.

Flowchart 13.3: Aguilera model of crisis balancing factor

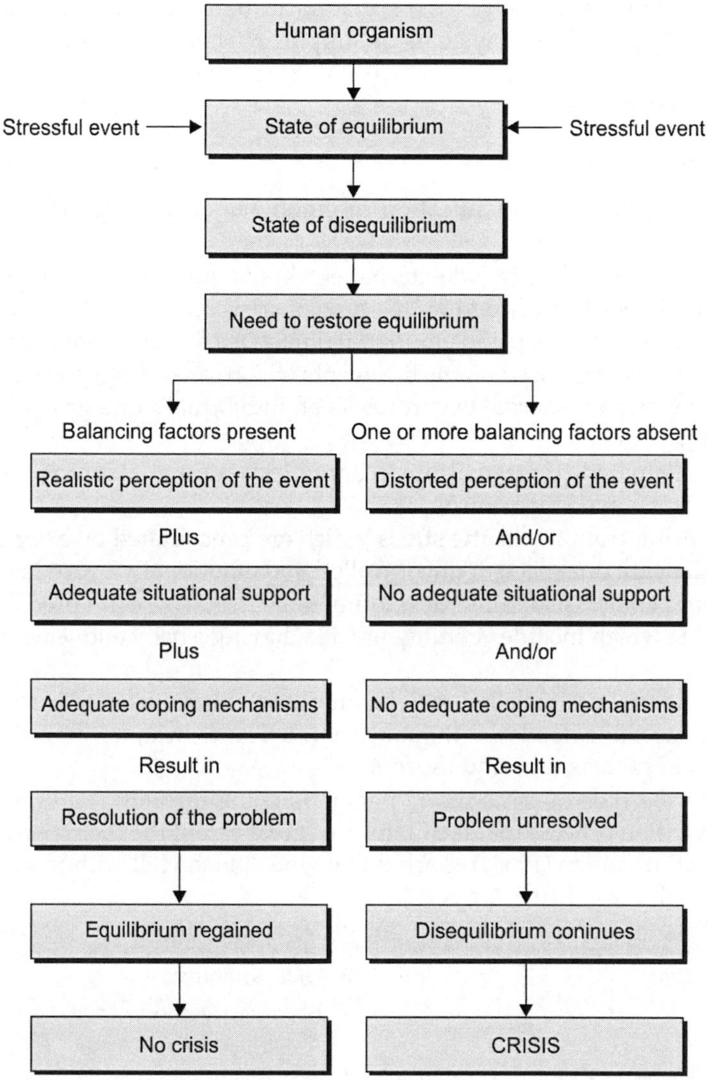

1. **Individual's perception of the event:** If the event is perceived realistically, the individual is more likely to draw on adequate resources to restore equilibrium. If the perception of the event is distorted, attempts at problem-solving are likely to be ineffective and restoration of equilibrium goes unresolved.

2. Availability of situational supports: Aguilera states, 'Situational supports are those persons who are available in the environment and who can be depended on help to solve the problem.' Without adequate situational supports during a stressful situation, an individual is most likely to feel overwhelmed and alone.

3. The availability of adequate coping mechanisms: When a stressful situation occurs, individuals draw on behavioral strategies that have been successful for them in the past. If these coping strategies work, a crisis may be diverted. If not, disequilibrium may continue and tension and anxiety may increase.

When the individual perceives the situation to be overwhelming and is unable to use the usual coping skills and systems of support effectively, the stress and discomfort continues to escalate. As a result, the individual is unable to regain balance without significant external intervention.

Types of Crisis

Baldwin (1978) developed a classification of emotional crises that includes six types of crisis:

1. **Dispositional crisis:** Also called external crisis is an unexpected or sudden event that impairs ones integrity. Included in this type of crisis are loss of a job, death of a loved one or relative and physical and emotional illness of a family member or an individual.
2. **Situational crisis:** It is based on the life events which can be both positive and negative. This occurs when an external event upsets an individual's or a group's psychological equilibrium.
3. **Crisis of anticipated life transitions:** That reflects normal life transitions over which the person may have little control.
4. **Crises resulting from traumatic stress** which are precipitated by external stressors or situations that are unexpected, uncontrolled and emotionally overwhelming.
5. **Maturational crisis:** Also called developmental crisis. These are predictable events in a person's life which includes getting married, having a baby and leaving home for the first time.
6. **Adventitious crisis:** Also called social/community crisis. Included in this category are: natural disasters like floods, earthquakes or hurricanes, war, terrorist attacks, riots and violent crimes such as rape and murder.

(Identifying the type of crisis that a person is going through is an important step of the crisis intervention process that facilitates to a great extent the therapist's work with the person in crisis. But Caplan (1964) reported that when person left without intervention, the crisis situation will resolve in 5–6 weeks).

Box 13.15: Signs and symptoms of crisis

Emotional symptoms	Physical symptoms
• Depression • Anxiety • Scattered, unfocused thinking • Self-doubt • Loss of motivation • Lack of patience or irritability	• Headaches and loss of appetite are common • Stomach and digestive upset • Joint pains • Fatigue and other somatic symptoms are often related to depression.

Because of the severity of these emotional symptoms leads to following consequences including:

- Avoidance of relationships
- Poor life decisions
- Chronic physical pain
- Insomnia
- Self-confidence issues.

Crisis Intervention

Definition

Crisis intervention refers to the methods used to offer immediate, short-term help to individuals who experience an event that produces emotional, mental, physical, and behavioral distress or problems.

Goals of Crisis Intervention

Rapoport (1970) has discussed four main goals for crisis intervention:

1. Relief of symptoms.
2. Restoration to the optimal level of functioning that existed before the present crisis.
3. Understanding of the relevant precipitating events that contributed to the state of disequilibrium.
4. Identification of remedial measures that can be taken by the client or family those are available from community resources.

General Principles

- Crisis lasts only for 5 weeks
- Deal not just with individual client but with family
- Crisis intervention deals with wide range of human problem
- It is not self-limiting for future
- Crisis intervention should focus upon present problem giving wide range of solution
- Teach more adaptive/coping mechanism to cope with future problems and crisis
- Crisis intervention should be reality oriented
- Crisis intervention should serve as a stepping stone to a long-term process.

Process of Crisis Intervention: The Role of the Nurse

Clients may need to address issues quickly, but may not tolerate frequent sessions. They may not respond to interventions, and may require an extended amount of time to resolve issues. A multidisciplinary approach may facilitate resolution because it provides support and a learning opportunity for both client and nurse.

The process of crisis intervention according to Aguilera (1997) contains five steps same as like nursing process are:

1. Assessment

Assessment of a client during crisis intervention depends on following factors, such as:

- Determining crisis severity
- Assessing client's perception.

Determining crisis severity: The first factor in the assessment process is to determine the severity of the crisis and to identify the degree of disruption the client is experiencing.

Recognizing the magnitude of physical, emotional, social, and spiritual components of a crisis is essential to helping clients, as well as to intervening such that additional complications do not develop.

- Is the individual anxious, depressed, fearful, confused, disoriented, suicidal, or homicidal?
- Is the crisis due to an interpersonal or intrapersonal issue?
- Does the crisis involve one person, several people, or a community?
- Is this a criminal situation with actual or potential harm or lethality?

Assessing client's perception: The second factor involves assessing the client's perception of the event. Two major approaches may be used:

1. **Symptom-focused approach:** Focuses on the emotions of the client.
2. **Constructivist self-development theory (CSDT):** Focuses on one's relationship with oneself and one's relationship with others. With CSDT, identifying a threat can help clients connect to their experiences on an emotional level and make sense of their feelings.
    - Are the client's perceptions realistic or distorted?
    - Does the client see the situation as a threat to self-esteem, well being, intimacy, self-control, or ability to trust?

2. Nursing Diagnosis

Examples of nursing diagnoses for clients experiencing a crisis may include the following:

- Disturbed thought process
- Risk for emergency situation like suicide, violence
- Anxiety
- Fear
- Ineffective coping
- Impaired verbal communication
- Risk for injury
- Dysfunctional grieving
- Disabled family coping.

3. Planning

With information gained through the assessment process and the formulation of one or more nursing diagnoses, several specific interventions are proposed.

Connoly and Chandler (1997) state that individuals must learn to ask for help and realize the potential for growth during a crisis. They should be involved in the choice of alternate coping methods and encouraged to make as many arrangements as possible by themselves. If significant others are involved, their needs and reactions must also be considered. The nurse should identify strengths and resources of all persons providing support.

4. Intervention

Therapeutic intervention depends on pre-existing skills, the creativity and flexibility of the nurse, and the rapidity of the person's response.

- The nurse helps the person establish an intellectual understanding of the crisis by noting the relationship between the precipitating factor and the crisis.
- He or she also helps the client explore coping mechanisms, remember or recreate successful coping devices used in the past, or devise new coping skills.
- Reducing immobility caused by anxiety and encouraging verbalization of feelings is an immediate goal of the nurse.
- An attempt is also made to establish new supportive and meaningful relationships and experiences.
- Follow reality oriented approach.
- Establish a positive working experience.
- Provide adequate support.
- Handle the feelings gently.
- Utilize the external support system.
- Clarify the problem.
- Displaying acceptance and attempting to establish a positive relationship.
- Encouraging the client to discuss present feelings, such as denial, guilt, grief, or anger.
- Helping the client to confront the reality of the crisis by gaining an intellectual as well as emotional understanding of the situation.
- Explaining that the client's emotions are a normal reaction to the crisis.
- Avoiding false reassurance.
- Set limits on destructive behavior.
- Assisting the client in seeking help with the activities of daily living until resolution occurs.
- Use the crisis intervention techniques.

The therapeutic techniques commonly used by nurses performing crisis intervention are explained in the box below.

Box 13.16: Techniques of crisis intervention

Abreaction:
The release of feeling that takes place as the individual talks about emotionally charged areas. E.g. the nurse encourages abreaction by asking the patient how he feels about his situation recent events and significant people involved in the crisis.

Catharsis:
Allowing clients to vent feelings and thoughts may be one of the most therapeutic strategies you can use. In order to do this, you need to provide a safe and accepting environment. In doing so you are saying that you accept the client's feelings and thoughts. This strategy is most often used with individuals who have struggled to get in touch with their feelings or thoughts.

Clarification:
Encouraging the patient to express more clearly the relationship between certain events in his life.

Manipulation:
It is a way of influencing the client, using the client's emotion, wishes or values to his benefit in the therapeutic process.

Contd...

Contd...

Suggestion:
Nurse will suggest the client and it influences an individual so that he/she accepts an idea or belief, particularly and that he/she feel better. E.g. nurse influence the client to see him/her as a confident, calm hopeful, empathetic leader who can help the client feel optimistic and in the will feel anxious.

Reinforcement behavior:
Giving the client positive response to adaptive behavior.

Support of defenses:
Encouraging the use of healthy adaptive behavior and discourages those which are maladaptive or unhealthy.

Raising self-esteem:
Helping the client to regain the feelings of self-worth, active participation, communicates effectively, accepts his feelings with respect.

5. Evaluation

Reinforcement is provided whenever necessary while the crisis work is reviewed and accomplishments of the client are emphasized. Assistance is given to formulate realistic plans for the future, and the client is given the opportunity to discuss how present experiences may help in coping with future crises.

Box 13.17: More to know!!

The six-step model of crisis intervention:

Developed by James (2008).This model provides a useful framework from which to work when confronted with crisis situations in a shelter setting.

- **Assessing:** Assessment is an important part of each of the six-steps of crisis intervention. The first three steps of this model are usually more passive listening activities than actions. When safety considerations are presented that concern anyone's potential to be hurt or killed you need to take action immediately. The final three steps are largely action behaviors on your part even though listening is always present along with assessment as an overarching theme.
- **Listening:** Involves attending, observing, understanding and responding with empathy, genuinesss, respect, acceptance, nonjudgmental, and caring. It is essential to establish an environment that provides individuals with 'psychological first-aid' which is defined as the establishment of safety of the client, reducing stress-related symptoms, providing rest and physical recuperation and linking clients to critical resources and social support systems is an essential part of the helping process.

The first three steps of the six-step model are:

- **Defining the problem:** The first step is to define and understand the problem from the client's point of view.
- **Ensuring client safety:** It is necessary that you continually keep client safety at the forefront of all interventions. Ensuring safety means constantly assessing the possibility of physical and psychological danger to the client as well as to others. This step is a fluid one in that assessing and ensuring safety is a continuous part of the process of crisis intervention.
- **Providing support:** It is important that you communicate to the client that you care about her. The support given may be emotional as well as instrumental and informational.
  - **Acting:** Steps 4, 5, and 6 involve acting strategies.
- **Examining alternatives:** Alternatives are examined from three possible perspectives. The first is supporting the individual to assess their situational supports or those people known to the client in the present or past who might care about what happens to the client. The second perspective is helping the client identify coping mechanisms or actions, behaviors, or environmental resources that she might use to help her get through the present crisis. The third perspective is assisting the client to examine her thinking patterns and if possible find ways to reframe her situation in order that the client's view of the problem will be altered which will in turn lessen the client's anxiety level.

Contd...

Contd...

- **Making plans:** The client is supported to make a plan that is very detailed and outlines the persons, groups and other referral resources that can be contacted for immediate support; provide coping mechanisms and action steps which are concrete and positive for the client to do in the present. Planning is about getting through the short-term in order to achieve some sense of equilibrium and stability.
- **Obtaining commitment:** In this last step, the issues of control and autonomy are also important to the process. This step involves asking the client to verbally summarize the plan. In some incidents where lethality is involved the commitment may be written down and signed by both individuals. The goal is to enable the client to commit to the plan and to take definite positive steps designed to facilitate them moving towards re-establishing a pre-crisis state of equilibrium. The commitments made by the client need to be voluntary and doable.

Modes of Crisis Intervention Program

- Mobile crisis program
- Telephone counseling and hotline.

Case example: Wendy called the crisis line from her neighbor's home. When the counselor answered the phone call she heard was sobbing. The counselor responded in a very calm voice, encouraging the caller to take some deep breaths.

The counselor reassured the caller that she was listening and she wanted to be able to provide support for her. She began asking close ended questions trying to determine whether the caller was safe or not. 'Are you in a safe place right now? Do you have children? Are the children with you? Are you alone with your children? Where is your partner right now? Do you need a safe place to stay? As Wendy was able to answer the questions she began to calm down more and was able to explain her situation.

- Disaster response and critical incident stress debriefing
- Crisis counseling.

Geriatric Consideration

A geriatric patient with a psychiatric emergency almost always poses an assessment challenge. Coexisting medical disorders and medical treatments often influence psychiatric presentation. Therefore, a thorough review of systems, a complete physical examination, and appropriate laboratory tests are imperative in this age group.

A medically-oriented evaluative approach may be more effective than a traditional psychiatric one. The clinician must ask short and simple questions in a straightforward manner and repeat them as necessary. He or she should speak clearly and slowly to geriatric patients. Due respect should be given to such patients by addressing them properly, usually formally. Further, the clinician should always consider a collateral source of history within the framework of confidentiality.

Common geriatric emergencies include delirium, delirium with dementia, depression, and psychosis. Delirium is a medical emergency that has a potentially fatal outcome if not treated in time. Physical symptoms, generally related to a hyperadrenergic state, and acute cognitive and perceptual changes are hallmarks of delirium.

Fluctuating consciousness, extreme attentional deficits, memory disturbance, disorganized thinking, and hallucinations are to be expected in some combination. The onset is acute and the course turbulent. Delirium may be comorbid with a pre-existing dementia. As soon as the clinician suspects delirium, he or she should initiate a thorough evaluation of etiology. Adverse drug interactions or an anticholinergic syndrome are present in some cases.

Intoxication secondary to an unintentional overdose (related to cognitive impairment) may also be associated with delirium. Depressed elderly patients may exhibit somatic symptoms and pseudodementia and may under report their suicidality. Suicidal risk is high. Depression may be related to a general medical condition and medication. Depression and psychosis may also be part of a dementing illness. Aggression is sometimes associated with psychosis. The etiology of such cognitive and behavioral change is often unclear.

14 Legal Issues in Mental Health Nursing

'Forensic' is derived from Latin and comes from the same root as the word forum. The Forum was the public space in ancient Rome where judicial and other public business was debated and decided.

Originally, forensic psychiatrists were part of an obscure and small group of 'alienists' who were dedicated to the study of mental conditions and their treatment among prisoners. At present, they form a part of an established and recognized group of super-specialists who have made deep incursions into the workings of the law and are transforming the practice of psychiatry.

Forensic psychiatry is a subspecialty of psychiatry, which in turn, is a medical specialty. It is commonly defined as 'the branch of psychiatry that deals with issues arising in the interface between psychiatry and the law' (Gutheil, 2004).

INDIAN LUNACY ACT (ILA), 1912

The Indian Lunacy Act (ILA), Act 4 of 1912, was based largely on the earlier English Lunacy Act of 1890. The act extends to the whole India except the state of Jammu and Kashmir. The IL A had eight chapters.

Chapter-I Preliminary information
Chapter-II Procedure for admission
Chapter-III Care, treatment and discharge
Chapter-IV Proceeding of lunacy in presidency town
Chapter-V Proceeding of lunacy outside presidency town
Chapter-VI Establishment of asylums
Chapter-VII Expense of lunatics
Chapter-VIII Rules.

Chapter-I Preliminaries Information

Some of the basic information given in this chapter includes:

- **Lunatic:** 'An idiot or person of unsound mind'. Defectiveness of reasoning, whether partial or complete, was considered as unsoundness of mind.
- **Asylum:** For lunatics established or licensed by the central or any state government.
- **Relative:** Includes any person related by blood marriage or adoption.

- **Cost of maintenance:** In an asylum includes the cost of lodging, maintenance, clothing, medicine and care of a lunatic and any expenditure incurred in removing such lunatic to and from an asylum together with any other charge specified in this behalf by the State Government in exercise of any power conferred upon it by this, Act.
- **District court:** The principal civil court of original justification in any area outside the local limits for the time being of the presidency towns.
- **Medical officer:** Means a gazetted officer and includes a medical practitioner declared by general or special order of the state government to be a medical officer for the purpose of this act.
- **Reception Order:** Order made by magistrate.

Chapter-II Procedure for Admission into Asylum

Voluntary Admission

According to ILA, the admission may be voluntary i.e. any person who is major can go to the asylum and apply in writing for admission. The medical officer incharge with the consent of at least two boards of visitors can admit the patient.

Reception Order

Reception order is issued by magistrate or a police officer in the presidency town for the detention of a lunatic in an asylum.

Patient Admitted on Petition

An application for a reception order shall be made by petition by relative/guardian accompanied by a statement of particulars to the Magistrate within the local limits of whose jurisdiction the alleged lunatic ordinarily resides, shall be in the form prescribed and shall be supported by two medical certificates on separate sheets of paper, one of which certificates shall be from a medical officer.

Transfer of Lunatics

From one asylum to another in the same state or other shall be with the consent of the state government.

Escape and Recapture

Every person received into asylum under such order as is required by this act may be detained these in until he is removed or discharged as authorized by the law and in case of escape, may police officers or by the person incharge of such asylum.

Reception and Detention of Criminal Lunatics

An order directing the reception of a criminal lunatic into any asylum which is prescribed for reception of criminal lunatics shall be sufficient authority for the reception and detention of any person named there in such asylum or in any other asylum to which he may be lawfully transferred.

Reception after Inquisition

A lunatic so found by inquisition may be admitted into an asylum in case of an inquisition or an order made by the high court or district court.

Chapter-III Care, Treatment and Discharge

The State Government shall appoint for every asylum not less than three visitors, one of whom at least shall be a medical officer. The Inspector-general of prisons (where such office exists) shall be a visitor *ex-officio* of all the asylums within the limits of his jurisdiction.

Three of the visitors of any asylum, of whom one shall be a medical officer, may, by order in writing, direct the discharge of any person detained in such asylum, and such person shall thereupon be discharged.

A lunatic detained in any asylum under a reception order, made on petition, shall be discharged if the person on whose petition the reception order was made so applies in writing to the person incharge of the asylum.

In case of patient admitted through police, he can be discharged if the family members agree in writing to take proper care of him and if the board of visitors is convinced that the client is to be discharged. In case of criminal lunatics on advice of board of visitors, those who are fit to stand for trial will send to court. Those who are transferred from prison will be handed over to prison.

Chapter-IV Proceeding of Lunacy in Presidency Town

The court may upon application by order direct an inquisition whether a person subject to the jurisdiction of the court who is alleged to be lunatic is of unsound mind and incapable of managing himself and his affairs. Application for such inquisition may be made by any relative of the alleged lunatic or by the advocate general.

There, a lunatic has been engaged in business the court, may if it appear to be for the lunatic benefit the business premises should be disposed of the same.

Chapter-V Proceeding of Lunacy Outside Presidency Town

Whenever any person not subject to the jurisdiction of any of the courts is possessed of properly and alleged to be a lunatic the district court person, within whose jurisdiction such person is residing may, upon application.

Chapter-VI Establishment of Asylums

Certain regulators are laid down for keeping the patients in various cells recreation standard diet and medical checkup and these parameters are checked up periodically by board of visitors.

The board of visitors is authorized to evoke the license of asylum if it is not satisfied with its functioning.

Chapter-VII Expense of Lunatics

When any lunatic is admitted to a licensed asylum under a receptions order and no engagement has been taken from the friends or relatives of the lunatic the cost of maintenance is to be paid by the government to the person incharge of such asylum.

Chapter-VIII Rules

- The state government may make rule for all or any of following purpose namely.
- To prescribe forms for proceeding under this act other than a proceeding before a high court.
- To regulate, case, treatment and discharge of criminal lunatic.
- To prescribe condition subject to which asylum may be licensed.
- All rules made shall be published in the official gazette.
- To detain two or more lunatics in any place not being an asylum shall be punishable important which may extend to 2 years or with both.

INDIAN MENTAL HEALTH ACT (1987)

The Mental Health Bill became the Act on 22nd May, 1987. Later, the Government of India issued orders that the act came in force with effect from April 1, 1993 in all the states and Union territories of India. The Act has ten chapters:

Chapter-I	Preliminary information
Chapter-II	Mental health authorities
Chapter-III	Psychiatric hospitals and nursing homes
Chapter-IV	Admission and detention in psychiatric hospitals
Chapter-V	Inspection, discharge, leave of absence and removal of mentally ill
Chapter-VI	Judicial inquisition
Chapter-VII	Liability to meet cost of maintenance of mentally ill
Chapter-VIII	Protection of human rights of mentally ill
Chapter-IX	Penalties and procedure
Chapter-X	Miscellaneous.

Chapter-I Preliminary Information

- **'Cost of maintenance':** In relation to a mentally ill person admitted in a psychiatric hospital or psychiatric nursing home, shall mean the cost of such items as the state government may, by general or special order, specify in this behalf.
- **'District Court':** Means, in any area for which there is a city civil court, that court, and in any other area the principal civil court of original jurisdiction, and include any other civil court in which the state government may, by notification, specify as the court competent to deal with all or any of the maters specified in this act.
- **'Licensed psychiatric hospital":** Also called 'licensed psychiatric nursing home' means a psychiatric hospital or psychiatric nursing home as the case may be licensed, or deemed to be licensed, under this act.
- **'Medical Officer':** Means a gazetted medical officer in the service of government and includes a medical practitioner declared, by a general or special order of the State government.
- **'Mentally ill person':** Means a person who is in need of treatment by reason of any mental disorder other than mental retardation.
- **'Mentally ill Prisoner':** Means a mentally ill person for whose detention in, or removal to, a psychiatric hospital, psychiatric nursing home, jail or other place of safe custody.

- **'Minor'**: Means a person who has not completed the age of eighteen years.
- **'Psychiatric Hospital':** Also called 'psychiatric nursing home' means a hospital or, as the case may be, a nursing home established or maintained by the government or any other person for the treatment.
- **'Psychiatrist':** Means a medical practitioner possessing a post graduate degree or diploma in psychiatry, recognized by the Medical Council of India.
- **'Reception Order':** Means an order made under the provisions of this act for the admission and detention of a mentally ill person in a psychiatric hospital or psychiatric nursing home.
- **'Relative':** Includes any person related to the mentally ill person by blood, marriage or adoption.

Chapter-II Mental Health Authorities

These authorities will regulate and coordinate the mental health services under Central and State Government, respectively.

Chapter-III Psychiatric Hospitals and Nursing Homes

It lays down the guidelines for establishment and maintenance of psychiatric hospitals and nursing homes. In addition, there is a provision for a Licensing Authority who will process applications for licenses. No private psychiatric hospital or nursing home will be allowed to function without a valid license, which has to be renewed every 5 years.

There is also a provision for an Inspecting Officer who will inspect the psychiatric hospitals and nursing homes to prevent any irregularities. There is a provision for separate hospitals for:

- Those under the age of 16 years
- Those addicted to alcohol or other drugs which lead to behavioral changes
- Mentally ill prisoners
- Any other prescribed class or category.

Chapter-IV Admission and Detention in Psychiatric Hospitals

Admission on Voluntary Basis

Any person (not being a minor), who considers himself to be a mentally ill person and desires to be admitted to any psychiatric hospital or psychiatric nursing home for treatment, may request the medical officer incharge for being admitted as a voluntary patient (in case of minor the guardian can apply).

On receipt of a request, the medical officer-incharge shall make such inquiry as he may deem fit within a period not exceeding 24 hours and if satisfied he may admit the patient.

Admission under Special Circumstances

Any mentally ill person who does not, or is unable to, express his willingness for admission as a voluntary basis, may be admitted on an application made in that behalf by a relative or a friend of the mentally ill person if the medical officer incharge is satisfied that in the interests of the mentally ill person it is necessary so to do.

Reception Orders

- **Reception orders on petition:** The medical officer of the psychiatric home where the mentally ill person is undergoing treatment finds, that the mentally ill person is suffering from mental illness and requires treatment for more than six months, or it is necessary in the interests of the health and personal safety of the mentally ill person or for the protection of others that such person shall be detained in a psychiatric hospital or psychiatric nursing home. He may write an application to the Magistrate within the local limits of whose jurisdiction the psychiatric hospital or, as the case may be, psychiatric nursing home is situated.
- **Reception order on production before magistrate:** Every officer incharge of a police station may take or cause to be taken into protection if any person found wandering within the limits of his station that he has reason to believe to be so mentally ill, shall take into protection.

  The person who is taken into protection shall be produced before the nearest magistrate within a period of 24 hours.

Admission as In-Patient after Inquisition

If any District Court holding an inquisition under this chapter regarding any person who is found to be mentally ill, is of opinion that it is necessary so to do in the interests of such person, it may by order direct that such person shall be admitted and kept as an in-patient in a psychiatric hospital or psychiatric nursing home.

Admission and Detention of Mentally Ill Prisoner

This section directing the reception of a mentally ill prisoner into any psychiatric hospital or psychiatric nursing home shall be sufficient authority for the admission of such person in such hospital or such person may be lawfully transferred for detention therein.

Chapter-V Inspection, Discharge, Leave of Absence and Removal of Mentally Ill

Inspection

Appointment of Visitors

The State Government or the Central Government, as the case may be, shall appoint for every psychiatric hospital and every psychiatric nursing home, not less than five visitors, of whom at least one shall be a medical officer, preferably a psychiatrist and two social workers.

The board of visitors should visit the hospital at least once a month and at least 3 members of them should be present.

Discharge

- Discharge on voluntary basis
- Discharge under special circumstances
- Discharge in respect to reception orders.

Leave of Absence

An application for leave of absence on behalf of any mentally ill person (not being a mentally ill prisoner) undergoing treatment as an in-patient in any psychiatric hospital or psychiatric nursing home may be made to the medical officer incharge.

Every application shall be accompanied by a bond, with or without sureties for such amount as the medical officer incharge may specify, undertaking:

- To take proper care of the mentally ill person.
- To prevent the mentally ill person from causing injury to himself or to others.
- To bring back the mentally ill person to the psychiatric hospital, or as the case may be, psychiatric nursing home, on the expiry of the period of leave.

The total number of days for which leave of absence may be granted to a patient under this sub-section shall not exceed sixty days.

Chapter-VI Judicial Inquisition

This chapter deals with the judicial inquisition regarding the alleged mentally ill person possessing property, custody of his person and management of his property. If the court feels that the alleged mentally ill person is incapable of looking after both himself and his property, an order can be issued for the appointment of a guardian. If, however, it is felt that the person is only incapable of looking after his property but can look after himself, a manager can be appointed.

Chapter-VII Liability to Meet Cost of Maintenance of Mentally Ill

This chapter deals with the liability to meet the cost of maintenance of mentally ill persons detained in psychiatric hospitals or nursing homes. The relatives are liable to pay the cost of maintenance of the client. If the patient does not have any family or relatives the hospital/ government will take charge of the client.

Chapter-VIII Protection of Human Rights of Mentally Ill

This chapter is aimed at the protection of human rights of mentally ill persons.

Chapter-IX Penalties and Procedure

If the psychiatric nursing home /hospital are not fulfilling the requirements, they are liable to pay penalty.

Chapter-X Miscellaneous

This chapter includes the miscellaneous rules and regulations related to the care of a psychiatric client.

RIGHTS OF MENTALLY ILL CLIENTS

When a patient is admitted in psychiatric hospital, he may be deprived of the freedom to leave the hospital, and also to maintain certain legal rights. The rights are sometimes defined by state law and nursing personnel should know the law in the state in which they practice. The important legal rights are as follows:

- Unless the person is declared incompetent, he maintains the right to vote, to manage his financial affairs and to execute legal documents.
- Right not to be denied the basic necessities of life in the name of treatment.
- Right to treatment doctrine and not guilty by reasons of insanity and committed crimes.
- Voluntary patient has a right to refuse treatment. For example, electroconvulsive therapy (ECT) and psychosurgery.
- An involuntary patient cannot sign the bill and transfer his property by making will.
- Right to receive mail and contact with relatives, friends by using telephone.
- Right to have visitors for reasonable time.
- Right to have human and physical environment, and sufficient qualified staff personnel to look after them.
- Right not to be subjected to unnecessary mechanical restraints.
- Right to confidentiality of records.

LEGAL RESPONSIBILITIES OF MENTALLY ILL

Criminal Responsibility

McNaughton's Rule

In 1843, Daniel McNaughton shot and killed Sir Robert Peel's (British Prime Minister) secretary Edward Drummond. It was shown that McNaughton suffered from a number of delusions of persecution and that killing had been inspired by these delusions, and the judge directed the jury to find him not guilty. After lot of a debate in the House of Lords, the famous McNaughton's Rules were formulated in England.

This law is slightly modified in many countries even now. In India, McNaughton's rules have been adopted by section 84 of Indian Penal Code (IPC) of 1860 states that 'Nothing is an offense which is done by a person who, at the time of doing it by reason of unsoundness of mind, was incapable of knowing the nature of the act or that what he is doing was either wrong or contrary to law.'

The Law generally classifies criminal lunatics into three classes:

1. An under-trial who cannot stand trial because of mental illness; guilty but insane.
2. Criminals who later become mentally ill.
3. A class II 'criminal lunatic' is acquitted under the law but is detained in a mental hospital (asylum) for further treatment.

Civil Responsibility

- **Marriage:** Under Hindu Marriage Act (1955) a marriage between two parties, either of whom was of unsound mind at the time of marriage is considered void. Divorce can be obtained on the ground of unsoundness of mind for a specific continuous period.
- **Adoption:** Under the Hindu Adoptions and Maintenance Act (Act 78 of 1956), any hindu male 'who is of sound mind and is not a minor' can adopt a child, with the consent of his wife unless she has been declared to be of unsound mind' (Section 7).

Similarly, any hindu female 'who is of sound mind', is not a minor, and is not married, can adopt a child. If she is married, 'then her husband is dead, or has renounced the world, or ceased to be a hindu, or has been declared to be of unsound mind' (Section 8).

In addition, the person capable of giving in adoption of a child should be of sound mind.

- **Witness:** Under the Indian Evidence Act 1872, an insane person is not competent to give evidence if he is prevented by virtue of his 'lunacy' from understanding the questions put to him and giving rational answers to them (Section 118).

  However, such a person can give evidence during a lucid interval on discretion of the judge (and the jury).
- **Testamentary capacity:** Testamentary disposition is regulated by the Indian Succession Act (Act 39 of 1925). If the person is suffering from mental illness at the time of making his will and if he does not have the mental capacity to understand the consequences of the act, his will becomes invalid.
- **Transfer of property:** Under the Transfer of Property Act, 1882 (Section 7), only persons competent to contract, are authorized to transfer property.
- **Contract:** Under the Indian Contract Act, 1872 (Section 11), every person to be competent to contract must be a major and of sound mind.

  A person is said to be of sound mind for the purposes of a contract, if at the time of making a contract he is capable of understanding it and of forming a rational judgment as to its effect upon his interests.
- **Driving:** It is important that advice be given regarding driving if there is likelihood that driving can be impaired by the nature of illness, prescribed medication and/or misuse of alcohol or drugs.

THE NARCOTIC DRUGS AND PSYCHOTROPIC SUBSTANCES ACT (NDPSA), 1985

Drug dependence in India is dealt in law under Narcotic drugs and psychotropic substance Act (NDPSA). The Act was enacted on 16th September, 1985. It replaces the earlier Opium Acts and Dangerous Drugs Act. The act includes narcotic drugs like opium, poppy, heroin, cannabis, cocaine, coco and all related synthetic 'drugs' and psychotropic substances, e.g. major and minor tranquilizers, barbiturates, etc.

In this act, if a person produces, possesses, sells, transports, imports or uses any narcotic drugs or psychotropic substances, he or she shall be punishable with rigorous imprisonment for not less than 10 (may extend up to 20) years with a fine of not less than 1 lakh rupees (may extend up to 2 lakh).

For repeated offence, the punishment is rigorous imprisonment for not less than 15 (may extend up to 30) years and a fine of not less than 1.5 lakhs (may extend up to 3 lakh).

ROLE OF NURSE IN LEGAL/FORENSIC PSYCHIATRY

- **Standard care:** The nurse has to maintain the standardized patient care by knowing the policies and procedures of an organization.
- **Legal duty:** If nurse observes an action which may harm to the patient, she has to act immediately and protect the patient from injury.

- **Confidentiality:** Confidentiality relates to the responsibility of the nurse to keep all information, records and correspondence, confidential and to allow access to those who take care of the patient.
- **Informed consent:** Nurse should explain each procedure to the patient and relatives before doing it. She must allow the patient and relative to express their views and answer to any questions which need to be clarified.
- **Malpractice:** The term malpractice is often used interchangeably with negligence to define the acts of a professional person that are called into questions because of the lack of due care.
- **Intentional torts:** Intentional torts are when others interfere in an individual's privacy, mobility, property or personal interests.
- **Battery:** The intentional touching of another without the consent of client.
- **Assault:** An intentional act which places fear in another that an immediate battery (violent beating) is about to be committed on him/her.
- **False imprisonment:** An intentional act which prevents an individual from moving about wherever he wants to be.
- **Defamation:** Publication of a false statement about an individual made either verbally or in some other form to the third person.

  This damages his reputation. Violation of privacy-revealing personal information about an individual which may be little him or interfere with his personal private life.
- The nurse must know policy and routines of the institution and procedures of admission, discharge and leave of absence for mentally ill.
- She should know and protect the legal rights of a mentally ill.
- The nurse has to act as an advocate for mentally ill to obtain their needs.
- Psychiatric nurse has to ensure rehabilitation of the patient in the community.

15 Community Mental Health Nursing

The community mental health programme is considered as one of the landmark changes in psychiatry, shortening hospitalization. Caring for clients near their homes, and providing alternatives to in-patient care are positive, well accepted objectives of this movement.

DEFINITION

'Community mental health is the process of raising the level of mental health among people in a community and reducing the number of those suffering from mental illness.'

Evolution of Community Mental Health

- Born in 1963, the community psychiatry movement has been hailed as the fourth psychiatric revolution.

  The *first revolution* was the age of enlightenment following the middle ages, when mental illness was viewed as a consequence of sin and witchcraft. The *second revolution* was the development of psychoanalysis and the third one is the development of *psychopharmacology*.
- The *community psychiatry* concept has its antecedents in Clifford Beers' (1908) mental hygiene movement and Adolf Meyer's recommendation (1913) of establishment of treatment centers in the community.
- The period between 1955 and 1980 was an era of deinstitutionalization in USA and other Western countries.
- In 1975, the World Health Organization (WHO) recommended the delivery of mental health services through Primary Health Care (PHC) system as a policy for the developing countries.
- In India, attempts to develop models of psychiatric services in the primary health centre, (PHC) setting were made nearly simultaneously at PGI, Chandigarh in 1975 (Raipur Rani block of Ambala district, Haryana) and National Institute of Mental Health and Neurosciences (NIMHANS), Bengaluru in 1976 (Sakalwara in Karnataka).
- The basic model of community mental health was defined by Gerald Caplan in 1967.

Characteristics of Community Psychiatry

- Responsibility to a population for mental health care delivery.
- Treatment close to the patient in community-based centers.
- Provision of comprehensive services.
- Multidisciplinary team approach.

- Providing continuity of care.
- Emphasis on prevention as well as treatment.
- Avoidance of unnecessary hospitalization.

Community Mental Health Nursing

It is defined as the synthesis of community nursing and public health practice to promote, maintain and conserve the health of population aggregates in the community, with particular emphasis on mental health.

Importance/Aims/Goals of Community Mental Health Nursing

- To provide preventive, promotive, mental health services
- To implement continuity of care
- To screen population at risk and referral services
- To mobilize family support system in providing patient care
- To provide crisis intervention services
- Assist individual to develop a sense of independent living
- Organize mass health awareness
- Consultation and mental health education services
- Encourage community participation
- Protect clients from residual effects from home
- Provide care at home
- Arrange training programs for school teachers, community leaders regarding mental health services
- Long-term care.

Community Mental Health Team

The community mental health team includes:

- Psychiatrists (including child psychiatrist)
- Clinical psychologist
- Psychiatric social workers
- Psychiatric nurses
- Necessary administrative helps
- Clerical staff
- Occupational and recreational therapist for inpatient and partial hospitalization programmes
- Links to welfare workers, clergy
- Family agencies, school and other human service groups are also maintained.

NATIONAL MENTAL HEALTH PROGRAMME (NMHP)

Mental health is an integral component of health with this aim in mind, an expert group was formed in 1980.

The Government of India has launched the National Mental Health Programme (NMHP) in 1982, keeping in view the heavy burden of mental illness in the community, and the absolute inadequacy of mental health care infrastructure in the country to deal with it.

The National Mental Health Programme (NMHP) appeared almost simultaneously with the National Health Policy (1993).

The Objectives of NMHP

- To ensure availability and accessibility of minimum mental health care for all in the foreseeable future, particularly to the most vulnerable and under privileged sections of population.
- To encourage application of mental health knowledge in general health care and in the social development.
- To promote community participation in mental health services development, and to stimulate efforts towards self-help in the community.

Aims

- Prevention and treatment of mental and neurological disorders and their associated disabilities.
- Use of mental health technology to improve general health services.
- Application of mental health principles in total national development to improve quality of life.

Strategies

- **Center to periphery strategy:** Establishment and strengthening of psychiatric units in all district hospitals, with outpatient clinics and mobile teams reaching the population for mental health services.
- **Periphery to center strategy:** Training of an increasing number of different categories of health personnel in basic mental health skills, with primary emphasis towards the poor and the underprivileged, directly benefiting about 200 million people.

Components of NMHP

There are three components of the program they are as follows:

1. Treatment subprogramme
2. Rehabilitation subprogramme
3. Prevention subprogramme

Treatment Subprogramme

At Village and Subcenter Level

Multipurpose workers (MPW) and health supervisors, under the supervision of medical officer, to be trained for:

- Management of psychiatric emergencies.
- Administration and supervision of maintenance treatment for chronic psychiatric disorders.
- Diagnosis and management of grand mal epilepsy, especially in children.

- Liaison with local school teacher and parents regarding mental retardation and behavior problems in children.
- Counseling in problems related to alcohol and drug abuse.

At Primary Health Center

Medical officer, to be trained for:

- Supervision of MPW's performance
- Elementary diagnosis
- Treatment of functional psychosis
- Treatment of uncomplicated cases of psychiatric disorders associated with physical diseases
- Management of uncomplicated psychosocial problems
- Epidemiological surveillance of mental morbidity.

At District Hospital

- There should be at least 1 psychiatrist attached to every district hospital as an integral part of the district health services.
- The district hospital should have 30–50 psychiatric beds.
- The psychiatrist in a district hospital was envisaged to devote only a part of his time in clinical care and greater part in training and supervision of non-specialist health workers.

Mental Hospitals and Teaching Psychiatric Units

These are the higher centers for psychiatric care and the activities include:

- Help in care of 'difficult' cases.
- Teaching
- Specialized facilities such as occupational therapy units, psychotherapy, counseling and behavior therapy.

Rehabilitation Subprogramme

The components of this subprogramme include:

- Maintenance treatment of epileptics and psychotics at the community levels.
- Development of rehabilitation centers at both the district level and the higher referral centers.

Prevention Subprogramme

The prevention component is to be community based, with the initial focus on prevention and control of alcohol-related problems. Later, problems such as addictions, juvenile delinquency and acute adjustment problems such as suicidal attempts are to be addressed.

The other approaches designed to achieve the objectives of the NMHP include:

- Integration of basic mental health care into general health services.
- Mental health training of general medical doctors and paramedical health workers.

THE DISTRICT MENTAL HEALTH PROGRAMME (DMHP)

The District Mental Health Programme (DMHP) was started in 1995 as a component of NMHP. The prototype of the District Mental Health Programme was the Bellary District Programme (in Karnataka). Started in 1985, it caters to a population of 1.5 million. District hospital psychiatry units have been opened in every district of Kerala and Tamil Nadu.

Components

- Training for all workers in the mental health team at the identified nodal institutes in the state
- Public education in the mental health to increase awareness and reduce stigma
- Providing valuable data and experience at the level of community to the state and center for future planning, improvement in service and research.

NMHP and 10th Five Year Plan

- The 10th five year plan was launched, with a plan to extend the DMHP to 100 districts.
- It also emphasizes the need to broaden the scope of existing curriculum for undergraduate training in psychiatry and to give more exposure to psychiatry.
- An essential list of psychotropic drugs was also being prepared.
- The emphasis of NMHP, 1982 was primarily on the rural sector. It is being realized that the urban mental health needs also need to be addressed under the ambit of NMHP.
- During the 11th five year plan, an allocation of ₹ 1000 crore (₹ 10 billion) has been made for the NMHP.
- The current focus is on establishing centers of excellence in mental health, increasing intake capacity and starting postgraduate courses in psychiatry.
- Modernization of mental hospitals and upgradation of medical college psychiatry departments.

INSTITUTIONALIZATION AND DEINSTITUTIONALIZATION

Institutionalization

Institutionalization is the process of committing a person to a mental hospital. In western countries especially in Europe and America institutionalization began as early as 17th century itself. During this period it was just custodial rather than curative.

Purpose of Institutionalization

- Prevention of self-harm and to others
- Rapid diagnosis and evaluation
- Management of the symptoms and emergency situation
- Decreasing the maladaptive behaviors.

Issues of Institutionalization

- Overcrowding in institutions
- Inadequate staffing
- Unable to adjust with independent living
- Failure to cure most of the mental illnesses.

Deinstitutionalization

The withdrawal of the individual with mental illness from institutions and the subsequent plan to provide care at community setup.

Aims

- To reduce population size of mental institutions
- To remove institutional processes from mental hospitals that may create dependency, hopelessness and other maladaptive behaviors.

Positive Effects of Deinstitutionalization

- Integrating family and social system in the care of patients
- Better care would be provided to mentally ill in their home communities with adequate social support
- Helps to develop independent living among the clients.

Negative Effects of Deinstitutionalization

- The stigma towards mentally ill still in most of the communities so that adequate support system is not available in many of the communities.
- Because of the above issues patients are often returned to the hospitals, stabilized and discharged again follow a cycling pattern of this.
- Emergency department use by acutely ill patient increased dramatically.
- Homelessness among patients increased.

MODEL OF COMMUNITY MENTAL HEALTH—PREVENTIVE PSYCHIATRY

Caplan discussed three levels of preventive intervention from the public health model to mental illness and disturbance.

Levels of Prevention

The prevention for psychiatric disorders follows the same principles as in case of other disorders and has been divided into:

- Primary prevention
- Secondary prevention
- Tertiary prevention.

Goals of Preventive Psychiatry

Decrease the onset (incidence), duration (prevalence and residual disability of mental disorders).

Primary Prevention

- The goal of primary prevention is to prevent the onset of a disease or disorder there by reducing its incidence
- Complete screening and diagnostic evaluation
- Health education to vulnerable groups/high risk group.

Secondary Prevention

- Secondary prevention is defined as early identification and prompt treatment
- Lowering the intensity and severity of the illness
- Increasing the supportive system
- Crisis intervention
- Referral to higher level.

Tertiary Prevention

- Lowering the disability and relapse
- Increasing the self-esteem
- Occupational training
- Prepare for self/re-employment and home bound employment.

Role of Community Mental Health Nurse in Preventive Psychiatry

Community mental health nursing is the application of knowledge of psychiatric nursing in preventing, promoting and maintaining mental health of the people, to help in early diagnosis and case and to rehabilitate the patients after mental illness.

Nurse plays an important role in primary, secondary and tertiary prevention of mental illness.

Nurses Role in Primary Prevention

Nurse play a major role in identifying high-risk groups and preventing the occurrence of mental illness in them. Some of these measures includes:

- Providing antenatal care and educating the mother to be regarding the adverse effects of irradiation, certain drugs and prematurely.
- Ensuring timely obstetrical assistance to safeguard against the ill effects of anoxia and injury to the newborn at birth.
- Providing destroy correction to infant suffering from metabolic disorders.
- Correcting endocrinal disorders.
- Planning and implementing training programs for the mentally and physically handicapped children like the blind, deaf, mute, etc.
- Identifying the problems of scholastic performance and emotional disturbance among school going children and giving timely intervention.
- Teaching the family members adaptive coping techniques.
- Counseling adolescents and retired persons passing through transitional crisis, brave families to accept the loss, etc.
- Educate the teachers and parents on maintaining a healthy environment at school and home.
- Keep contact with voluntary agencies.
- Interaction with social welfare personnel.

Nurses Role in Secondary Prevention

Nurses play an important role:

- Early diagnosis and case finding
- Early referral

- Screen programs
- Early and effective treatment for the patient and if necessary family members
- Mental health education
- Crisis intervention
- Consultation services.

Nurses Role in Tertiary Prevention

- Social reintegration of the discharged chronic mentally ill back into the community.
- Vocational rehabilitation and job placement for the mentally restore.
- Re-equipping the mentally restored with daily living care abilities.
- Administration of medication at the doorstep of the mentally ill.
- Utilizing the resources of the family and community for the rehabilitation of the mentally restored.

Box 15.1: Existing mental health services and manpower in India

No. of government mental hospitals	= 37
No. of mental hospital beds	= ~19000
Private psychiatric hospital beds	= 2000–3000
General hospital psychiatry unit beds (GHPU beds)	= 4000–5000
Psychiatric beds in India per 10, 000 population	= 0.25
Psychiatrists (qualified) in India	= ~3500
Clinical psychologists in India numbers	= ~1000
Psychiatric social workers numbers	= ~1000
Psychiatric nurses in India numbers	= 800–900
Postgraduate centers	= ~40 (very few of 140 medical colleges have a psychiatry department)

Community Facilities Available for Psychiatric Patients

Day Hospital/Centers

This facility is organized on a day time basis. The patient receives a full range of treatment, services, and returns home at the end of the day. The concept introduced by DE Cameran in 1946, is now being used in rehabilitation and psychiatric care.

A day hospital is staffed by trained psychiatrist and other team members. In India only a few day care centers are available for mentally ill. The family feels relief for few hours in a day and develops coping energy for the rest of the time when the patient is at home. The patient develops discipline and routine.

Halfway Home

It is a transition facility for psychiatric patients who no longer need the full services of a hospital but are not yet ready for a completely independent living. They need supervision for medication and for carrying on domestic activities. If they are still in job, they will leave for to job and come back to this halfway house. Medical facilities are regularly provided.

Group Homes

These homes belong to hospital or rented by 15–20 mentally ill recovering patients. These are patients stay together, meet their financial commitments and like in a society like other members. They try to provide moral emotional and social support to each other. If the one or the members is leading towards release, others try to help him by providing support.

Foster Homes

It is a home in which a patient recovering from a mental disorder is placed in voluntary family by a social agency for family care. The family is paid by the agency. Placement may be temporary or permanent. The patient gets a home like environment.

Sheltered Workshop

It is a work oriented rehabilitation facility with a controlled working environment to fulfill the individual's conational goals. In this workshop ex-long-term mentally ill patients can utilize their experience and abilities by relearning. This helps the patient to make progress towards a normal living and economic independence.

Self-help Groups

Self–help groups in the community will help the individual as well as members of the family. Alcoholic anonymous groups, drug addiction groups, groups of patients with mental retardation are a few of the examples.

MENTAL HEALTH AGENCIES

The mental health agency called a local management entity manages services for mental health developmental disability. Drug and alcohol abuse and now does that mostly through contracts with private providers rather than a staff of its own. They are of following types:

- Government
- Voluntary agencies
  - National
  - International

Government Mental Health Agencies

Psychiatric care and rehabilitation in India is partly hospital based and largely confined to the government mental hospital. Some of them are:

- NIMHANS, Bengaluru
- The Central Institute of Psychiatry, Ranchi
- Institute of Mental Health, Chennai
- Govt. Mental Health Center, Thiruvananthapuram
- Govt. Mental Health Center, Calicut
- Vidyasagar Institute of Mental Health and Neurosciences, New Delhi
- Mental Health Center, Christian Medical College (CMC), Vellore
- All India Institute of Medical Sciences, Department of Psychiatry, etc.

National Agencies

Some of the national agencies related to mental health services are as follows:

- SCARF (Schizophrenia research foundation), Chennai

- Medico Pastoral Association (MPA), Bengaluru
- AA group (Alcoholic Anonymous) group in many part of the country
- TT Krishnamachari Foundation, Chennai
- MS Chellamuthu Trust, Madurai, Tamil Nadu
- Paripurnata, Kolkata, West Bengal
- Sneha (Chennai), Saarthak, Delhi–is a Mental Health Institution and Prerna (Mumbai) work on suicide prevention activities
- Bapu Trust (Pune) women's mental health
- Ashagram in Madhya Pradesh.

International Agencies

- World health organization (WHO) development of community based mental health program.
- World federation of mental health (WFMH)
  - Promotes mental health and optimum function
  - Heighten public awareness about importance of mental health
  - Improve the care and treatment of those suffering from mental illnesses.

Psychiatric Nursing Organizations

- Indian society of psychiatric nurses
- The disability network of India
- Kerala state mental health authority

MENTAL HEALTH ISSUES OF SPECIAL POPULATION

Children and Adolescents

Untreated mental illness, mental disabilities and developmental disabilities in children have major outcomes in terms of personality development and mental disorders in adult life.

There are several types of child abuse, but the end result will be the emotional disturbance in the child. The common forms may be *emotional abuse* (in the form of shaming, humiliating, threatening, limited physical contact with the child etc), child neglect (failing to give a child's basic needs), physical and sexual abuse.

Psychiatric Disorders in Adolescence

- Antisocial
- Affective disorders
- Somatization disorders
- Alcohol and drug abuse
- Poor job performance
- Unstable interpersonal relationships
- Accident proneness
- Low academic achievement.

The genesis of deviant behavior in children and adolescents can be traced back to, more than any other single factor, the decay of parenting, which in then is a direct consequence of the declaim of family basic building block of civilized society.

The institution of the traditional family rests on four pillars.

1. Shared values
2. Shared goals
3. Shared emotional concern
4. Shared activities.

Women

The daily newspapers carry news of female infanticide.

- Rape
- Wives fortuned for not bringing enough dowries
- Discrimination against women
- Denial of their basic rights.

Problems in Women

- Female literacy and mental health.
- Women and common mental disorder
  - For example, depression
- Chronic mental illness
  - Anxiety
  - Depression
  - HIV
- Suicide and self-harm
- Mentally ill women and their marriages
- Other psychosis.

Rehabilitation of Women

Usually the women brought for rehabilitation are more often accompanied by their parents than their spouse, even if they are married. The focus of rehabilitation has to be on activities of daily living (ADL), performance of domestic chores, parenting skills, interpersonal relations within family.

Elderly

Problems of elderly people include:

- Mental illness associated with physical illness
- Handicap or disability
- Deflect of visual, hearing
- Hypertension
- Diabetes mellitus
- Cardiovascular disorders
- Osteoarthritis

- Abuse (physical, emotional and sexual)
- Neglect caregiver's refusal
- Financial exploitation.

Psychiatric Illness

- Nonorganic psychosis (43%)
- Organic psychosis (22%)
- Neurosis (17%)
- Alzheimer's disease
- Dementia
- Anxiety
- Depression.

Care of Elderly

- Public health sector
- Geriatric medicine as a special area of health care hospitals
- Old age homes in India 354 in 1997
- Urban lenders
- Medical and recreational facilities
- Family is still the primary source of care.

Victims of Violence and Abuse

Family violence is an act of action performed by a family member to get the decided conformity from the other members and when it carries a negative emotional component.

Types

- Physical violence (94%)
- Verbal and psychological violence (75%)
- Quelty to loved ones (12%)
- Abuse from in-laws (5%).

Problems

- Family violence
- Physical symptoms due to battering
- Psychological symptoms
- Child abuse
- Wife abuse
- Elder abuse
- Rape and sexual assault.

HIV/AIDS

Psychiatric Aspects

- Disorders around the time of seroconversion
- Discovery of serostatus

- Asymptomatic and early symptomatic phases of infection
  - Adjust mental disorders
  - Suicide
- Disorders of symptomatic phase and aids
  - Delirium
  - HIV-associated cognitive/motor complex (AIDS dementia complex)
  - Psychotic disorders(organic mood syndrome)
  - For example, mania, euphoria, grandiose, delusions, schizophrenia.
- Neurological aspects
- Neurological problems
  - For example, headache
  - Meningeal irritation.

Nursing Care

- Safe environment
- Structured activity schedule
- Emotional support
- Therapeutic communication
- Attention to nutrition
- Sleep to feel comfort.

Physically Handicapped

The problems of the physically have many facets, varied in nature and poses differing attitudes at various level in society.

The handicapped individuals often develops the feelings of insecurity, anxiety, depression, negative self-concept, isolation, frustration, unemployment, mobilization, difficulties, economical dependency, poor socialization, substance abuse and homelessness. Lacks of cohesive family bond has led to violence and health hazard of various levels.

Many need assistance in physical and vocational rehabilitation. Based on the assessment of their residual vocational capacities, they may be assisted in:

- Developing their work skills in suitable traders by means of formal or informal training.
- Arranging essential rehabilitation aids with a view to enhancing their physical functioning and thereby increasing their work capacities.
- Securing suitable employment/self-employment/home bound employment for them
- Utilizing their own resources to the extent possible, for their carrier development and their integration in the society through individuals/group counseling, guidance, adjustment training and social adjustment.

The physically disabled requires not only vocational rehabilitation but also medical and educational and social rehabilitation.

16 Miscellaneous

PSYCHIATRIC NURSING PROCESS

INTRODUCTION

The nursing process is an interactive, problem-solving process. It is systematic and individualized way to achieve outcome of nursing care. The nursing process respects the individual's autonomy and freedom to make decisions and be involved in nursing care.

The nurse and the patient emerge as partner in a relationship built on trust and directed toward maximizing the patient's strengths, maintaining integrity, and promoting adaptive response to stress.

In dealing with psychiatric patients, the nursing process can present unique challenges. Emotional problems may be vague, not visible like many physiological disruptions. This can also show different symptoms and arise from a number of causes. Similarly, past events may lead to very different form of present behaviors.

Many psychiatric patients are unable to describe their problems. They may be highly withdrawn, highly anxious, or out of touch with reality. Their ability to participate in the problem-solving process may also be limited if they see themselves as powerless.

Nursing process aims at individualized care to the patient and the care is adapted to patient's unique needs. The following steps for nursing process are:

- Assessment
- Nursing diagnosis
- Outcome identification
- Planning
- Implementation
- Evaluation.

Assessment

Individualized care begins with a detailed assessment as soon as the patient is admitted. In the assessment phase, information is obtained of the patient in a direct and structured manner through observation, interviews and examination. Initial interview includes an evaluation of mental status. In such cases, where the patient is too ill to participate in or complete the interview, the behavior of patient exhibits to be recorded and reports from family members if possible, can obtained.

Assessment is a systematic way of identifying the clients actual or potential health problems. Even when the initial assessment is complete, each encounter with the patient involves a continuing assessment. The ongoing assessment involves what patient is saying or doing at that moment.

When the nurse investigates a patient's specific behavior, it is valuable to explore the following:

- Situation that precipitated that behavior
- What the patient was thinking at that moment?
- Whether that behavior makes any sense in that context?
- Whether the behavior was adaptive or dysfunctional?
- Whether a change is needed?

If the nurse has to interview the patient, she should select a private place, free from noise and distraction and interview should be goal directed. Although, the patient is a regarded as a source of validation, the nurse should also be prepared to consult with family members or other people knowledgeable about the patient.

This is particularly important when the patient is unable to provide reliable information because of the symptoms of psychiatric illness. She should gather information from other information sources, including health care records, nursing rounds, change of shifts, nursing care plans and evaluation of other health care professionals.

Nursing Diagnosis

After collecting all data, the nurse compares the information and then analyses the data and derives a nursing diagnosis.

A nursing diagnosis is a statement of the patient's nursing problem that includes both the adaptive and maladaptive health responses and contributing stressors. These nursing problems concern patient's health aspects that may need to be promoted or with which the patient needs help. A nursing diagnostic statement consists of three parts:

1. Health problems
2. Contributing factors
3. Defining characteristics.

The defining characteristics are helpful because they reflect the behavior that are the target of nursing intervention. They also provide specific indicators for evaluating the outcome of psychiatric nursing interventions and for determining whether the expected goals of the nursing care were met. For example, If a patient is making statements about dying, he is isolative, anorexic, cannot sleep and wants to die. Then, the nursing diagnosis can be:

- Helplessness related to physical complaints, as evidenced by decreased appetite and verbal cues indicating despondency.
- Fatigue related to insomnia, as evidenced by an increase in physical complaints and disinterest in surroundings.
- Social isolation related to anxiety, as evidenced by withdrawal and uncommunicative behavior.

Outcome Identification

The psychiatric mental health nurse identifies expected outcomes individualized to the patient. Within the context of providing nursing care, the ultimate goal is to influence the health outcomes and improve the patient's health status. Outcomes should be mutually identified with the patient, and should be identified as clearly and determine the effectiveness and efficiency of their interventions.

Before defining expected outcomes, the nurse must realize that patient often seek treatment with goals of their own. These goals may be expressed as relieving symptoms or improving functional ability. The nurse must understand the patient's coping response and the factors that influence them. Some of these difficulties in defining goals are as follows:

- The patient may view a personal problem as someone else's behavior.
- The patient may express a problem as feeling, such as 'I am lonely' or 'I am so unhappy'.

Clarifying goals is an essential step in the therapeutic process. Therefore, the patient-nurse relationship should be based upon mutually agreed goals. Once the goals are agreed on, they must be stated in writing. Goals should be written in behavioral terms, and should be realistically described what the nurse wishes to accomplish within a specific time span. Expected outcomes and short-term goals should be developed with short-term objectives contributing to the long-term expected outcomes. Example of short-term goals:

- At the end of the two weeks, patients will stay out of bed and participate in activities.
- At the end of the one week, patient will sleep well at night.
- At the end of the one week, patient will eat properly and maintain weight.

Planning

As soon as the patient's problems are identified, nursing diagnosis made, planning of nursing care begins. The planning consists of:

- Determining priorities
- Setting goals
- Selecting nursing actions
- Developing/writing nursing care plan

In planning the care the nurse can involve the patient, family, members of the health team. Once the goals are chosen the next task is to outline the plan achieving them. On the basis of an analysis, the nurse decides which problem requires priority attention or immediate attention.

Goals stated indicates as to what is to be achieved if the identified problem is taken care of. These can be immediate short-term and long-term goals. The nursing action technique chosen will enable the nurse to meet the goals or desired objectives. For example, the short-terms for a depressed patient is 'to pursue him or her to take bath'. The nursing action may be 'the nurse firmly direct the patient to get up and finish her/his bath before 8 o'clock. On persuasion the patient takes bath. This is an example of selection of the nursing action. Writing or recording of the problems, goals, and nursing actions is a nursing care plan.

Implementation

The implementation phase of the nursing process is the actual initiation of the nursing care plan. Patient outcome/goals are achieved by the performance of the nursing interventions. During the phase, the nurse continues to assess the patient to determine whether interventions are effective.

An important part of this phase is documentation. Documentation is necessary for legal reasons because in legal dispute 'if it was not charted, it was not done'. The nursing interventions are designed to prevent mental and physical illness and promote, maintain, and restore mental and physical health. The nurse may select interventions according to their level of practice.

She may select counseling, wilieu therapy, self-care activities, psychological interventions, health teaching, case management, health promotion and health maintenance and other approaches to meet the mental health care needs of the patient.

To implement the actions, nurses need to have intellectual, interpersonal and technical skills. Nursing actions are of two types:

1. **Dependent nursing actions :** Actions derived from the advice from the psychiatrist. For example, giving medicines.
2. **Independent nursing actions:** This is based on nursing diagnosis and plan of care, pursuing the patient to attend to personal hygiene.

Evaluation

The continuous or ongoing phase of nursing process is evaluation. Nursing care is a dynamic process involving change in the patient's health status over time, giving rise to the need of new data, different diagnosis, and modifications in the plan of care.

When evaluating care, the nurse should review all previous phases of the nursing process and determine whether expected outcome for the patient have been met. This can be done by checking–have I done everything for my patient? Is my patient better after the planned care?

Evaluation is a feedback mechanism for judging the quality of care given. Evaluation of the patient's progress indicates what problems of the patient have been solved, which need to be assessed again, replanted, implemented and re-evaluated.

APPENDICES

APPENDIX 1

Psychiatric History Collection Format

1. **Identification Data**
   - Name :
   - IP Number/Client ID :
   - Age :
   - Sex :
   - Address :
   - Education :
   - Occupation :
   - Income :
   - Religion :
   - Marital status :
   - Date of admission :
   - Date of care started :
   - Date of care ended :
   - Diagnosis :
2. **Informant**
   - Name of informant :
   - Relation with patient :
3. **Presenting Chief Complaints**
   - According to patient :
   - According to informant :
4. **History of Present Illness**
   - Onset : Acute/subacute/insidious.
   - Duration : Weeks/months/years.
   - Precipitating factor :
   - Relieving factor :
5. **Treatment History**
   - Drugs, ECT, psychotherapy, family therapy, etc. :
6. **Past Psychiatric History and Medical History**
   - Hospitalization :
   - Substance use :
   - Surgical procedures/accidents/head injury/DM, etc. :
7. **Family History**
   - Genogram :
   - Family composition :

8. **Personal History**
   - **Perinatal History**
     - **Antenatal Period** : **Uneventful/eventful**
     - Birth : Full term/premature/postmature
     - Delivery : Normal/instrumental/caesarean
     - Birth cry : Immediate/delayed
     - Birth defects :
     - Postnatal complications :
   - **Childhood History**
     - Primary caregiver :
     - Feeding : Breastfed/Artificial
     - Age at weaning :
     - Developmental milestones : Normal/delayed
     - Behavior and emotional problems
   - **Educational History**
     - Age at beginning of formal education :
     - Academic performance :
     - Relationship with peers :
     - School phobia :
     - Reason for termination of studies :
   - **Play History**
     - Games played, relation with playmates
   - **Emotional Problems during Adolescence**
     - Running away from home/smoking/drug abuse, etc.
   - **Puberty**
     - Age at menarche :
     - Appearance of secondary sexual characteristics
     - Anxiety related to puberty :
     - Regularity, duration of menstrual flow :
     - Masturbation :
   - **Obstetrical History**
     - LMP :
     - Number of children :
     - Termination of pregnancy and menopause, etc. :
   - **Occupational History**
     - Age at starting work :
     - Reason for changing job :
     - Current job satisfaction :
     - Present income :
     - Whether the job is appropriate to client's background
   - **Sexual and Marital History**
     - Type of marriage :
     - Duration of marriage :

- Number of marriage :
- Interpersonal and sexual relations :
- Details of spouse and children :

- **Premorbid Personality**
  - Interpersonal relationships :
  - Use of leisure time :
  - Predominant mood : Optimistic/pessimistic
  - Attitude towards self and others :
  - Attitude to work and responsibility :
  - Religious beliefs and moral attitudes :
  - Fantasy life :
  - **Habits:** Eating pattern/sleeping pattern/elimination/sleeping pattern/use of drugs/ tobacco, etc.

APPENDIX 2

Mental Status Examination

- **General Appearance and Behavior**
  - **Appearance:** Looking one's age/older/younger
  - **Level of grooming:** Normal/shabbily dressed/over dressed/idiosyncratically dressed
  - **Level of cleanliness:** Adequate/inadequate/overtly clean
  - **Level of consciousness:** Fully conscious and alert/drowsy/stuporous/comatosed
  - **Mode of entry:** Came willingly/brought using physical force
  - **Cooperativeness:** Normal/more than so/less than so
  - **Eye to eye contact:** Maintained/difficult/not maintained
  - **Psychomotor activity:** Normal/increased/decreased
  - **Gestures:** Normal/exaggerated/odd
  - **Posture:** Normal/catatonic
  - **Other movements:** Stereotypes/tremors, etc.
  - **Other catatonic phenomena**
  - **Conversion and dissociative signs**
  - **Hallucinatory behavior**

  Inference
- **Speech**
  - **Initiation:** Spontaneous/speaks when spoken to/minimal/mute
  - **Reaction time:** Normal/delayed/shortened/difficult to assess
  - **Rate:** Normal /slow/rapid
  - **Productivity:** Decreased/increased
  - **Volume:** Normal/increased/decreased
  - **Tone:** Normal variation/monotonous
  - **Relevance:** Fully relevant/sometimes off target/Irrelevant
  - **Stream:** Normal/circumstantial/tangential
  - **Coherence:** Fully coherent/loosening of association
  - **Others:** Rhyming/echolalia/neologism, etc.

  Inference
- **Mood**
  - **Subjective**
  - **Objective**

  Inference
- **Thought**
  - **Stream:** Normal/pressure of thought/thought block/flight of ideas, etc.
  - **Form:** Normal/formal thought disorder
  - **Content:** Ideas/delusions/obsessional/compulsive phenomena

  Inference

- **Perception**
  - **Hallucinations:** Auditory/visual/olfactory/gustatory/tactile
  - **Somatic passivity**
  - **Illusions**
  - **Depersonalization and derealization**

  Inference
- **Cognitive Function**
  - **Consciousness:** Conscious/cloudy/comatosed
  - **Orientation:** Time/place/person
  - **Attention:** Normally aroused/aroused with difficulty
  - Digits forward, digits backward
  - **Concentration:** Normally sustained/sustained with difficulty/distractible 100-7/40-3/20-1
  - Name of month (backwards)
  - Name of weekdays (backwards)
  - **Memory:** Immediate
  - **Recent** (recent happenings–Last meal, visitors, etc.)
  - **Remote:** Personal events/impersonal events/illness-relate events
  - **Intelligence:** Arithmetic ability/mental arithmetic/written sums
  - **Abstraction:** Normal/concrete, interpretation of proverbs/similarities between paired objects/dissimilarities between paired objects.

  Inference
- **Insight**
  - **Awareness of abnormal behavior/experience** : Yes/maybe/ no
  - **Attribution to physical causes** : Yes/maybe/ no
  - **Recognition of personal responsibility** : Yes/maybe/no
  - **Willingness to take treatment** : Yes/maybe/no

  Inference
- **Judgment**
  - **Personal** : Intact/impaired
  - **Social** : Intact/impaired
  - **Test** : Intact/impaired

  Inference

APPENDIX 3

Case Study Format

1. **Identification Data**
   - Name :
   - Age :
   - Sex :
   - Address :
   - Education :
   - Occupation :
   - Income :
   - Religion :
   - Marital status :
   - Date of admission :
   - Date of care started :
   - Date of care ended :
   - Diagnosis :
2. **Informant**
   - Name of informant :
   - Relation with patient :
3. **Chief Complaints**
   - According to patient :
   - According to informant :
4. **Present Psychiatric History**
   - Onset : Acute/subacute/insidious
   - Duration : Weeks/months/years
   - Precipitating factor :
   - Relieving factor :
5. **Treatment History**
   - Drugs, ECT, psychotherapy, family therapy, etc. :
6. **Past Psychiatric History**
   - Hospitalization :
   - Substance use :
   - Surgical procedures/accidents/head injury/DM, etc. :
7. **Family History**
   - Genogram :
   - Family composition :

8. **Personal History**

- **Perinatal History**
  - Antenatal period : Uneventful/eventful
  - Birth : Full term/premature/postmature
  - Delivery : Normal/instrumental/cesarean
  - Birth cry : Immediate/delayed
  - Birth defects :
  - Postnatal complications :
- **Childhood History**
  - Primary caregiver :
  - Feeding : Breastfed/artificial
  - Age at weaning :
  - Developmental milestones : Normal/delayed
  - Behavior and emotional problems
- **Educational History**
  - Age at beginning of formal education :
  - Academic performance :
  - Relationship with peers :
  - School phobia :
  - Reason for termination of studies :
- **Play History**
  - Games played, relation with playmates
- **Emotional Problems During Adolescence**
  - Running away from home/smoking/drug abuse, etc.
- **Puberty**
  - Age at menarche :
  - Appearance of secondary sexual characteristics
  - Anxiety related to puberty :
  - Regularity, duration of menstrual flow :
  - Masturbation :
- **Obstetrical History**
  - LMP :
  - Number of children :
  - Termination of pregnancy and menopause, etc. :
- **Occupational History**
  - Age at starting work :
  - Reason for changing job :
  - Current job satisfaction :
  - Present income :
  - Whether the job is appropriate to client's background
- **Sexual and Marital History**
  - Type of marriage :
  - Duration of marriage :

- Number of marriage :
- Interpersonal and sexual relations :
- Details of spouse and children :

• Pre-morbid Personality
- Interpersonal relationships :
- Use of leisure time :
- Predominant mood : Optimistic/pessimistic
- Attitude towards self and others :
- Attitude to work and responsibility :
- Religious beliefs and moral attitudes :
- Fantasy life :
- Habits: Eating pattern/Sleeping pattern/Elimination/Sleeping pattern/Use of drugs/tobacco, etc.

Mental Status Examination

(A) General Appearance and Behavior

- **Appearance:** Looking one's age/older/younger
- **Level of grooming:** Normal/shabbily dressed/over dressed/idiosyncratically dressed
- **Level of cleanliness:** Adequate/inadequate/overtly clean
- **Level of consciousness:** Fully conscious and alert/drowsy/stuporous/comatosed
- **Mode of entry:** Came willingly/brought using physical force
- **Cooperativeness:** Normal/more than so/less than so
- **Eye to eye contact:** Maintained/difficult/not maintained
- **Psychomotor activity:** Normal/increased/decreased
- **Gestures:** Normal/exaggerated/odd
- **Posture:** Normal/catatonic
- **Other movements:** Stereotypes/tremors, etc.
- **Other catatonic phenomena**
- **Conversion and dissociative signs**
- **Hallucinatory behavior**

Inference

(B) Speech

- **Initiation:** Spontaneous/speaks when spoken to/minimal/mute
- **Reaction time:** Normal/delayed/shortened/difficult to assess
- **Rate:** Normal/slow/rapid
- **Productivity:** Decreased/increased
- **Volume:** Normal/increased/decreased
- **Tone:** Normal variation/monotonous
- **Relevance:** Fully relevant/sometimes off target/irrelevant
- **Stream:** Normal/circumstantial/tangential

- **Coherence:** Fully coherent/loosening of association
- **Others:** Rhyming/echolalia/neologism, etc.

Inference

(C) Mood

- Subjective
- Objective

Inference

(D) Thought

- **Stream:** Normal/pressure of thought/thought block/flight of ideas, etc.
- **Form:** Normal/formal thought disorder
- **Content:** Ideas/delusions/obsessional/compulsive phenomena

Inference

(E) Perception

- **Hallucinations:** Auditory/visual/olfactory/gustatory/tactile
- **Somatic passivity**
- **Illusions**
- **Depersonalization and derealization**

Inference

(F) Cognitive Function

- **Consciousness:** Conscious/cloudy/comatosed
- **Orientation:** Time/place/person
- **Attention:** Normally aroused/aroused with difficulty
- Digits forward, digits backward
- **Concentration:** Normally sustained/sustained with difficulty/distractible 100-7/40-3/20-1
- Name of month/(backwards)
- Name of week days/(backwards)
- **Memory:** Immediate
- Recent (recent happenings–Last meal, visitors, etc.)
- **Remote:** Personal events/impersonal events/illness-relate events
- **Intelligence:** Arithmetic ability/mental arithmetic/written sums
- **Abstraction:** Normal/concrete, interpretation of proverbs/similarities between paired objects/dissimilarities between paired objects.

Inference

(G) Insight

- **Awareness of abnormal behavior/experience** : Yes/may be/ no
- **Attribution to physical causes** : Yes/may be/ no
- **Recognition of personal responsibility** : Yes/may be/no
- **Willingness to take treatment** : Yes/may be/no

Inference

(H) Judgement

- **Personal** : Intact/impaired
- **Social** : Intact/impaired
- **Test** : Intact/impaired.

Inference

Physical Examination

- Head :
- Eye :
- Ear :
- Nose :
- Face, neck, throat :
- Chest :
- Abdomen :
- Extremities :
- Genitalia :
- Back :
- Vital signs :

Laboratory Investigations

Sl. No.	Name of the test	Patient value	Normal value	Remarks

Medications

Sl no.	Name of the drug	Dose	Route	Action	Indications	Contraindications	Side effects	Nurses responsibility

Review of Literature

- Anatomy and physiology
- Definition
- Epidemiology
- Etiological factors
- Psychopathology
- Clinical features
- Investigations
- Treatment
- Nursing management

Sl No.	Book Picture	Patient Picture

Process Recording

Place:

Date and Time:

Objectives of Interview:

(1)

(2)

(3)

Person	Verbatim	Nonverbal communication	Inference

Summary: List of inferences.
Care plans made according to inferences.
Any special difficulties faced during the inference.
Techniques used to overcome the difficulties.

Nursing Care Plan

NANDA approved Nursing Diagnosis according to priority.

Assessment	Nursing diagnosis	Nursing goal	Planning	Implementation	Evaluation
Subjective data Objective data					

Psychoeducation

Conclusion

Bibliography

APPENDIX 4

Geriatric Assessment Form

Identification data

- Date of visit : ……………………………………
- Place of living : ……………………………………
- Name : ……………………………………
- Age : ……………………………………
- Sex : ……………………………………
- Marital status : ……………………………………
- Address : ……………………………………

Source of information (informant) Reliability
Chief complaints (If any)
Family history
Family composition/family health history/family functioning
HPI or current health status

Past Medical History

General state of health

- General growth
- Date of most recent physical exam (Pap, Mammo, PSA, stool examination, CXR, HIV)
- Fatigue, Stresses, Allergies

Past illnesses

Past surgical history

Falls

Stage of Adult Development

- Major areas of functioning
- ADLs
- IADLs
- Muscle power and coordination
- How does he/she view health?
- Does the client have any sexual concern or problems?
- What will the patient need to regain or maintain functional ability?

Socioeconomic Assessment

- Place of birth
- Place of residence

- Occupation (early days)
- Current source of financial support
- Is he/she satisfied or not?
- How many contacts does he/she make in a day?
- Who visit him/her?
- What are the living arrangements?
- Is there any need for modification of the arrangements?
- How much independence does he/she possess?
- Hobbies:

Habits

Sleep/elimination/exercise/nutrition/use of substances/sexuality

Physical Examination (Follow Format of Physical Examination)

- General
- Vital signs
- HEENT
- Respiratory
- Cardiac
- Gastrointestinal
- Genitourinary
- Musculoskeletal
- Neurologic
- Psychologic (attitude/activity level/communication/attention and concentration/memory)

Summary

Impression

APPENDIX 5

Admission Procedure Form

A. History Collection

- Demographic data
- Chief complaints/present complaints
- Present psychiatric history/nature of current episode
- Past psychiatric history
  - Past medical history
  - Past surgical history
  - Obstetrical history (female)
  - Family history
  - Personal history

B. Methods of Admission

- Voluntary base: If major/minor
- Under special circumstances: Relatives/Police/Magistrate
- Psychiatric emergency methods
- Criminal (prison) patient

C. Conclusion

Discharge Procedure Form

A. History Collection

- Demographic data
- Chief complaints/present complaints
- Present psychiatric history/nature of current episode
- Past psychiatric history
  - Past medical history
  - Past surgical history
  - Obstetrical history (female)
  - Family history
  - Personal history

B. Methods of Discharge

- Voluntary base: If major/minor
- Under special circumstances: Relatives/police/magistrate
- Psychiatric emergency methods
- Criminal (prison) patient

C. Prognosis

D. Conclusion

APPENDIX 6

Assisting in Therapies

- Name of the therapy :
- Identification data :
- Diagnosis :
- Indications :
- Objectives :

Role of Nurse

Preorientation phase	Orientation phase	Working phase	Termination

Signature of Student **Signature of Supervisor**

Date: **Date:**

APPENDIX 7

Nurse's Assessment on Electro convulsive Therapy (ECT)

Name

- Age
- Sex
- Ward
- Unit
- Diagnosis
- IP/OP number
- Date of admission
- Physical condition
- Course of ECT recommended
- ECT administration : 1st
  2rd
  3rd
  4th
  5th
  6th
  7th
- Date of assessment
- Chief complaints on admission

Assessment before ECT

- Temperature
- Pulse
- Respiration
- BP
- Premedication

Assessment during ECT

- Parameters of current
- Voltage
- Duration
- Type of ECT : Direct/Modified
- Application of electrode : Unilateral/bilateral
- Type of seizure produced :
- Temperature
- Pulse
- Respiration
- BP

Assessment after ECT

- Temperature
- Pulse
- Respiration
- BP

Status of patient after ECT:

Complication of ECT:

Bibliography

1. Ahuja Niraj. A short text book of psychiatry. 6th edition. New Delhi: Jaypee brothers medical publishers; 2006. 35-56.
2. FA Devis, Nursing care plan, 9th edition
3. Kaplan HI and Sadock BJ (1997), 'Comprehensive textbook of psychiatry', Vol- I, 6th edition, Williams and Wilkins Publications, New Delhi, Page 23–31.
4. Lalitha K.,(2007), Mental health and psychiatric nursing, an Indian perspective. Ist edition. VMC book house, Bangalore. Page no. 421-427.
5. Sreevani. R. A guide to mental health and psychiatric nursing. 2nd edition. New Delhi: Jaypee brothers medical publishers; 2007.85–96.
6. Townsend C Mary. Psychiatric mental health nursing. 5th edition. Philadelphia: F.A. Davis company; 2007. 434–440.
7. url:https/www.currentnursing.com

Index